LECTURE NOTES ON
GERIATRICS

D1395707

LECTURE NOTES ON
GERIATRICS

NICHOLAS CONI
MRCP, FRCP(C)

WILLIAM DAVISON
TD, FRCP(E)

STEPHEN WEBSTER
MD, MRCP

*Associate lecturers, Faculty of
Clinical Medicine, University of
Cambridge, and Physicians to the
Department of Geriatric Medicine*

FOREWORD BY
SIR JOHN BUTTERFIELD
OBE, MD, DM, FRCP

*Regius Professor of Physic,
University of Cambridge*

Master of Downing College, Cambridge

SECOND EDITION

BLACKWELL SCIENTIFIC PUBLICATIONS

OXFORD LONDON EDINBURGH
BOSTON PALO ALTO MELBOURNE

© 1977, 1980 by
Blackwell Scientific Publications
Editorial Offices:
Osney Mead, Oxford OX2 0EL
8 John Street, London WC1N 2ES
23 Ainslie Place, Edinburgh,
  EH3 6AJ
52 Beacon Street, Boston, Mass.
  02108, USA
667 Lytton Avenue, Palo Alto,
  California 94301, USA
107 Barry Street, Carlton
  Victoria 3053, Australia

First published 1977
Second edition 1980
Reprinted 1984, 1986 (twice)

Printed in Great Britain at
Billing and Sons Limited,
Worcester

DISTRIBUTORS

USA
  Blackwell Mosby Book Distributors
  11830 Westline Industrial Drive
  St Louis, Missouri 63141

Canada
  The C.V. Mosby Company
  5240 Finch Avenue East,
  Scarborough, Ontario

Australia
  Blackwell Scientific Publications
    (Australia) Pty Ltd
  107 Barry Street
  Carlton, Victoria 3053

British Library
Cataloguing in Publication Data
Coni. Nicholas
  Lecture notes on geriatrics. - 2nd ed
  1. Geriatrics
  I. Title   II. Davison, William
  III. Webster, Stephen
  618.9'7 RC952

ISBN 0-632-00566-1

CONTENTS

FOREWORD TO THE FIRST EDITION

I am very pleased to commend to students of British Medicine, of all ages, these 'Lecture Notes on Geriatrics'.

The authors are a close-knit team providing the regular geriatric services to the elderly in and around Cambridge and, this being the inaugural year of the Clinical School, Coni, Davison and Webster are also accepting day-to-day responsibility for teaching their subject. Their book is being published soon after a Secretary of State for Health and Social Security has reported that over half the patients in acute hospital beds in England are over 65 years of age. So this crisp and compact manual is timely, and in my view timely for several other good reasons.

Good medical care and teamwork

First, the authors remind us that we should consider the whole patient and indicate why this is particularly important in geriatric cases. This assertion is not intended to imply that doctors and specialists in other fields are guilty of shortcoming in this fundamental aspect of good medical care. But it is a reminder to us all of an ideal to which we should re-dedicate ourselves with each new patient for whom we accept responsibility. Furthermore, valuable resources may be wasted if we do not adopt this holistic approach.

Second, the authors stress not only the resulting interdisciplinary nature of good care for so many medical cases, they also emphasize the role and responsibilities the medical profession must accept, integrating the various elements available. This integrative theme is particularly germane in the present climate following the recent reorganization of the National Health Service and points the way out of most of the organizational dilemmas which appear to beset us so much, so soon after that major upheaval.

Thirdly, and this it seems to me follows directly, current medical teamwork will rarely, perhaps never, be without social and personal health education components. In such circumstances geriatricians and general physicians must have much more contact than they did with those who work outside the hospital and clinic. Geriatricians have wider contacts and more experience in these matters than most of us and can help and guide us.

Regarding health education, I admit that there may be little health educational content for the elderly patient apart from teaching a general understanding of the use of any drugs prescribed—it is usually too late for much prevention—but there are often important health educational points for the family. Is this the kind of old age they want for themselves? Are they taking any steps now to secure a better, healthier old age than this elderly, ailing relative?

The clinical challenge of geriatrics

Until recently, the geriatric wards were regarded as burdensome, unrewarding and full of insoluble or unworthy clinical problems. The authors of this present book have brushed aside that image and presented the clinical picture of modern geriatric practice clearly and precisely. The chapters on diseases in the various body systems are excellent statements of today's realities with which medical students will be grappling from the moment they become pre-registration house officers. The coincidence of several disease processes in old age makes treatment more complex. This is a challenge to the doctor intent on good medical care for his elderly patients using the extensive therapeutic armoury of drugs.

The research and recruitment challenges of geriatrics

Undeniably, Medicine has its fashions. In the thirty years since I qualified there have been three waves of intellectual activity in clinical medicine which have attracted many, if not most, of the ablest minds, and three of which have had periods of much less appeal. There are no prizes for sorting the following alphabetical list into the appropriate groups: cardiology, general practice, geriatrics, immunology, psychiatry and renal medicine. There can be no doubt the intense interest in cardiology, renal medicine and immunology can be traced to research developments —Cournand's cardiac catheter, Richard's micropuncture of the renal glomerulus, McFarlane Burnet's immunological hypotheses.

It is my view that this present publication may excite students' interest and thus prepare the ground for the recruitment of able young investigators into the field of gerontology—a Cinderella subject at the moment, awaiting patiently the appearance of those research developments—which will be the vehicle for countless projects, Ph.D.'s and M.D. theses in the field and carry innumerable young people off to the glittering ball of professional success (and one not ending at midnight, either).

Conclusions

To the intending readers of this book, I can give the following assurances. It gives an excellent and broad overview of the subject of geriatrics. It forms a well-balanced and useful basis for revision for students approaching their Finals, a revision which, through its multiple authorship, will almost certainly be rewarding for most practitioners and, I believe, many specialists. The style is lucid, the reading is easy and the subject matter practical: in how many other books does one find lecture notes for the general practitioner's own lecture to lay groups in the very first chapter?

But, most of all, I believe and hope this book may encourage more interest and recruitment into the field we must all practise now, and where, therefore, we must of necessity follow the masters, especially experienced and enthusiastic ones like Coni and his colleagues, Davison and Webster.

Cambridge, 1976   W. J. H. BUTTERFIELD

PREFACE TO THE SECOND EDITION

Despite the economic ice age afflicting health care in the United Kingdom and many other countries, several heartening circumstances encourage us to offer a second edition of Lecture Notes on Geriatrics. Considerable advances continue to be made in this rapidly developing field, dictating some alterations in emphasis and content. A number of modifications are prompted by the welcome feedback received in the form of letters from colleagues near and far. Finally, the gratifying sales of the first edition at home and overseas make this second edition a necessity.

PREFACE TO THE FIRST EDITION

There is a danger that the current economic and political difficulties which beset the health and social services may blind us to the far greater crisis which is imminent. It is the vast and still growing burden of disease and disability in our increasing population of elderly people which threatens to overwhelm these services in the closing quarter of the century. The doctors and nurses of the future must be prepared both emotionally and intellectually to meet this challenge, whatever field of practice they subsequently enter. 'We are all geriatricians now' is a frequent claim, and indeed it is true that except for those specializing in paediatrics and obstetrics, all the professionals working in our health service will find they will spend the major part of their working lives looking after elderly patients. It is important therefore that they should have been taught to do it properly. General practice, general medicine and surgery, gynaecology, orthopaedics, urology, psychiatry and ophthalmology are all increasingly concerned with the diseases of old age. Fortunately, examiners for qualifying and higher examinations are beginning to realize this. Yet, there is still a comparative dearth of books on geriatric medicine aimed primarily at the undergraduate medical student.

It is intended that this book will help to fill the gap. In addition, it is hoped that it will be of value to general practitioners and general physicians who are being called upon more and more to provide a comprehensive geriatric service. Those chapters which are concerned with the organizational aspects of geriatric care are necessarily somewhat parochial in outlook. Nevertheless they may enable planners and medical administrators overseas to adopt what is best in the British system, and to avoid some of the pitfalls which have emerged. The clinical sections are also intended to help those studying for the membership examination, and the text has been designed to provide a source of information for nurses, health visitors and other professionals concerned with the care of the elderly. We also offer it as a practical guide to house physicians and registrars on joining the geriatric department. This book is in no sense a textbook of medicine, but is complementary to the many excellent ones available. In general, only those diseases showing a predilection for old age, or presenting special features in old age, are considered in any detail. Many other conditions which affect old and young alike are therefore only mentioned cursorily or are omitted altogether. To facilitate revision each chapter is intended to be reasonably complete. This inevitably leads to a certain amount of repetition, but repetition is an essential part of the learning process.

Furthermore, many of the ethical and logistic problems which beset us are left unanswered because they are at present unanswerable. We very much hope that our readers will be stimulated into thinking for themselves about the difficult questions raised by the demography of ageing and into providing some of the solutions.

Finally, geriatrics permits a greater diversity of method and emphasis than any other hospital specialty. The authors accept responsibility for the views expressed in this book, but realize that they will not necessarily be shared by all their readers!

ACKNOWLEDGMENTS

We have pleasure in recording our gratitude to our colleagues on the consultant staff of Addenbrooke's, too numerous to name individually. Whenever we have sought their wisdom and expertise, they have responded generously, patiently, and ungrudgingly. We are also indebted to the Department of Medical Illustration and Photography for preparing a number of the figures, and to the Cancer Bureau of the East Anglian Region for access to their records. Many of the tables are based on statistics contained in the Registrar General's Reports, The Hospital Inpatient Enquiry and in *Social Trends*, published by the Central Statistical Office. Some of the data in Chapter 2 is taken from 'The Elderly at Home' by Audrey Hunt, HMSO, 1978.

CHAPTER 1 · THE AIMS OF
GERIATRIC MEDICINE

It is not enough for a great nation to have added new years to life. Our objective must be to add new life to those years.

JOHN F. KENNEDY

'We are all geriatricians now' is commonly said by physicians and surgeons whatever their background or training. Quite so! We are all involved to a greater or lesser degree in the medical treatment of the elderly sick. Special skills and attitudes are essential to the successful practice of geriatrics and all students need to be able to recognize and manage the more common diseases of the elderly and be familiar with the *modus operandi* of the geriatric department.

Geriatric medicine has been defined as that branch of general medicine concerned with the clinical, preventive, remedial and social aspects of illness in the elderly. It is a very rewarding field of practice for the clinician—rich in pathology and offering enormous therapeutic opportunities. Regrettably it is a field which received scant attention from the medical fraternity (with a small number of notable exceptions —including Galen and Charcot) until the second half of this century. Although the elderly are the major users of the National Health Service (NHS) in Britain, it does not take their special needs sufficiently into account. Priorities within the hospital service ought to be redirected towards this group. Community medical and domiciliary services also require re-orientating towards the needs of the elderly. The present generation of older folk tends to have a low expectation of positive health and reluctantly seeks medical advice or help from the social services. The onus must be on the community as a whole to take the initiative in encouraging old people to seek the advice and help they need. On humanitarian grounds doctors have special responsibilities to give unhurried, sympathetic and helpful consultations to elderly patients. Furthermore, it is only by means of careful, detailed medical consultations that the doctor can bring maximum benefit to his patients and make optimum use of available resources.

Table 1.1. Aims of Geriatric Medicine

---

1 Maintenance of health in old age by high levels of engagement* and avoidance of disease.
2 Early detection and appropriate treatment of disease.
3 Maintenance of maximum independence consistent with irreversible disease and disability.
4 Sympathetic care and support during the terminal illness.

---

* See text for explanation of the use of this term.

The enabling approach

The aims of geriatric medicine are to enable elderly people to lead full and active lives and to reduce to a minimum the period of pre-death dependence. 'Allow them to die with their boots on' as one student so aptly put it. This enabling approach to permit the elderly to achieve the maximum capability allowed by their physical, mental and social disabilities is the core of good practice in geriatrics. A holistic approach is desirable in all branches of medicine but in geriatric practice it is absolutely essential. The patient's outlook and social environment affect function just as surely as her age and illness. Modern geriatric medicine is a dynamic affair in which the patient's needs are assessed in detail by a multidisciplinary team. An appropriate plan of medical treatment, rehabilitation and social work is then drawn up, promulgated and brought about to allow the elderly person to enjoy a life as near normal as possible.

Orientation towards the patient's needs

The central person is the patient. Her co-operation is essential to the success of the entire enterprise. The geriatric team needs to know a great deal about her to be able to act effectively. The problem list will have more than a few medical diagnoses on it. Often there will be problems of housing, finance and interpersonal relationships with the patient's family and social circle. More than most hospital doctors the geriatrician is interested in the patient's attitudes, her loves, her hates and her fears; he is interested in the patient's house—the layout, furnishings, fixtures, fittings, and what the neighbours think—do they really care or is their concern a façade adopted because society expects it?

Whole person diagnosis

Geriatrics is general medicine in its broadest sense and is fully a multidisciplinary affair. In a word, geriatrics is diagnosis; not just a medical diagnosis but a whole person diagnosis. It is multifactorial and the various facets of the patient's problem need a properly co-ordinated team approach. However, full and proper medical diagnosis is necessary in all cases because this is the keystone on which medical treatment depends.

Often it is difficult to elicit a satisfactory history. Important facts may be left out and the sequence of events may become fragmented. Persistent careful questioning of the patient, her relatives and others may be required to draw out the necessary information. Mental confusion is commonly present in association with serious physical illness in the elderly and indeed the patient may be totally incoherent. Further difficulties may arise because of the inability to decide which changes are due to age and which to disease, and because of the usual concurrence of several diseases. Successful geriatric practice demands meticulous clinical examination and appropriate investigations to detect all the pathology present, followed by an assessment of priorities for treatment. Thorough treatment of all that it is reasonable to treat then takes place simultaneously or in logical sequence.

Geriatrics is team-work

Effective team-work depends on an effective team and an effective team leader. Geriatric medicine is not for the egocentric doctor, bent on doing his own thing in his own way without much heed to the needs, hopes and ambitions of others. In geriatrics the doctor has a crucial leadership role. The team consists of everyone coming into contact with the patient—doctors, nurses, physiotherapists, occupational therapists, social workers, clerical staff, catering staff, gardeners—yes, literally every one of these can influence the patient! Given good leadership the influence of the team will be wholly beneficial. Given poor leadership the individuals in the team will each go his own way and pull in a different direction. Parataxis develops and chaos results. Morale sinks and treatment potential dwindles.

Doctor as team leader

The doctor must accept the key leadership role in the geriatric team. His role is essential to the making of a proper medical diagnosis and to the prescription of appropriate medical treatment. He needs help from his team in many of his decisions. 'Is it worthwhile attempting more medical treatment in this case?' 'Should this patient be admitted?'

'Should that patient be discharged to that home set-up?' These questions are best decided by the team on a consensus basis but with the doctor as leader accepting the final burden of responsibility. Most clinical management decisions affect more than just the patient about whom the decisions are made. For example the use of a resource (hospital bed, day hospital place) for any patient must mean that this particular resource is not available to another patient. A good team allows sensible, humane, balanced decisions to be made to the overall benefit of the community and with maximum relief to individual patients. Furthermore, the team offers support, encouragement and opportunities for growth in understanding for all its members.

Care in the terminal illness

The management of the dying patient also requires a team approach. Good medical and nursing care will aim to secure full relief from distressing physical and mental symptoms, especially anxiety, pain, vomiting and insomnia. Other members of the team, in collaboration with the patient's relatives and friends, can help to sort out personal, domestic and legal problems. Peace at the last is the aim. Frenetic medical and nursing activity is not indicated but rather the minimum technical intervention necessary to allow a comfortable death. An atmosphere of quiet, relaxed stillness and the ready availability of someone to talk to is important. Empathy and compassion are essential qualities in all members of the geriatric team.

Preventive geriatrics

In the past most illness in old age was regarded as inevitable but there is increasing evidence that a great deal of it is essentially preventable. Of course many go into retirement already ill or disabled on account of chronic disease contracted earlier in life. Chronic bronchitis, ischaemic heart disease, arthritis are all common examples. In addition many have affective disorders of near life-long duration (especially women with anxiety and depression). Others by contrast enter retirement fit and apparently well provided for but without any clear sense of purpose. Long periods of time without the personal resources for using it become a burden. A previously active, happy person used to grappling with the manifold problems of a busy family life becomes bored and apathetic when she feels no longer needed. She becomes less and less reactive to environment—people and things—she becomes increasingly 'disengaged'.

Social engagement

A highly engaged person is constantly involved in a wide range of activities—mental and physical, at work or in social intercourse. She has available lots of different kinds of material which she uses for her activities—for example, books, the radio, writing materials and household equipment. She is in more or less regular communication with a whole range of other people—her family, friends and neighbours. At most times of the day she can be seen to be taking an interest in herself and her environment.

By contrast large numbers of elderly people spend a large proportion of every day doing nothing. Retirement from paid work or the routine round of looking after children and home may be 'the end of the world' so far as they are concerned. They find the unwanted leisure of later life the most difficult burden to accept. This problem bears hardest on those of low educational status, who read and write (if at all) only as a necessity and perhaps have no appreciation of art, literature, politics, current affairs or music.

Initially they may keep themselves occupied with simple physical tasks but gradually these too are abandoned. Lack of drive associated particularly with early dementia and mental depression accelerates the process of disengagement.

The better-educated person possessing sufficient drive should have much less difficulty in using her new-found leisure to develop her personality more fully. Furthermore, she has an excellent opportunity to be more involved in local affairs and voluntary work and thus make a significant contribution to the common good. Pre-retirement counselling and preventive geriatrics have as a goal the maintenance of high levels of 'engagement' (reactivity to the environment) and thereby the maintenance of positive health at all stages of life including retirement and old age. The real positive opportunities of later life need emphasis.

'Rest equals rust'

Inactivity, mental or physical, is what the retired should guard against. It is necessary throughout life to present the mind and body with sufficient challenge to keep fit. The cycle of activity—interest, effort, rest, restoration and hence the capacity for more effort—is the key to success. Regrettably in people of middle age and beyond the cycle is frequently—no interest, apathy, rest, a sense of weariness and a capacity for doing very little. Much of the benefit of geriatric re-ablement courses stems from the realization that the elderly patient like everyone else must make an effort to become fit and stay fit. 'Rest equals rust' is a useful aphorism. It is most unfortunate that we are unable to distinguish between the sensation of tiredness due to work and the tiredness due to lack of activity. However, all but the most heavily blinkered can recognize the difference between activity and inactivity (engagement and disengagement) and this will point the way to a possible improvement in vitality.

Under-reporting of illness

It is well established that there is gross under-reporting of ill health in the elderly. Presumably this is because older people (and their relatives) ascribe each and every decrement in health and mobility to 'just old age'. Thus the illnesses known to the family doctor are only half the story. There is a lot more that he does not know about unless he sets to, to find out. This is a worthwhile object because much of the illness and disability can be alleviated by quite simple means. Even when diseases are found for which there is no definite treatment (e.g. senile dementia, inoperable cancer), the knowledge gained will allow better overall management including domiciliary support.

Furthermore, sick elderly people will be found causing insuperable difficulties for younger supporting relatives. Left as it is, such a situation is bound to collapse and be brought to the attention of the family doctor as a crisis. The older person will then be admitted to hospital as an emergency but never be able to return home because the relatives, not unreasonably, will utterly refuse to take on the burden. This phenomenon of rejection by relatives is predictable but can be avoided or at least postponed by timely intervention on the part of the family doctor—but only if he knows what to do to relieve the situation. If he is in doubt as to what to do the local geriatrician is there to help him. Timing is all-important and the specialist should be consulted early rather than late.

Screening in the elderly

Sociomedical screening by the primary care team is a 'must' for preventive geriatrics. Contact with the patient is initiated by the family doctor. An age/sex register of the practice will allow all the elderly to be identified. This register may be compiled from the Family Practitioner Committee lists and matched against the Register of Electors. Allowing for death and removal this would be accurate to over 95 per cent. Those at risk (the over-75's, especially the housebound, the recently bereaved, recently discharged from hospital and those living alone) should be visited systematically by the practice health visitor and asked to co-operate in a health check. Most old people will readily agree and be delighted that someone is taking a special interest in them. The health visitor conducts an interview and a simple examination by the doctor (preferably in the surgery) follows and is supplemented by routine blood and urine testing. Most old people can be brought to the surgery by car. The others—with more severe disablement—can be examined at home.

Screening the over-75's in general practice can yield a rich harvest of conditions for which medical action is required—ranging from a course of oral iron for anaemia to major surgery. Referral to specialist practitioners may be indicated—especially chiropody. Almost all patients will feel that they have benefited by the health check and advice given even if no serious pathology is detected. In this age group 75 per cent might be found to have significant disability, 30–40 per cent will be found to live alone and 20–25 per cent to be housebound. 'Age Concern' England (The National Old People's Welfare Council) asserts that most elderly people want visits from their doctor. Doctors who have visited find it a worthwhile venture, provided that they do not fall into the trap of assuming that all the disability they see is due simply to ageing, and as a result fail to seek out and treat remediable disease. It cannot be over-emphasized that disability is due to disease and not to old age. Social support may also be required, but calling in the community nurse and the home help service is no real substitute for diagnosing and treating the old lady with hypothyroidism, osteomalacia, iron deficiency anaemia or whatever.

Table 1.2. Screening the elderly in general practice

Common findings
1 Mental depression.
2 Deafness.
3 Chronic bronchitis.
4 Foot defects.
5 Hip disease.
6 Anaemia.
7 Dementia.
8 Blindness.
9 Anxiety state.
10 Cardiac failure.
11 Diabetes mellitus, osteomalacia, hypothyroidism.
12 Faecal impaction.

Health in retirement

Doctors are often asked to give talks on keeping fit in later life; following is a guide.

KEEPING FIT IN LATER LIFE

1   A reason for being alive, a sense of purpose, concern for others. 'Thinking outside yourself.'

2   Purposeful activity, mental and physical. Quite vigorous too! Structured day to include attention to personal hygiene and appearance, regular meals, periods of both rest and work together with opportunities for social interaction.

3   Suitable environment, housing, ambient temperature at least 18·3°C, avoid freezing bedroom! Accessible amenities, shops, library, church, club etc.

4   Accident prevention especially falls—stairs, trailing wires, pets, 'slip mats', fires—the open hearth and the paraffin heater. Beware the stranger at the gate—villains and confidence men. Use of door chain, peephole with fish-eye lens etc.

5   Adequate diet in terms of calories, protein, vitamins and essential elements like calcium and iron (see Chapter 3). An ordinary mixed diet gives all the necessary foodstuffs but elderly people are often rather low on vitamins and essential elements so stress the need for fresh fruit and vegetables and a pint of milk daily.

6   Finance—generally the more money the better. State retirement pension always set below the poverty line. Will not cover the essentials of food, rent, fuel, clothes, maintenance of house and its contents. Supplements essential—rent and rate rebates, fuel allowance, allowance for the registered blind etc. If in doubt consult the local Social Security department.

7   Self-discipline—perhaps the most difficult of all. Weight loss does wonders for the heart and joints. Smoking is bad for everyone other than tobacco merchants. Inebriation (drugs as well as alcohol) leads to accidents.

8   Medical care—no panacea for a faulty life-style. Medicine often worse than the malady. Doctors have important but limited role. Each individual is captain of her own fate—keeping fit at any age is essentially a personal problem.

CHAPTER 2 · THE ELDERLY

Happy the year, the month that finds alive a worthy man
in health at seventy five.

SAMUEL TAYLOR COLERIDGE, 1772–1834

The aged in society

The aged in society are defined legally, socially and culturally in ways
which differ from time to time and from country to country. In English
law in 1899 the word 'aged' was interpreted as meaning not below 50
years! There is no similar definition of 'the elderly' but today for
government retirement pension purposes in the UK 60 years for females
and 65 for males is the rule. Other countries have different statutory
retirement ages. These fixed retirement ages produce a somewhat
arbitrary cut-off point in the lives of most people and beyond these
ages most will engage in little or no paid employment. Furthermore,
the proportion of older people remaining economically active has been
falling steadily in all industrialized nations (Table 2.1) at the same time

Table 2.1. Men still in paid employment (UK)

Year	Age 65–69 years	70–74 years
1921	80%	53%
1961	40%	21%
1976	25%	14%

Includes substantial part time work.

as the total number reaching retirement age has been increasing (Fig.
2.1). In times of unemployment the older worker is much more likely
to be made redundant.

9

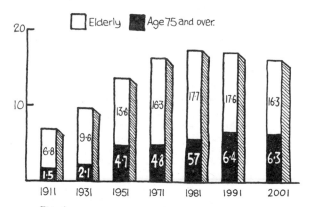

Elderly as a percentage of the total population.
Males aged 65 and over. Females aged not less than 60.

Fig. 2.1

Elderly not a homogeneous group

Whatever cut-off point is used for retirement there is a marked tendency
for everyone above that age to be referred to as elderly or even old
rather than just retired. Within this group of elderly people, however,
will be found great diversity of intellect, physical strength and stamina.
Indeed, almost any quality which is measured shows a bigger diversity
in older people than in the young. So that, although the basic needs of
purposeful activity, food, housing, finance and social intercourse, can
be regarded as essential to all, the details of provision for these necessities together with the additional needs of social support and medical
treatment will vary enormously.

The important point is that the elderly are not a race apart—they are
people. 'They are us yesterday and we are them tomorrow', wrote
Marjory Warren. This description of the elderly by one of the pioneers
of British Geriatric Medicine reminds us that the needs of the elderly
today are similar to ours. Tomorrow they are identical.

Demography of ageing

Britain, along with other industrialized countries, has experienced (and
is still experiencing) dramatic changes in the population structure

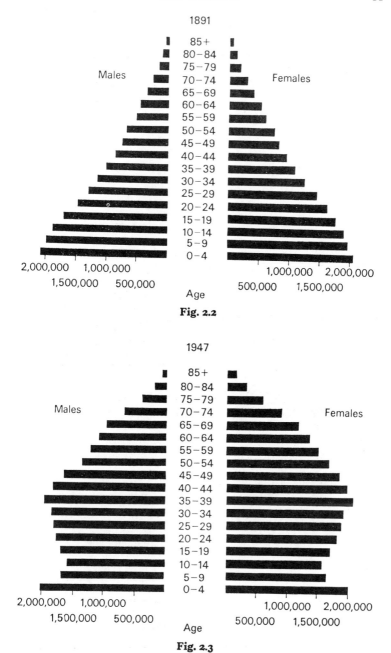

1891

	85+
	80-84
	75-79
Males	70-74
	65-69
	60-64
	55-59
	50-54
	45-49
	40-44
	35-39
	30-34
	25-29
	20-24
	15-19
	10-14
	5-9
	0-4

Females

2,000,000   1,000,000
      1,500,000   500,000

1,000,000   2,000,000
500,000   1,500,000

Age

Fig. 2.2

1947

85+
80-84
75-79
Males   70-74   Females
65-69
60-64
55-59
50-54
45-49
40-44
35-39
30-34
25-29
20-24
15-19
10-14
5-9
0-4

2,000,000   1,000,000
      1,500,000   500,000

1,000,000   2,000,000
500,000   1,500,000

Age

Fig. 2.3

leading to an increase in the number (both absolute and relative) of elderly persons (Figs. 2.2, 2.3, 2.4).

These changes have taken place more rapidly than we have been able to cope with satisfactorily. This is especially true in terms of the lack of agreement on a suitable role for the elderly in society, and the lack of a significant shift in national wealth towards this group. Looked at from almost any angle the field of ageing would appear to be underprovided.

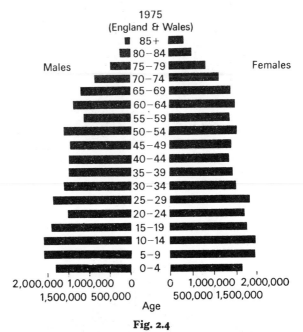

Fig. 2.4

In underdeveloped countries the proportion of over 65's is usually less than 5 per cent of the total population—rather as it was in Britain at the beginning of this century. In 1976 in the UK 17·1 per cent of the population was over retirement age—a spectacular increase in a comparatively short space of time. This change has come about because of the fall in birth rate to less than half of the high levels of Victorian times together with a marked fall in death rate of younger people— mostly as a result of the virtual elimination of the infectious diseases as a cause of death. Thus a much higher proportion of people live on into old age, i.e. have an increased expectation of life. On the other hand the increase in life expectation for those who attain retirement has changed very little (Figs. 2.5, and 2.6).

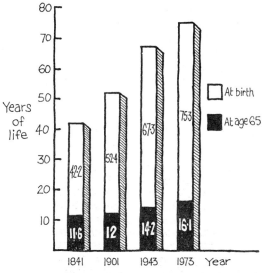

Expectation of life. Females (England)

Fig. 2.5

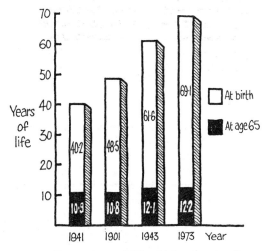

Expectation of life. Males (England)

Fig. 2.6

'The old old'

The elderly make much heavier demands on health and social services
than do the young and the oldest of the elderly make the heaviest
demands of all. The over-75's have by far the highest incidence of
hospital admission and their average duration of stay is very much
longer. (Table 2.2) The incidence of chronic illness rises as a function

Table 2.2 Hospital discharges in 1974 expressed as percentage of the
age group population and showing duration of stay in days. (All departments excluding psychiatry and maternity). England and Wales.

Age group	Discharge Rate	Duration of stay Median	Mean
15–44	6·9	4·1	7·0
45–64	8·7	8·2	12·8
65–74	13·4	11·4	20·8
75+	20·7	14·5	41·2

of age (Fig. 2.7). Currently the young old (below 75) are much more
numerous than the old old (over 75). However, by the year 2001 we
may expect the population over age 75 in the UK to have increased by
40 per cent. By then we may expect 1·8 million over 85, an increase of
50 per cent.

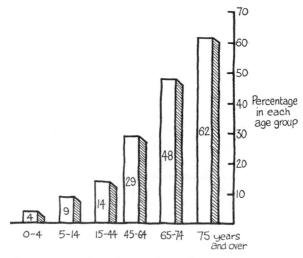

Persons reporting long-standing illness (England and Wales 1972)

Fig. 2.7

Furthermore, it should be noted that at age 75 there are almost two women for every one man and by age 85 over three women for every man. These statistics justify the statement that the problem of old age is a problem of old women. This problem is not entirely due to nature. Some of it must be attributed to the inherently unhealthy life style of British men coupled with their propensity for engaging in life-threatening activities at work, at play and on the battlefields of the world.

Major shift in demand for services

These demographic changes of ageing, especially the 40 per cent increase in the over-75's due to take place within the professional lifetime of the students reading this book, will have a profound influence on health and welfare services. There will be a radical shift in the kind of demands made on the personal social services, on the local authority provision of special housing and residential homes and also, of course, on the health services we aim to provide.

RESPONSE TO THE NEW DEMANDS

This new situation requires a new look at the way we deploy resources of finance, housing, social services, medical and nursing care. Current estimates suggest a need, nationwide, for a three-fold increase in the home help services and in the meals on wheels service, a five-fold increase in sheltered housing and a seven-fold increase in the availability of chiropody to the elderly. Presumably the increased numbers of the very old will increase all of these needs still further. Already the demand for medical and nursing services is seemingly insatiable. For example, in the hospital service, patients over the age of 65 years, representing just over 14 per cent of the population, occupy 56 per cent of all non-psychiatric beds. The majority are in Departments of Geriatric Medicine but they also account for:

> 36 per cent of all trauma and orthopaedic beds
> 42 per cent of all general surgical beds
> 49 per cent of all ophthalmology beds
> 50 per cent of all general medical beds
> 80 per cent of all general practitioner beds

By the year 2001 on current trends elderly males could occupy 75 per cent and elderly females 90 per cent of all acute general hospital beds (excluding maternity)!

New patterns of care

New patterns of care are emerging which (hopefully) will allow us to cope with the new situation. The properly run geriatric department has a major (but not exclusive) role in coping with the rapidly rising tide of elderly sick persons. Most sections of health and social services are involved. The major burden will be borne outside of hospitals and similar institutions, because that is where over 90 per cent of the elderly are.

Main emphasis on enablement

By enablement we mean to make able, to strengthen, to supply with means and opportunities. Modern patterns of care concentrate on enabling the elderly person to care for herself and to achieve self-fulfilment through purposeful enjoyable living. This requires resources of money, housing, education and leisure activities to be made available so that the elderly have at least a sporting chance to live independently. More important still, it requires a special attitude of mind to encourage all care practitioners to accept enablement as a valid goal and work towards it. Where increasing age, frailty and disability require that more assistance be given it should be given on this enabling basis. For example, if residential care proves to be necessary then the pattern of care within the home should encourage maximum self-realization and achievement (engagement) more than has hitherto been the case.

Too often in the past care has been a matter of the carer bestowing care on the cared for—a process which rapidly erodes the old person's resolve and ability to care for herself; a process virtually guaranteed to produce increasingly dependent clients! The logistics of the current problem of caring for the elderly dictate that the client must do the maximum of which she is capable. The support role of doctor, nurse, social worker, relative or whatever is to enable the elderly person to achieve this.

Role of the newly retired

Faced as we are with people retiring earlier and for longer, society needs to identify a positive role for these very large numbers of relatively fit and active, younger elderly people. Furthermore, it is clear that a very large increase in manpower will be needed to support the increasing numbers of very frail, very old people at the other end of the retirement scale. It is tempting to suggest that the needs of these two sub-groups of the elderly might to a considerable extent be complementary. That is to say social service by the fitter younger elderly to help support the less fit, older elderly.

This sort of role for the newly retired is one to be encouraged since it provides valuable, purposeful activity for those in retirement possessed of energy and ability and also provides an increased level of service to the many frail, disabled old people who are unable adequately to fend for themselves. Already a great deal of supportive work for the dependent old is given by the more recently retired. Let us hope that further development of this type of activity can be achieved.

Role of the young

The young have a considerable contribution to make to the welfare of the elderly. Young people helping through the agencies of youth groups (e.g. Youth Action), school and university social service schemes or contributing on an individual basis all have important roles to play. The benefits are two-way. The old people benefit directly by the provision of services (shopping, redecorating, simple household repairs). The young people benefit by giving their services, by a feeling of satisfaction for a job well done and by a deepening awareness of the problems associated with old age and its attendant disabilities. Lastly the young value the insights into a bygone age given by the elderly. Descriptions of horse-drawn transport make a refreshing change from present-day supersonic jetliner travel.

Attitudes towards the elderly

Society's attitudes towards the elderly are often ambivalent. For example, there is a sizeable gap between the expressed concern for the needs of older people and action actually taken to meet those needs. This is evident at all levels. At family level it is not uncommon to hear children, grandchildren, neighbours or friends insist that 'something must be done' but so often, in these cases, the expectation is that someone else will do it. Happily, although the grumble is there, it is rare for the family to renounce their elderly relatives. However, the feelings of ambivalence make good care more difficult to achieve. At regional and national level there is shock and indignation when poor standards of care are exposed. Yet it is at just these managerial levels that a rearrangement of priorities of money, staff and buildings would allow for vastly improved standards of care for the aged.

Many people harbour feelings of hostility towards the elderly in general while enjoying extremely good relationships with the elderly of their own family or social circle. These people might accept low standards of provision in housing, pension, social service and medical care for the elderly in general but are shocked to see their own kith and kin suffering as a result. In the fairly recent past ambivalent attitudes like these were more readily understandable in socioeconomic terms. Generally speaking, the influential and relatively 'well-to-do' managerial and professional classes could reassure themselves that, without recourse to statutory help, they and their relatives could secure good housing, an adequate income and appropriate levels of medical and nursing care for their elderly. This can be true now, in Britain, for only a very small percentage of the population, so that enlightened self-interest should help raise the general levels of provision for the elderly.

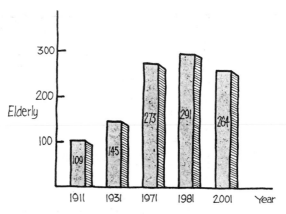

Elderly per thousand working population.
(England and Wales).

Fig. 2.8

Resentment and antagonism may be due to the lack of a clearly defined role for the elderly in society (Table 2.3). Much of this is due to the economic dependence of the old (Fig. 2.8). Thus old people as a group may arouse feelings of distaste—being thought of as a social and economic drag on society. In a world orientated towards acquisitiveness, the ever-increasing demands for material wealth make essential the

Table 2.3. Low status for elderly in Western Society

No positive role
Too numerous
Rapid social change
Rising unemployment
Materialism

concept of an infinitely expanding economy. Clearly the unproductive elderly have no place here!

Fortunately the expectations of today's old have been shaped by their experiences at an earlier age when standards of living were very much lower. Overall standards of living have been rising *pari passu* with the increasing numbers of pensioners in society. These factors have allowed the wage earners to enjoy very much higher living standards than the pensioners without the latter feeling at all aggrieved. Indeed the wage earners (and the politicians) often express a desire for higher standards of living for the elderly than the elderly do for themselves. Here again there is ambivalence. 'They (the pensioners) should get at least an extra £10 each week.' Not an unreasonable suggestion you might think, but if ten million pensioners are eligible (a figure likely to be reached by 1991) £10 × 10 × 52 = £5,200 million extra money has to be found annually from somewhere. This is where the difficulty comes. What do we sacrifice to make that extra money available? These problems are difficult enough in a buoyant economy, but when the chill winds of industrial recession blow across the land, the gap widens between sympathy and action.

Attitudes of doctors and nurses

Due to improvements in health and welfare more people live through to old age. This is one of the benefits of a high standard of living and something of which we should be proud. Yet many doctors and nurses complain that they have too many old people to look after! Ambivalence again. Dedicated to health and welfare but irritated by the demographic changes brought thereby.

'Old age is a losing game' they say. Well of course it is. The whole of life is a losing game in this sense. Whatever we achieve, whoever we are, our life span is limited. Sooner or later we fall sick and inevitably we die. After the age of puberty the liability to die increases as the years go by. Nevertheless, sickness in old age does not necessarily mean that medical treatment is of no avail. On the contrary, many illnesses in the elderly are successfully and simply treated, and some have a less serious prognosis than in the young; e.g. carcinoma of the breast, hypertension and lymphatic leukaemia.

'Geriatrics is not a specialty' they say. True in a sense, false in another sense. True in the sense that many modern medical specialties focus on a single group of diseases (oncology, immunology, venereology), others on the diseases of a single system or organ (neurology, nephrology, cardiology). Geriatric medicine by contrast has to grapple with multiple illness over a wide range of medicine. In this sense it might be described as a generality rather than a specialty. On the other hand the successful practice of geriatric medicine requires a special body of knowledge, special techniques of investigation and treatment, a special pattern of organization and an appropriate philosophy—all to be applied most conscientiously and with exactitude. In this sense geriatrics obviously is a specialty and a taxing, fascinating and worthwhile specialty at that.

OVERPROTECTIVE ATTITUDES

Many people working with the elderly are hampered in their work by overprotective attitudes towards the client. Doctors and nurses are liable to become so caught up in the patient's problems that they find rational decisions difficult to make. For example the patient may regard the hospital as a haven of rest and security after the daily battle for survival at home. Although the patient's medical and nursing needs may be comparatively modest an overprotective staff can quickly induce her to be totally dependent upon the hospital. By taking the short-term view the staff and the patient gain some satisfaction but the long-term results are disastrous for patient and staff alike. The hospital resource is left giving 'tender loving care' for the few, rather than medical investigation and more energetic treatment for the many. An increasingly lengthy waiting list for admission then gives silent testimony to the failure of the hospital system to work. The patient cared for in this overprotective way suffers a gradual and irreversible disintegration of personality due to loss of personal responsibility and self-esteem and a whittling away of areas of free choice as a result of being treated in hospital. Unfortunately the overprotective doctor or nurse may see the apathetic, crumpled, shuffling figure as justification for the decision to let her stay in hospital, rather than an indictment of an overprotective system of care, producing unwanted dependence in a patient who could have regained some degree of independence.

THE AUTHORITARIAN APPROACH

This is commonly used by the doctor or nurse—keeping the patient at a distance, issuing orders but not much given to listening to the patient or allowing a meaningful discussion to develop. It is a very poor approach to the problems of our elderly patients. Admittedly we do feel we know what is best for a particular disease or symptom complex and we are irritated by the patient who expresses views on treatment contrary to our own. Yet why should we be so rigid with patients, when we know full well that knowledge (and fashion) change rapidly in medicine; to the extent that the correct treatment for a disease today may be the antithesis of what it was a year or two ago! Furthermore, with increasing knowledge this treatment will almost certainly change again in the not too distant future. Medicine and surgery simply abound with examples of this phenomenon, e.g. absolute bed rest for patients with myocardial infarction, a low residue diet for spastic colon and diverticular disease and colectomy for autointoxication.

Another aspect of the authoritarian approach is to treat the patient as a child. The generation gap and frequently an educational gap between patient and doctor may make communication difficult. The doctor feels and behaves as if he is superior to the patient, yet a more full awareness by the doctor would allow him to recognize the differences and difficulties inherent in the consultation but without the biased value judgement.

If brain damage exists in the patient the temptation for her attendants to treat her as a child is even greater. Some essentially kind, but ill-informed practitioners (not just doctors) cause a great deal of misery by treating their elderly patients as if they were children. For example, an old lady of eighty suffering from a stroke and struggling to gain her independence is not helped by being scolded in front of other patients by one of the nurses saying 'You're a naughty girl, wetting yourself; you ought to be ashamed.' An enfeebled elderly person is an adult and must be treated as an adult.

Family relationships

There is no doubt that the services provided by families for their aged parents are of overwhelming importance and dwarf the provisions of the statutory social services. Where children exist they give much more support than is popularly believed. The misconception must be due to the sharp impact on the social conscience when the young (in those rare cases) abdicate their duties towards the old.

The major source of support for the younger elderly man is his wife but women, of necessity have to be more self-reliant. As frailty and bereavement supervene, children and others take on extra responsibility by visiting or by sharing accommodation with the elderly person. Nevertheless the number of very old people (especially women) living alone must give cause for concern. (Table 2.4).

Table 2.4. Living arrangements age 65 plus (age 85 plus) UK percentages 1976

Living with	Men	Women	All
Self	16 (30)	39 (50)	30
Spouse	62 (31)	32 (5)	44
Spouse+child	11 (4)	3 (1)	7
Self+child	3 (11)	9 (20)	6
Self+other	8 (25)	17 (24)	13

For the most part, children do take the care and support of their elderly relatives very seriously indeed. Daughters especially can carry an enormous burden of responsibility, day in day out for year after year without complaining. However, when the unremitting toil and moil eventually causes the supporting relative to turn for help her pleading must not fall on deaf ears. Furthermore, 25 per cent of the elderly have no children at all and so are especially vulnerable in times of illness or other crisis. In other cases, although there are children, they may live at a distance or be otherwise quite unable to help.

Because it is now known that supporting relatives do so much for the aged, there is a danger that where supporting relatives exist they will be expected to carry an undue burden. Many of the children of our very old patients are themselves elderly and cannot be expected to cope with a limitless task. Doctors and others must be fully aware of the need to look for and relieve social strain of this nature. Domiciliary support services, a temporary stay in a residential care home or a short-term admission of a sick person to hospital when appropriate can maintain the problem within tolerable bounds. This is absolutely vital to allow adequate care for the elderly. Regular services, like help with shopping, housework (including maintenance of house and garden) and social visits, are best performed by relatives with some help from friends, neighbours and voluntary services. Short-term crisis work also is usually well coped with by relatives with similar assistance. The statutory social services cannot hope to cater for all these needs but they can do a great deal, by helping in critical areas, to allow maximum overall care to be provided by relatives and others.

The corollary of all this is that the elderly who lean most heavily on the social services and become long-term residents in institutions (including hospitals) are likely to be those who live alone, have no children or have very little contact with their children. Currently about 6 per cent of the elderly are in institutions of some sort including the hospitals. This small percentage imposes very heavy burdens on these institutions so that a further small percentage shift towards institutional care would be insupportable given the present provision for this type of care. A further 12 per cent of the elderly are enabled to manage in their own homes by support from the various agencies already mentioned. It is crucial that these domiciliary services continue and be augmented by the use of additional resources or a redeployment of existing resources.

Some 15 per cent of elderly women and 5 per cent of elderly men have never married. Surprisingly, proportionately as many of these single old people live with others as do the widowed. Mostly the single live with siblings but often with more distantly related or unrelated people. A remarkably high proportion (50 per cent) of very old women live alone. The majority of elderly men are still married (75 per cent) whereas the women are mostly widowed (or single) (Table 2.5). Of those very old people with no spouse, 36 per cent of men and 44 per cent of women live with some relative or other person.

Table 2.5. Marital status age 65 plus (and age 85 plus) UK percentages 1976

	Men	Women	All
* Single	6 (13)	13 (11)	10
Widowed	19 (51)	49 (83)	38
Married	75 (36)	38 (6)	52

* includes divorced, separated.

Interpersonal relationships

Personality is another factor to be reckoned with in the care of the elderly. Where good interpersonal relationships exist even old people living alone enjoy much support from children, friends and neighbours. Furthermore, care practitioners of all grades are keen to help them. On the other hand, a difficult personality can drive away help that would otherwise be readily available. The life-long cultivation of a good personality would seem to be a counsel of perfection but it certainly eases the stresses and strains when things go awry in old age. 'To be needed, be helpful to others, to be wanted, be nice to people' are the somewhat platitudinous guidelines for growing old gracefully with the hope of receiving help as and when it is required.

CHAPTER 3 · DEPRIVATION

'Some misguided enthusiasts have believed that by lengthening life, they would confer a priceless boon to the human race, forgetting that it is not the length of day which makes us love the summer, but the brightness of the sun, the beauty of the flowers, the singing of the birds.'

EDMUND GOLDSMID, 1885

Introduction

The title of this chapter might well be considered to be alarmist. However, it is not our intention to argue that all old people are deprived, but it must be accepted that old age is rarely a period of social or economic expansion. The limitations in life-style which occur at this time of life, can result in even well-supported and financially comfortable people feeling relatively underprivileged, when comparisons are made with the standard of living they enjoyed in their youth. This relative deprivation is especially likely to occur in times of inflation such as prevail at the present.

It is sadly true that the elderly of our society include amongst their number some of the most deprived members of our community. These unfortunate old people are especially likely to become patients of departments of geriatric medicine. Their admission to hospital will occur because of one or other of the following two combinations of problems.

(a) disabilities caused by deficiencies in their environment, or

(b) a breakdown being caused by their medical disabilities, making it impossible for them to continue their struggle against their hostile environment.

Examples

1 A patient illustrating group (a) would be an elderly person who has become hypothermic due to inadequate heating and sub-standard housing.

2 A patient illustrating group (b) would be an elderly person with arthritic hips who can no longer cope with the difficulties presented by an outside toilet, and is forced to be incontinent.

Both crises could obviously have been avoided but, long-term social neglect leads frequently to urgent hospital admission.

However, in medicine, and especially in geriatric practice, it is rare for situations and sequences of events to be simple. Crises will have multifactorial origins, and a patient deprived in one way will probably also be underprivileged in others. The major causes of deprivation are:

1   Financial
2   Social

The great difference between these, is that the 1st is relatively easily corrected—needing mainly money. Correction of the 2nd is more difficult and may require changes in attitudes of the community, and will need self-sacrifice.

Financial deprivation

People in general tend not to realize the expensive aspects of old age. The assumption is frequently made that costs are reduced as age proceeds. In some instances this is a correct assessment—for example, a mortgage is normally completed in advance of retirement but for the 50 per cent of the population who are not owner-occupiers rent must be paid as before. Similarly, massive outlay for expensive domestic appliances is not expected in old age. These will have already been acquired or conversely with a reduced income, they will never be within grasp. However, because of failing health and strength the need for such labour saving devices will become greater, as the possibility of buying them recedes. Mechanical breakdown of the appliances may present the previously fortunate owner with an insurmountable bill.

Causes of financial deprivation

Financial deprivation occurs in two main varieties in old age.

1   The chronic poor—whose situation worsens with retirement and mounting disabilities.
2   The new poor—'distressed gentle-folk'—who suffer withdrawal of services and facilities, which they are no longer able to replace.

The chronic poor

These people will not only lack money, but also will suffer from many of the manifestations of long-term financial deprivation. Their housing is likely to be substandard and poorly equipped with modern aids. Many will lack the necessary knowledge for obtaining their entitlements, or of making the maximum advantage of what they can afford. Those who with skill and fortitude have learned to maintain high standards on a low budget, will find it increasingly difficult to maintain them when physical disabilities restrict their activities.

Examples

1 Osteoarthritis of hips and knees makes 'shopping around' for bargains difficult. The resulting use of the nearest shop, or dependence on errand-runners may lead to the use of convenience foods, which are usually expensive and of poor nutritional value.
2 Failing vision due to cataracts, makes sewing and darning impossible. Clothes therefore have to be replaced more frequently and choice is reduced as in example (1).
3 Dyspnoea secondary to a macrocytic anaemia will mean that it is no longer possible to walk to save bus fares, when visiting the surgery for an inappropriate repeat prescription for ferrous sulphate!

The members of this group are likely to be totally dependent on their State retirement pension, which for a couple, is currently about half the minimum recommended wage and for a single person is far less. The fact that approximately one third of those drawing the retirement pension also find it necessary to draw supplementary benefits, clearly demonstrates its inadequacy. The problem is probably even greater, as the elderly are notorious for their reluctance to apply for such aid, and their ignorance of how to obtain it.

The new poor

Generally, these are people who have planned well for their old age from a previous position of financial security. Their planning may not have taken into account the fact that this period was going to extend for as long as 30 years. Furthermore unexpected external economic disasters may confound their monetary calculations. Such risks become increasingly common during periods of inflation and recession.

The members of this group are likely, in addition to their dwindling savings, to have an occupational pension as well as the state provision. They may also be eligible for assistance from charities connected with their previous occupation. Also they are not excluded from obtaining supplementary benefits whilst still holding certain assets, such as a house.

A recent hopeful development is the introduction of index-linked pension schemes which attempt to keep up with inflation.

Manifestations of financial deprivation

Deficiencies in the provision of the basic needs of shelter, warmth and food are the most serious manifestations of poverty. It is unfortunately true, to the shame of our society, that it is the elderly who most frequently lack some or all of these essentials for a reasonable standard of living.

POOR HOUSING

About 7 per cent of elderly people in this country lack the basic amenities of running hot water, a bathroom and an indoor toilet. Seven per cent may not seem high, but this represents approximately 350,000 people, which is slightly more than the entire population of a city the size of Hull. A further 20 per cent lack two of the previously mentioned essentials, which is equivalent to the entire population of Birmingham.

INADEQUATE HEATING

A recent survey showed that 30 per cent of elderly subjects admitted to not being sufficiently warm in the winter. As old people are sometimes unable to appreciate that they are cold (see Chapter 16) this is probably an underestimate of the size of the problem.

Half of the victims of hypothermia are in receipt of supplementary benefits whereas only one-third of all people of pensionable age claim. It is therefore clear that poverty plays an important role in its causation.

Only one-quarter of all the elderly have central heating compared with one-third of all other households. Seventy-five per cent of old people have living-rooms colder than the minimum set by the Parker Morris housing standards (18·3°) see Fig. 3.1.

POOR NUTRITION

Subclinical malnutrition rather than severe undernutrition is the main dietary problem of old age. Clear-cut deficiency diseases are rare but many elderly people may have a reduced resistance to disease and stress because of their poor dietary intake.

In a national survey conducted by the Department of Health and Social Security (DHSS) 25 per cent of the subjects had a daily energy intake of less than 2,000 calories (8·4 MJ). More than half the survey participants took less than the recommended amounts of vitamin C or D (see Fig. 3.2).

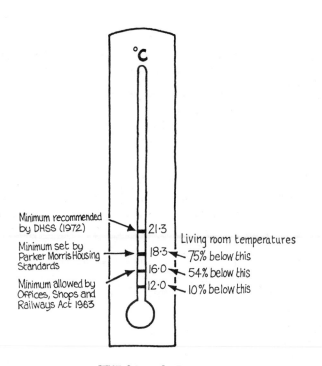

Minimum recommended by DHSS (1972) — 21·3

Living room temperatures

Minimum set by Parker Morris Housing Standards — 18·3 ← 75% below this

— 16·0 — 54% below this

Minimum allowed by Offices, Shops and Railways Act 1963 — 12·0 ← 10% below this

THE COLD OLD

Fig. 3.1

A BALANCED DIET FOR OLD AGE

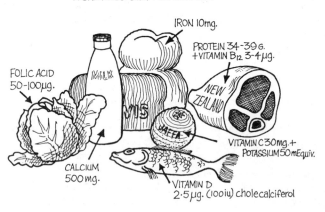

IRON 10mg.

PROTEIN 34-39 G. + VITAMIN B₁₂ 3-4 μg.

FOLIC ACID 50-100μg.

VITAMIN C 30mg. + POTASSIUM 50 mEquiv.

CALCIUM 500 mg.

VITAMIN D 2·5 μg. (100iu) cholecalciferol

Recommended energy intake 1900-2350 Kcals (7·9-9·8MJ)

Fig. 3.2

Although 62 per cent of elderly people admit to worries concerning the cost of food there are many other possible causes for nutritional deprivation:

1 Dementia
2 Depression
3 Physical disabilities
4 Ignorance

The medical complications of financial deprivation

All of the following conditions may arise as a direct consequence of financial deprivation. They can conveniently be divided into those due to inadequate heating and poor housing and those due to poor nutrition. It should not be forgotten that many of the medical conditions described also have other causes.

The complications of inadequate heating and poor housing

1 HYPOTHERMIA
2 LOSS OF MOBILITY
3 SPHINCTER DISTURBANCES
4 ACCIDENTS
5 SUSCEPTIBILITY TO ILLNESS
6 RESISTANCE TO DISCHARGE FROM HOSPITAL.

1 HYPOTHERMIA

In the majority of cases the patient's environment will have played a significant role (see Chapter 16 for details on aetiology and management of hypothermia).

2 LOSS OF MOBILITY

In severely cold weather and with inadequate heating facilities, the only chance that an old person has of keeping warm is to remain in bed, permanently clothed. The price paid for keeping warm in this way may be very high, even to the extent of complete loss of mobility and independence. It is surprising how short a period in bed is required for some arthritic joints to become fixed, and for contractures to develop, and pressure sores to develop.

Disabled people in unsuitable accommodation may have their mobility severely limited. If not housed on the ground floor patients with strokes or arthritis may be prisoners in their own homes. When there are multiple changes in floor levels between rooms they may be restricted to living in a single room.

3   SPHINCTER DISTURBANCES

If the lavatory is inconveniently sited its use will present a disabled
person with enormous problems. Consequently less frequent visits
will be made or makeshift alternative arrangements tried. Adherence
to the former plan will lead to constipation, then faecal impaction
with the ultimate loss of bladder and rectal control. The alternative
plan will result in accidents with spillage of urine or trauma to the
victim. Either way a bad situation will become worse and an independent
life at home may be made impossible.

4   ACCIDENTS

In 1971 4,000 people over the age of 65 years died in accidents in their
own homes. The majority, 3,431, of these deaths resulted from falls.
The elimination of the risks inherent in old and neglected buildings,
would avoid many of the accidents. Particular dangers are the stairs,
which are often poorly lit and have worn carpeting—497 elderly people
died from falls on their stairs in 1971. Falls due to uneven floors and
worn, awkward steps caused 352 deaths. Even without serious injury,
a fall often causes serious loss of confidence. The results of these
episodes are frequently seen when such patients are admitted to hospital
for much needed rehabilitation after a period of immobility.

5   SUSCEPTIBILITY TO ILLNESS

A recent paper has demonstrated a relationship between extremes of
weather and death from various illnesses (pneumonia, bronchitis,
myocardial infarction and strokes). If a person's housing is poor and
inadequately heated the effects of changes in the weather are likely to
be more pronounced.

6   RESISTANCE TO DISCHARGE FROM HOSPITAL

A patient admitted to a geriatric ward on making a good recovery will
usually wish to return home. However, her relatives, neighbours and
even some doctors and social workers may attempt to prevent her
discharge. These workers may be *so* appalled by the patient's home
conditions that it offends and embarrasses them to realize the extent of
that person's long-standing neglect and deprivation. The final decision
must, however, be made by the patient, who may well prefer independence in squalor rather than the neat regimentation offered by an
institution or the upheaval of moving to unfamiliar council accommodation.

The complications of poor nutrition

1 SCURVY
2 OSTEOMALACIA
3 HYPOKALAEMIA
4 ANAEMIA

1 SCURVY

Approximately half our elderly population take less than the recommended amount of Vitamin C (30mg) in their daily diet. In fact, the situation may be even worse, ascorbic acid is easily destroyed in cooking. Examination of the blood on routine admissions to a geriatric unit has shown the incidence of abnormal levels of ascorbic acid to be as high as 58 per cent. In contrast, only two definite cases of scurvy could be confirmed in 800 subjects studied in a national survey (there were also 2 other strongly suspected cases). As an overt clinical problem, scurvy is therefore not common, but when it does occur, it is usually found in widowers. The diagnosis may be initially suggested by the finding of sheet haemorrhages, usually on the legs and not to be confused with the very common senile purpura found on the hands. Follicular haemorrhages and stunted curled body hairs are further clues. Bleeding gums, however, do not occur in the edentulous. Painful joints and a refractory anaemia are other possible findings.

The diagnosis is best confirmed by estimation of the leucocyte ascorbic acid levels which are unfortunately not universally available. Other tests depending on urine collections, are unreliable and difficult to perform on elderly patients.

From the haematological and dietary evidence available, subclinical scurvy would seem to be much commoner. Although less dramatic than the fully developed disease, it may well be of considerable significance. The healing of leg ulcers, pressure sores and surgical wounds is thought to be delayed in the absence of adequate amounts of ascorbic acid. These problems are all too frequent in geriatric practice, and extra loading with vitamin C may be beneficial and may speed recovery.

2 OSTEOMALACIA

This is a condition which is more common in the elderly, than in the rest of the population in this country. Current survey findings indicate that about 50–60 per cent of the elderly take less than the recommended daily intake of vitamin D (100 international units). The main sources are fat fish (herrings, salmon and sardines) dairy products and fortified margarine. Because of cost, convenience or taste, many of these products are unavailable or unacceptable to the elderly.

Our knowledge of the metabolism of vitamin D is still incomplete but it is becoming increasingly evident that its endogenous production in the skin on exposure to sunlight is of great importance. The discrepancy between the incidence of dietary deficiency of vitamin D (up to 60 per cent) and the incidence of osteomalacia (4 per cent) in the same population indicates that there are serious gaps in our information about this condition. For clinical details see Chapter 9.

3 HYPOKALAEMIA

The finding of low serum potassium levels in old people admitted to hospital is common. Similarly, low dietary intakes of potassium have been reported in almost half of those elderly subjects studied in their own homes. Because hypokalaemia can cause confusion, depression and weakness, it is an important deficiency worthy of detection and treatment. Many patients will have been forced into a deficient situation by their poorly managed drug regimes, diuretics and purgatives being especially dangerous. Such preparations will often be taken in conjunction with a poor diet (less than 50 milliequivalents of potassium daily). Rich sources of potassium are citrus fruits, instant coffee and milk chocolate. These foods are rarely eaten by the elderly in significant amounts (See also Chapter 16).

4 ANAEMIA

Dietary deficiencies of iron, vitamin B_{12} or folic acid are undoubtably capable of producing anaemia. However in most anaemic elderly patients the aetiology lies elsewhere. Iron deficiency is mostly secondary to blood loss and B_{12} deficiency due to its malabsorption in pernicious anaemia. The incidence of folate deficiency in old age is high—up to 20 per cent of geriatric patients have a low red-cell folate level. The significance of this finding is not yet known but most of the deficient patients are not anaemic. For a fuller discussion of anaemia see Chapter 17.

The correction of financial deprivation

Many of the results of financial deprivation can be corrected by medical means. However, unless the basic social problems are solved the improvement may not be lasting. In some instances the situation may be worsened if the correct solution is not applied. For example a depressed or anxious person may consult her doctor. The general practitioner, feeling powerless when confronted by her social problems, may try to cure with a purely medical device. The antidepressant given, may then cause dangerous and unwanted side effects and make a bad situation worse by adding medical problems to social difficulties.

Where financial deprivation exists it can be corrected either by:
1 Providing extra money.
2 Supplying services or facilities not available because of relative poverty.

1 PROVISION OF EXTRA MONEY

To provide all old people with as much money as they would like is an impossible task. Individual needs and preferences obviously vary considerably but a pension system which forces one-third of its recipients to apply for supplementary benefits is clearly inadequate. Furthermore approximately one-sixth of pensioners are also eligible for extra payments, and do not apply. Half of our pensionable population have insufficient funds to maintain a minimum standard of living.

The Supplementary Benefits Commission

The Supplementary Benefits Commission (previously National Assistance Board) is the main source of additional grants. Extra money can be provided for such items as additional heating, special diets or laundry costs. Application is made on form SB1 obtained from any post office. Allowances are based on both need and extent of income, including income from capital. Allowances when granted are paid through special order books, which may be combined with the retirement pension book, and the money received from the nearest post office. Single payments may also be made to cover exceptional or unexpected costs, such as replacement of bedding or clothing.

Rent rebates and rent allowances

These are for council tenants, and tenants of unfurnished private accommodation. Application is made through the Town Hall or rent officer and refunds depend on income, number of people living in the accommodation and of the value of the rent.

War pensions

If any disability can be shown to have followed a war injury (including those to civilians) an additional pension may be available. The length of time between injury and claim is irrelevant, but a long delay obviously makes it more difficult to prove the cause of the disability.

Attendance allowances

These take the form of grants, made available to help cover the cost of care for people requiring considerable assistance, in personal functions and needing nursing care, or both. Although available for disabled people of all ages about one-third are taken for people over the age of 65 years. The first step in making a claim is completion of form DS2 obtained from the local social security office, a medical examination is then arranged at a later date.

Invalid Care Allowance

This is a maintenance benefit for potential breadwinners who are devoting their lives to caring for severely disabled relatives receiving an attendance allowance. At least 35 hours a week must be spent in caring for the disabled person and only those prevented from performing fulltime gainful employment are eligible.

Special disabilities

Special disabilities such as blindness will qualify for extra concessions and financial assistance. Arrangements for registration as a blind person are made through the local authority departments of the social service. Special registers are also kept for sufferers from other chronic disabilities such as epilepsy, chronic neurological disorders, arthritis and respiratory impairment. Registration is voluntary, but it might help when making further financial claims.

Charities

These are far too numerous to mention; but are related to professions, religious denominations or specific diseases. The Charity Commission keeps a national index and local authorities should list smaller, local, charitable funds. Usually only small grants are made for special well-defined needs, but regular payments are made in some instances.

Concessions

Discounts are often available to the elderly for a variety of services, e.g. fares, cinema tickets and hair care. Although a patronising method of providing help, they should be used when available. It would be better if the elderly had sufficient funds to pay the full economic price.

2   THE PROVISION OF SERVICES AND FACILITIES

Provision of suitable accommodation

In many instances, it will be found that the solution of an elderly
person's housing problem will also assist in difficulties with heating
and nutrition. There is therefore a considerable overlap between the
topics dealt with in this section and the preceding section and the
one which follows.

Home improvements

Home improvement grants will be available in many instances to
provide modern sanitation. Though the life expectancy of the property
is relevant, that of the applicant is not. Old people should therefore be
encouraged where possible to apply for such assistance. For the community this will be a worthwhile investment that will help to improve
the general housing stock, even if the prognosis of the elderly applicant
is poor. Other improvements can make life easier and safer in the elderly
person's home, e.g. handrails, conversion of steps to ramps and changing
the position of electrical sockets and switches. These can usually be
arranged by the local authority's domiciliary occupational therapy
service.

Improvements to heating

The availability of extra money for heating has already been mentioned.
The local authority social services department will also help in providing
more efficient and safer forms of heating, if these seem appropriate.
    Voluntary organizations in some areas will also help with insulation
improvements and local authority grants may be available for this
purpose. Local knowledge is normally required in order to locate
such help—social workers or the Age Concern organization will know
the necessary contacts.

Special housing

This usually takes the form of a small group of single bedroom flats,
bedsitters or bungalows built either by the local authority or housing
associations. A few private schemes also exist. The concept is commonly
described as sheltered housing, and the group is usually supervised by a
resident warden. It is not a new idea, but has many similarities to the
old almshouses system. The aim of such housing is to keep the elderly
person as independent as possible, by making the activities of daily

living as simple as possible. Also, it is easy to provide additional support such as home help, and meals-on-wheels to the residents of such sheltered housing, should it become necessary. The time needed for a home help to give support in a slum might be the same as the time taken to support three residents of separate modern purpose-built flats.

The number of sheltered housing units in the country is not precisely known, but it is certainly increasing. It is estimated that at the present time less than 1 per cent of the over 65-year-old population lives in such accommodation. As just over 5 per cent are thought to be in need of sheltered housing, the short fall in supply is obvious.

Where the operation of such schemes has been studied, it seems the majority of vacancies arise from the tenant's death. This therefore suggests that, given suitable housing, most old people can retain their independence and privacy right up to the time of death. Because of these results it is now increasingly the policy of those caring for the elderly, to argue in favour of more sheltered housing, with the necessary supporting services, rather than increasing the number of places in residential care.

Residential care

This topic is more fully dealt with in Chapter 4. Originally, this form of accommodation was conceived as providing hotel facilities for fit elderly people. However, because of the increasing disability of many of the residents now being accepted, and the greater awareness of the adverse effects of institutionalization, policy changes are occurring in the management of these homes. Many are being forced into providing nursing-home care, whilst others are attempting to divide their residents into small groups living as independently as possible in their own flats. Such a flat would consist of about six bedrooms, a common dining-room, lounge and kitchen.

The prevention and correction of poor nutrition

Dietary education

Dietary education is important throughout life. However, extra opportunities to increase dietary knowledge arise, when pre-retirement courses are held. Also dietary advice and demonstrations can be given in clubs run by and for the elderly, and also in local authority day centres and geriatric day hospitals.

Luncheon clubs

The great advantage of luncheon clubs is that they provide both food and contact with other people. They are usually run by the local authority or by a voluntary organization such as the Womens Royal Voluntary Service (WRVS) or Red Cross and may use the same kitchen as the meals-on-wheels service. The present rate of provision is 185,000 meals each week. A particularly attractive scheme is where the elderly diners join children in their school canteen—this gives much pleasure to the elderly, and increases the insight of the young into the problems of old age.

The major obstacle in running a luncheon club is lack of transport. It is unfortunately true that it is easier and cheaper to transport meals than people. Meals however, deteriorate during transport but people will often enjoy, and benefit from a ride around their neighbourhood taking them from home to luncheon club.

Meals-on-wheels

This is the commonly used name for the service which takes prepared meals to the housebound. Originally instituted by the WRVS it has, in many areas, been taken over or supported financially by the local authority. At present about 2 per cent of the elderly receive such meals although, it is estimated that 7 per cent would like to. Of the 119,500 who benefit from the meals-on-wheels service only 2 per cent receive meals on seven days a week—the majority have to manage with two or three visits from the service each week.

Because of the problems of bulk cooking and transport delays, the nutritional value of the delivered meal is often poor and, in addition, there is considerable wastage as the meals are often unacceptable to the clients. For these reasons in order to encourage the social benefits associated with eating together, more effort should be made to substitute luncheon clubs for the meals-on-wheels service wherever possible.

Social deprivation

Social deprivation is impossible to define. Social needs vary not only from person to person but day by day. There is therefore no physiological range or minimum daily recommendation. It is the loss of freedom to alter social contact according to need that leads to social deprivation.

Aetiological factors in social deprivation

1   ISOLATION

Thirty per cent of the elderly population live alone. Many of these people have done so all of their lives—either by choice or circumstance. Some will enjoy their apartness others will have grown to accept it. The success of adjustment is likely to be proportional to the duration of the period of isolation.

Isolation is not however, synonomous with living alone. An old person living with her family if neglected and actively resented may, in effect, be more isolated than a housebound widow living alone in a warden-controlled flat. Resentment occasionally reaches the pitch of 'granny-bashing'.

People living alone are clearly at risk of suffering from social deprivation. They are fortunately easily recognized but unwelcome help must not be forced upon them. But it is important that they be informed of the nature and availability of assistance.

2   PERSONALITY FAULTS

It is said that personality traits become more obvious with ageing. Faults are likely therefore to become more evident. Selfishness, greed and intolerance may all increase in the final years of people with such tendencies. They may therefore very effectively alienate themselves from their relatives and friends, at the very time that their help would be most needed.

Psychologists suggest that there are four broad patterns to ageing with the following resulting types (Fig. 3.3).

(a) 'Rocking-chair man'—happy with his past, contented with his present and unafraid of the future.

(b) 'Armoured man'—determined to live independently and for as long as possible whatever the odds and each new difficulty is accepted as a challenge.

(c) 'Angry man'—bitter because of the inequalities between youth and old age.

(d) 'Self-hating man'—wishing for death so as not to be a burden to anybody.

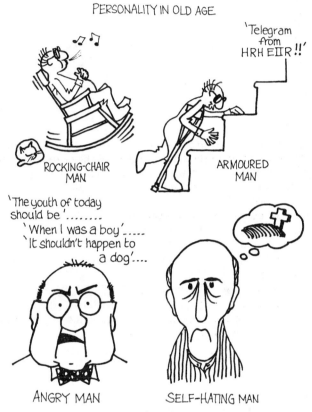

Fig. 3.3

The first example is usually loved and cherished, the second admired but the third and fourth are much less attractive and in extreme forms will be avoided by society in general.

3 DEPRESSION

Depression may not only result from social deprivation but may also be a potent ingredient in its causation. Contact with other people may be lost because of a general lack of motivation and withdrawal or be secondary to feelings of unworthiness sometimes found in victims of depression.

4 PARANOIA

Elderly people with this characteristic, sometimes due to a form of schizophrenia are likely to be unattractive to their neighbours and other potential helpers. The paranoid person's false accusations of persecution will eventually discourage even the kindest supporter. The deaf and partially sighted are particularly prone to the development of paranoia, probably due to the misinterpretation of poorly appreciated visual and auditory information.

5 DEMENTIA

Short-term memory loss in dementia makes meaningful conversation impossible. Apparently pointless repetition of the same question will cause immense frustration and annoyance to everyone. In the late stages of dementia the unkempt appearance and offensive smell of some victims will increase their unattractiveness. Constant failure to recognize even the closest relatives (husband, son) may occasionally so upset the unrecognized that they are unable to continue caring for the patient.

6 PHYSICAL DISABILITIES

Physical disabilities may lead to social deprivation either by restriction of mobility or by the reduction of attractiveness to others. Up to 20 per cent of elderly people are housebound and therefore very limited in their opportunities for contact with others. Many younger people, because of their own fears concerning illness and deformity and ageing, find the appearance of the elderly disabled an unacceptable threat to their own security and therefore avoid any contact with them. Problems associated with cramped living conditions, e.g. stale air and general untidiness also act as deterrents to visitors.

7 RETIREMENT

Retirement means more than the simple loss of a job; it means less contact with colleagues; it means loss of status, because people are often judged by the jobs they perform, it means reduction in usefulness, and it means a fall in income.

Although retirement, in most instances, is foreseeable it is rare for preparation to be undertaken. The result is frustration and disillusionment. A quarter of retired men freely admit to missing the companionship of work and even more—39 per cent will express a desire to return to work if only it were possible.

8 BEREAVEMENT

Early death is the only sure protection from bereavement which is therefore an inescapable experience for most people surviving into old age—especially women.

The death of a partner or close friend is obviously a traumatic event. The fact that over 50 per cent of the bereaved experience hallucinations —in the form of imagining the presence of the loved one is a good indication of its significance. Fortunately the majority are not disturbed by the hallucinations but others require reassurance of their common occurrence.

More serious is the marked rise in mortality amongst the survivors of bereavement, especially in the early stages, when death can occur up to 40 per cent more commonly than is normal. This phenomenon is perhaps one of the best examples of psychosomatic disease and illustrates the point that it is not restricted to the young and immature. Suicide in the elderly increases after bereavement, and is about $2\frac{1}{2}$ times more frequent in the year following the death of a close relative.

9 MIGRATION

As our society becomes more mobile from a social, mechanical and geographical point of view families are going to become more dispersed. Happily this is accepted and even encouraged by most families and the consequent loss of contact between the generations is accepted. Social crises do however become more likely and more easily precipitated.

Contact between relatives is probably better than expected as 30 per cent of elderly people are reported to have daily contact with a son or daughter or other close relative. A similar number have at least weekly contact.

Prevention and correction of social deprivation

Prevention is always preferred to correction, and is certainly the most realistic way of dealing with social deprivation. Mention has already been made of the difficulties in detecting the socially deprived as self-reporting is rare, and because of the nature of the defects, it is unlikely that others will easily notice the deprived person's needs. As in other situations, it is frequently the case that by the time the needs are realized the opportunity for improving the state of affairs has passed.

RE-EVALUATION OF RETIREMENT

Enormous changes in attitudes to work and our system of valuing
people's worth to society are needed. At present, success is measured
against increasing responsibility and monetary rewards and both are
expected to increase with age. However, ability to cope with new
situations does not improve with age, whereas experience with familiar
situations does, and is a valuable asset of the elderly. Successful
decision making therefore requires the problem solving abilities of the
young, plus the past experience of the old. To expect ageing persons to
perform both roles exposes them to unnecessary stress and causes poor
results. Social gerontologists are aware of this phenomenon, and
consider it one of the causes of industrial recession.

The pre-retirement phase of life can therefore be very difficult and
stressful. In addition the increasing fear of compulsory retirement and
unemployment may worsen the situation. Pre-retirement courses
should therefore aim to help with the winding down of work responsibilities and the stimulation of thoughts concerning retirement. Such
courses should start many years before employment ceases and spouses
should also participate.

Retired people need not only advice about the use of their increased
leisure time, but also they will need opportunities to do socially valuable
tasks for others. Provision of many of the services discussed in the rest
of this present chapter provide fit elderly people opportunities to help
others, for example, the provision and organization of transport services and day centres for the more frail elderly.

Another function for pre-retirement courses is the dissemination of
knowledge about ageing and health in old age. It is generally accepted
that puberty is made easier if the expected changes are known to the
individual and the same is true for ageing.

There is considerable evidence that carefully planned retirements
are the most successful, and our aim should therefore be to ensure that
everybody enjoys the same advantages. Large firms should therefore
be encouraged to run their own schemes, and smaller concerns should
be able to receive help from the educational services or from organizations such as Age Concern.

SOCIAL CLUBS AND DAY CENTRES

The main function of these organizations is the maintenance of a wide
circle of friends and social contacts. This becomes an increasingly
important function, for as ageing increases, death will begin to remove
friends and relatives at an increasingly rapid rate. Although complete

substitute relationships can rarely be made to compensate for loss due to death in old age, contact with a plentiful number of acquaintances will help. (The situation for young widows and widowers is quite different.) It should be remembered that a close husband–wife relationship may be all that is required in young and middle life, but this is a potentially dangerous situation in old age where bereavement can leave the survivor entirely alone.

Another function for these clubs and centres is that they provide worthwhile activities for the 'young old' to assist the 'old old'. In the first ten years of retirement, health and activity are usually maintained, and involvement in the organization of a club will provide many satisfying rewards, and it should also provide insight into one's own ageing process.

IMPROVEMENT OF TRANSPORT FACILITIES

This is closely linked with the above description of social clubs, as frequently those most in need of attending are the housebound. Because of their physical disabilities, they will be prevented from becoming members of a club if they cannot have access to suitable transport. Similar help will also be needed to assist visits to friends and relations, including those in hospital and residential homes.

Improvement in 'bus design would make it possible for the elderly to use public transport more readily. The payment of travel allowances would make it possible to afford taxi services. The 'young old' could help to provide transport for the older and frailer if they could receive help with their petrol costs.

VISITING SCHEMES

It should be the aim of every general practice to arrange a system of regular visits to the housebound on their list, and also those under exceptional stress such as occurs at the time of bereavement. These visits can be performed by the community nurse, health visitor or doctor, according to the patient's known and anticipated needs. The frequency of such visits will also be variable, but should be regular.

In addition, social visiting by the local authority social workers and volunteers organized by churches, professional bodies, clubs and work places should take place. Ideally, these volunteers should receive some guidance and training. Their task is difficult, tact is required, methods of introduction need to be learnt and skill is needed in detecting hidden needs and potential dangers. The professional workers and health visitors, doctors and social workers should all assist in the necessary training, and this initial contact should also make the reporting back of problems much easier and more efficient.

IMPROVEMENT IN TOWN PLANNING

The idea here should be flexibility and comprehensive mixing. In a truly mixed and complete community, it is easy for a person to move house according to accommodation requirement without separation from friends, neighbours and relatives. Such arrangements not only provide the most suitable accommodation according to the person's needs, but also ensure proper use of all available housing stock for the community. Under-usage of large family homes by widows and widowers is avoided and life for such people can be made easier by occupation of purpose-built flats or bungalows in the same district. The use of familiar clubs, pubs and churches can still be enjoyed and old social contacts maintained.

CHAPTER 4 · PATTERNS OF CARE

Warm baths, good food, soft sleep, and generous wine—
These are the rights of age, and should be thine.

Advice from Ulysses to his father, Laertes (HOMER)

The vast majority—about 94 per cent—of the elderly are living in private households, so that only 6 per cent are being cared for in institutions run by the Health and Social Services or in private nursing homes. A one per cent swing away from the community would add a catastrophic 17 per cent to the demand for institutional care. The 94 per cent living in the community fall into three overlapping groups— those who are independent, those who are supported by relatives or neighbours, and those who are supported by the community services.

The independent

These are the most able-bodied and, generally, the youngest among the old (Fig. 4.1) because, over the age of eighty, it is unusual to be sufficiently active to cope with the shopping as well as the housework and cooking.

Support from relatives

Many elderly and frail people live with their relatives, but some receive considerable support from them although living apart.

Those living with their relatives

Some of these are so disabled that they require considerable nursing. The skills required for home nursing are mostly self-taught, so teaching programmes for groups of relatives can be very worthwhile. These relatives are the unsung and unpaid heroes and heroines of the welfare state, and often, though themselves ageing and ailing, sacrifice their own health and leisure to provide a home and nursing care.

Other families are only too anxious to shrug off the responsibility for the care of their aged relatives on to the state and its servants. In a

45

highly industrialized and mobile society, it is becoming increasingly unlikely that when we grow old, our children will have settled down in the same village or town. Care cannot easily be provided by remote control.

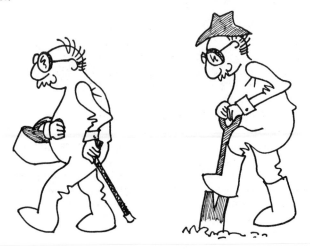

DEPENDENCE   1 Independence
Able to shop, perhaps even garden.
Home — little support required.

Fig. 4.1

Even when the children do live nearby, but give little support, it is too easy to criticize apparent indifference. It is impossible for the outsider to delve back into the murky recesses of family psychopathology. The lovable little twinkling eyed grandmother may have been a far from perfect wife and mother. Indeed, she may be reaping the harvest of a lifetime's selfish neglect of the rest of the family.

The army of daughters and nieces looking after chronically disabled old people deserves whatever the state can afford. The *Attendance Allowance* can be claimed by persons requiring considerable personal assistance (see Chapter 3). The geriatrician can also do a great deal through counselling to make the burden more tolerable. He can offer one or two *holiday admissions* a year to enable the supporting relatives to get away. (This should be anything but a holiday for the patient, because an attempt should be made to rehabilitate her and thereby increase her capacity for self care.) Alternatively, the doctor can provide *day hospital* care one or more days a week if this is preferred. Unfortunately, the hospital cannot compete with the one to one staff to patient ratio which an old lady may enjoy at home with her daughter, and the quality of care suffers accordingly.

Those living apart from their relatives

These old people may rely on numerous visits daily for help with getting out of bed, dressing, cleaning the house, cooking, lighting the fire, washing, and even with personal hygiene. Or it may simply be a question of doing the shopping and offering hospitality for Sunday lunch.

Support from the community services

A number of supportive services are provided by the social services and by voluntary organisations. These are designed to augment the help given by relatives and to provide for those without supporting relatives. The recipients are generally HOUSEBOUND and no longer independent (Fig. 4.2).

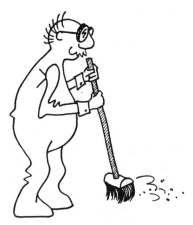

DEPENDENCE   2 Housebound
Capable of a little cooking and very light housework.
Home with support. May need rehousing.

Fig. 4.2

The aetiology of 'housebinding'

It is often easy to see why people become housebound. They may only be able to walk short distances, possibly with the help of a frame. They may lack the physical agility to cross the road in safety, or the mental agility to cope with shopping. Impairment of vision or hearing will add considerably to these difficulties. Sometimes, however, the condition seems to be almost deliberate. Social isolation (see Chapter 3) may produce a vicious circle leading to withdrawal from normal social intercourse and a reluctance to meet people, even singly. And sometimes it seems to be due simply to a dislike of fresh air and exposure to the elements. If this unwillingness to leave home can be overcome *day care* may provide a valuable way of expanding social contacts and relieving loneliness. This may be available one or two days a week at a *local authority day centre* or at one of the residential homes. (Some of these homes will also offer support to relatives by looking after an aged person who cannot be left on her own for the odd morning or evening.) Day care may also be provided by voluntary bodies at *luncheon clubs* and *over 60's clubs*. As well as the opportunity to meet others and make friends, attendance at these centres and clubs can bring other benefits such as a hot meal and various diversional activities and classes. Transport is usually necessary, but some local authorities provide mobile units for foot care, and in a few places there are mobile day units to serve rural populations. Passing mention should be made of the various holiday schemes arranged by voluntary bodies.

Domiciliary services

These bring assistance right into the home, to replace or supplement the help of family and friends. There are limitations to these services and in particular there are geographical variations in the scale of provision. It is usually difficult to provide attention during the nights and weekends.

The general practitioner

Mentioned for the sake of completeness, he clearly carries prime responsibility for the health and overall well-being of his patient. He is the leader of the primary care team.

The community nursing service

The community nurse can help in the supervision of drug regimes as well as giving enemas, injections and dressings. Less skilled tasks such as bathing may be carried out by auxiliaries. Twilight nursing involves settling the patient for the night and exceptionally night nursing may be arranged.

The health visitor

In addition to her nursing qualifications she has received special training in the social aspects of health. This enables her to offer advice concerning the overall welfare of her patients and to play a co-ordinating role in the deployment of the various services available.

The social worker

The social worker will visit by request to assess the needs of the client. He, or she, will be able to offer guidance and practical help as well as acting in a liaison capacity. Another aspect of the social worker's case-work is emotional support through counselling, for instance immediately following bereavement. He/she is also responsible for the assessment of applicants for residential care.

The hospital at home

This is a concept which has been pioneered in Paris and adopted with modifications elsewhere. It comprises an identifiable team of medical, nursing and rehabilitation staff who can deliver appropriate continuing care following discharge from hospital. In selected cases it offers the choice of avoiding hospital admission. It appears likely that the French model will require considerable adaptation before it can offer any great advantage over existing services in this country. Here, for example, in addition to the general practitioner and the community nurse, *domiciliary physiotherapy* is available in some localities; domiciliary *chiropody* is reasonably widespread; and the *domiciliary occupational therapist* can advise concerning adaptations around the house to make life easier and safer for the disabled. Equipment is available on loan from the local authority or the British Red Cross Society.

The home help

Home helps are an extremely valuable body of women employed by the local authority to cope with much of the housework, cooking and washing. Shopping and other extra tasks are often undertaken. (A *laundry service* may be provided by the local authority, but foul linen is usually only accepted by hospital laundries.)

Meals-on-wheels

These are organised by voluntary bodies such as the WRVS or by the social services department. A variation on this theme is the *cook-a-meal scheme* whereby a neighbour who is cooking for her own family will prepare an extra portion for which she is reimbursed and will carry it to the recipient.

The domiciliary care assistant

This is an experimental grade of staff whose task it is to perform the same range of simple personal services which are expected of their counterparts in residential homes. These include some assistance with dressing and bathing which would otherwise be given by a well intentioned relative.

The flying warden

An innovative scheme has been reported whereby an old person can summon a mobile warden by simply removing the plug from a small radio alarm transmitter installed in her own home. Pocket units are available for those liable to fall.

Voluntary services

Most of the help that old people receive comes from friends and neighbours. Often this is on a personal basis, but, failing this, assistance may be organized through co-ordinating bodies such as Age Concern. This organization has a network of village representatives, as well as offices in the larger towns which can answer many enquiries. Examples of the type of service they may be able to locate include:

Night sitters—a non-qualified night sitting service providing surrogate relatives in order to tide over social crises affecting persons who cannot be left alone at night.

Day sitters—to come in for a few hours during the absence of a relative.

Home care or good neighbours—untrained helpers who undertake personal tasks on a 'pop-in' basis perhaps four times a day.

Street wardens—who can be contacted in the event of any crisis affecting an aged person on their 'patch'. All these services are usually voluntary, but in some places are paid for by the social services department. Other activities include weekend meals, transport, day centres and luncheon clubs. Special provision for blindness and deafness are made by the social services department as well as by voluntary bodies.

The Church also participates in the care of the old in the community. A familiar example is the 'Fish' which is placed in the window to attract attention to the need for help within.

Rehousing

A question which often arises is whether the home itself should be changed. In other words, should application be made for rehousing? The old, it has been said, do not transplant readily, and the decision to change locality to be with, or near, the family may be taken in haste and regretted at leisure. Similarly, a move to another part of town into a convenient, warm old people's bungalow can appear to be tidy and humane, and reluctance can be difficult to understand. The fact is that the ramshackle, unheated, squalid house with the toilet the other side of the back yard may represent familiarity and security, and such moves are probably better made sooner rather than later if at all. A very valuable development has been the construction of *'sheltered housing'* usually consisting of warden controlled flatlets or bungalows. These flatlets are of modern design and the warden who supervises them is available to the residents at the press of a bell in case of emergency. In some places, complexes have been planned, comprising a residential home, sheltered accommodation, a day centre, and perhaps even a community hospital with a small day hospital on the same site. Such developments smack of the establishment of 'geriatric ghettoes', and there is no reason to suppose that segregation of the aged is desirable.

Finding accommodation for the homeless is always difficult, but in some places *boarding out schemes* have been organized in an attempt to match a frail elderly person with a suitable landlady, who will be paid something approaching the commercial rate for the job.

There are a number of housing associations (e.g. the Abbeyfield Society) who offer a variety of mixes of independence, companionship, and support.

Institutional care

It cannot be sufficiently emphasized that one of the fundamental aims of geriatric medicine is to avoid long-term institutional care. It is the basic tenet of our philosophy that our patients prefer us to help them remain in their own homes, than to herd them into institutions where they can be 'wrapped in cotton wool' and preserved in comparative comfort and safety for year after empty year. The staff may strive with dedication and usually a fair degree of success to make the quality of life as good as human ingenuity can make it, but loss of independence leads to loss of initiative and intellect and personality. Institutional care is also very expensive both in financial resources, which are scarce, and in human resources, which are scarcer still. It has been well said that people are looked after by people, not by beds and buildings. For once, therefore, humanitarian and economic considerations coincide.

It is ironic that so much geriatric accommodation is still situated in the old workhouse: and the workhouses were designed to deter those without, rather than to provide adequate amenities for those within. The object of today's geriatric service is to ensure that hospitals are used for the job they do best, which is mainly diagnosis and treatment, but also the longer-term care of those patients for whom no alternative pattern of care would be appropriate. It is essential that they care for this latter group of patients with humanity and compassion.

Local authority residential care

(Otherwise known as Old People's Homes, Welfare Homes, or Part III Accommodation.)

These homes provide hostel-type accommodation to those who have lost domestic competence—in other words are unable to maintain a home of their own (Fig. 4.3). It is usual to find that residents have

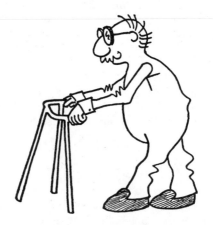

DEPENDENCE 3 Frailty

Walks, dresses, continent, "personally independent" but may need help bathing. Cannot maintain a home. Local Authority Residential Home – or relatives.

Fig. 4.3

their own rooms or share with one other person. There is generally a central dining room but a successful practice is the division of the home into small units of six to eight people having their own sitting room and kitchen facilities. A variable charge is made up to the full maintenance cost (£55-£60 per week in 1979), depending on the ability to pay. In theory the residents should be sufficiently mobile, perhaps with the help of a walking frame, to reach the lavatory or dining room without assistance. They should be capable of dressing themselves and should, in general, be continent although irreversible incontinence in an otherwise able-bodied person is not necessarily a disqualifying factor. Finally, the residents should be of sufficiently sound mind not to require constant supervision, although a variable degree of confusion may be tolerated. Most will require assistance with bathing.

These homes are the responsibility of the social services department of the local authority, and it has been suggested by the DHSS that places in them should be provided at a scale of 25 per thousand of the elderly population (65 and over). They are staffed by care assistants under the supervision of the officer in charge.

Hospital facilities

The activities of the hospital service can be divided into 'cure' and 'care'. What hospitals do best is active investigation and treatment, so the initial aim of admission to a geriatric ward is cure. Unfortunately, failure to achieve this goal is all too frequent in hospital practice, especially if the goal is broadened to encompass the restoration of activity as well as the successful treatment of disease. The outcome of survival without successful rehabilitation is a patient who remains dependent on continuing nursing care. If she is immobile and incontinent, she cannot be managed by the staff of a residential home, and can seldom be looked after by her relatives (Fig. 4.4).

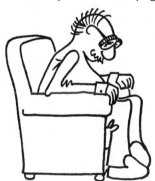

DEPENDENCE 4 Dependent
Chair or bedridden. Hospital or relatives.

Fig. 4.4

Mental frailty

Qualitatively, no other disability will so seriously threaten domestic competence as mental frailty. This leads to difficulty in handling money or forgetfulness in turning off taps or stoves. No other disability so strains filial affection as harbouring an aged in-law incapable of maintaining any kind of rational conversation, or worse, requiring constant supervision so that she cannot ever be left alone, or, most alienating of all, persistently incontinent.

Quantitatively, the importance of chronic brain disease is stressed in Chapter 8. The incidence rises linearly with increasing age, so this burden will increase steadily as the population ages.

Care of the mentally disabled

The psychiatric equivalent of the continuing care geriatric ward is to be found in the geriatric wards of the mental hospital, which house

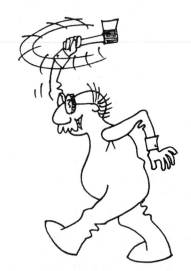

DEPENDENCE 6 Severe Dementia
Anti-social behaviour. Ambulant.
Mental Hospital.

Fig. 4.5

ambulant but demented patients, generally with anti-social conduct (Fig. 4.5). Those who are demented but also so physically handicapped that they need to be lifted out of bed and on to the chair or lavatory are properly the responsibility of the geriatrician. There is also a level of intellectual failure at which supervision by mentally trained nurses and psychiatrists is not really necessary, particularly where the behaviour is not anti-social. This category of patient is sometimes rather mis-leadingly referred to as the 'happy wanderer' (Fig. 4.6). In the absence

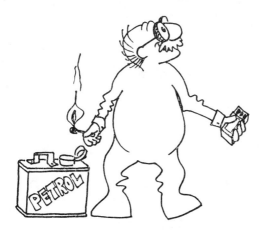

DEPENDENCE 5 Mental Infirmity
Mild dementia: the "happy wanderer."
Probably incontinent and needs supervision
Local Authority Residential Home for
Elderly Mentally Infirm – or relatives.

Fig. 4.6

of willing relatives, they are sometimes looked after in special residential homes for the 'elderly mentally infirm' (EMI) where a degree of incontinence is acceptable and where there is sufficient supervision to cater for a tendency to wander. Other authorities distribute these people among ordinary residential homes, and yet others have adopted a policy of attaching EMI wings to all newly built homes. It has been recom-mended that five places per thousand elderly (over 65) should be provided for the EMI, and 2.5 to three beds in psychiatric hospitals for the 'elderly severely mentally infirm' (ESMI), although at least twice this number is probably more realistic.

The interfaces

There are three principal frailties which develop in old age—physical, mental and social. They should not be thought of as mutually exclusive but as forming a kind of triangular continuum (Fig. 4.7). Physical, mental, and social factors often all co-exist in varying degrees, and may be interdependent. It is therefore not always clear to the family doctor, social worker, and relatives, whether help should be sought from the geriatrician, psychiatrist, or department of social services. If action is

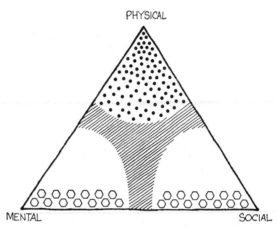

The three-cornered continuum of frailty: the Geriatric Department should accept responsibility for patients within the spotted area, but cannot be expected to accept those along the baseline area. There is a large central zone (hatched) which should be the object of constructive discussion rather than rejection.

Fig. 4.7

taken early enough (for instance, by referral to the geriatric out-patient clinic), wheels can be set in motion. If nothing is done, crisis is inevitable, but because it is multifactorial, it will be impossible to find a suitable and rapid solution. The resulting confusion and 'buck-passing' from one department to another, leads to frustration and resentment (Fig. 4.8).

Considerable controversy currently surrounds institutional provision for the frail elderly once they are no longer competent to maintain their own homes or live with their families. Continuing care geriatric and psychiatric hospitals are often remote, unhomely, and too rigidly subdivided into 'physical geriatrics' and psychiatry. They are also expensively staffed (comparatively speaking) with highly qualified nurses. Admission should therefore be restricted to those who are continuously dependent upon a high level of nursing care. Local authority residential homes, on the other hand, are staffed at a much lower level and do not employ nurses except coincidentally. They are sometimes structurally unsuitable, though perhaps elegant buildings, which, with minor modification, would make excellent Outward Bound Schools! The result is that the type of resident they can manage has to be so independent as to be by no means in need of institutional care. There is a growing body of opinion that there is no major role for

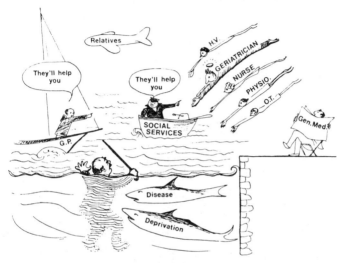

Fig. 4.8

residential care that fulfils anything less than a nursing home type of function, and that persons not needing this type of facility should be supported in their own homes. This major change towards a high-dependency resource has been taking place slowly but surely over the past decade. It is accepted in principle by many officers in charge, and will inevitably continue apace due to demographic pressure: it has profound implications on the numbers and type of staff required, as well as necessitating purpose-built accommodation.

The demarcation disputes between the different forms of institution represent an attempt to make the customer fit the institution, rather than the more appropriate exercise of adapting our institutions to meet the needs of the clients. And the clients are increasingly belonging to the 'grey area' or no man's land, between the hospital service and the social services. The typical candidate is in her 80s and is quite incompetent to continue to live alone, partly due to a significant degree of dementia, leading to confusion, restlessness and a tendency to wander. She also has physical disabilities and although her functional level will fluctuate from day to day, she can in general only walk short distances very slowly with her frame, and even then is liable to fall. She usually needs a fair amount of help or supervision with dressing and bathing. She is only partially sighted, and finds her hearing aid difficult to manage. Finally, she is incontinent of urine often and faeces when she becomes constipated. She does not in fact need nursing of a sophisticated kind, but she needs a considerable amount of the sort of care that would otherwise be provided by sensible, well intentioned relatives—provided that they were fit and active and more than one in number. The old 'joint user' establishment (part residential, part hospital) afforded the flexibility to cope rather better with this sort of person than our present segregated units, but were undesirable in other ways. Perhaps the answer is to upgrade our local authority homes structurally, expand them numerically to meet anticipated needs, and provide some nursing supervision as well as far higher staffing establishments. The financial implications are all too clear. Meanwhile, our endeavours must not culminate in dispute and rejection. They must aim to ensure that the most severely infirm are looked after in hospital (geriatric or psychiatric, depending on the main disability), that the next most severely infirm are looked after in residential homes, and that the most severely infirm thereafter receive the maximum amount of community support.

Indeed, the relative merits of domiciliary and institutional support are also coming under increasingly critical scrutiny. It may be better for the old person to remain in her own home, but it is becoming clear that it is not necessarily cheaper. In fact it is very expensive to deploy professional and other workers on a one-to-one basis in private homes, and to finance the inevitable car journeys between one client and the next. Domiciliary support for the very frail, therefore, may be more costly than institutionalization unless it is provided at such an inadequate level as to constitute neglect rather than care. Be that as it may, the allocation of a place in a residential facility to an old person less feeble than the above description should only ever be on a short-term basis, for instance as a form of crisis intervention.

The private sector

Private nursing homes run the complete gamut from the private equivalent of an old people's home (at 1979 prices about £40 to £50 per week) to the non-acute hospital with individual rooms and full nursing staff (anything over £200). In between is a large number of establishments of varying quality and with a varying amount of nursing cover, usually in the £50 to £100 range. In some parts of the country, they are too few in number to make a sizeable contribution to the care of the elderly, but in many popular retirement zones, they provide as many places as does the local authority. Inspections are carried out in order to maintain standards and the DHSS or the local authority may agree to support persons without means in these homes. It should be noted that persons in private nursing homes may also be eligible for the Attendance Allowance. Voluntary and religious bodies also run a number of homes, mainly of a residential character (Table 4.1).

Table 4.1. Institutional care (not hospitals) in England

Number of residents	Number of homes	Type
100,000	2,576	LARC
24,000	1,052	Voluntary sector
21,000	1,811	Private homes registered with LA SSD
24,367 Not all elderly	1,087	General medical, convalescent and geriatric private nursing homes registered with AHAs

CHAPTER 5 · THE GERIATRIC DEPARTMENT

> Every One Discharged Cured from this Infirmary be enjoined by the Chairman to give Publick Thanks in their Parish Churches.
>
> (from Orders for Inpatients, Westminster Hospital, 1720–1724)

Geriatric medicine has been a recognized specialty in the United Kingdom since the late forties. During the thirty or so years of its existence, the specialty has expanded enormously. It has established a pattern of practice which has achieved activity and independence for countless old people who would formerly have been consigned to chronic sick wards. It has transformed the chronic sick wards from the slum properties of the hospital service into places of hope and cheer. Its influence has spread to other countries where British-trained geriatricians have helped to pioneer hospital services for the elderly sick.

Unfortunately, geriatricians have been less successful in communicating this enthusiasm and know-how to colleagues in other medical specialities, and insufficient trainees are coming forward to feed the apparently insatiable appetite of the NHS for consultants in geriatric medicine. For this reason it is seriously questioned whether it is realistic for the DHSS to attempt to staff specialist geriatric units throughout the length and breadth of the country. Perhaps departments of geriatric medicine should exist only in special centres with a concentration of facilities for research and teaching. Elsewhere, hospital services for the aged could be provided by physicians who have acquired the necessary skills by undergoing training in these special departments but who are not restricted to the care of the elderly. Another alternative to the separate geriatric unit is the integration of geriatricians into general medical firms, so that geriatric expertise is available to all very elderly medical patients with multiple physical and mental disabilities, and to those looking after them. However the current debate is resolved, it is the purpose of this chapter to offer guidance on the management of a hospital service for the old.

The work of the physician in geriatric medicine involves him in four main roles:

1 Investigation and treatment of acute illness in the elderly

2 Providing medical leadership of the teamwork required for the rehabilitation and maintenance of activity of his patients
3 Determining the relative priorities of those irreversibly dependent patients referred to him with a view to long-term care
4 Teaching, research, and advising health authorities and other bodies concerning the needs of the old.

The assessment of the geriatric patient

More than any other hospital specialty, geriatric medicine is 'whole-person medicine'. It is a branch of medicine which can be pursued as academically as any other while always preserving a sense of proportion concerning the overall welfare of the patient. It therefore also demands common sense, compassion and patience. Each patient is assessed under the following main headings.

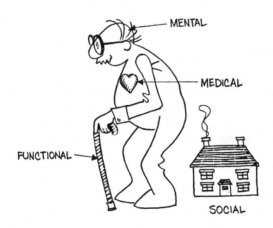

GERIATRIC ASSESSMENT

Fig. 5.1

1 Mental state

Although geriatrics is traditionally a branch of general medicine rather than psychiatry, no apology is made for placing this aspect at the top of the list. For one thing, the intellect is most conveniently assessed at the outset of the consultation, and for another, the interview cannot proceed if it is grossly impaired. The preliminary polite inquiries, such as 'How old are you?', 'How did you get here?', and 'Why have you come to see me?', will establish, without causing offence, whether the patient is correctly orientated and can give a reasonable account of herself, or whether more detailed questioning is necessary. It is usual to proceed to further probing, but it should be remembered that the detachment and realism which often accompany advanced years may make the name of the current occupant of 10 Downing Street a matter of little consequence! The name of the person who does the bulk of the housework is a better guide to social competence.

Furthermore, it cannot be sufficiently emphasized that the mental state is the single most important factor determining the potential quality of life. Even in someone physically well, significant dementia will make an independent life out of the question; and in the physically disabled, it will effectively prevent successful rehabilitation. It should be assumed, unless there is a reliable history of long-standing intellectual deterioration from a relative, that any apparent loss of mental function is due to a toxic confusional state rather than to irreversible dementia.

2 The diagnoses

The pathology is usually multiple, and some is active and some is inactive but nevertheless contributory to the overall picture. For example, the presenting illness is congestive cardiac failure, probably due to ischaemic heart disease, with uncontrolled atrial fibrillation and a superimposed chest infection. But a note must also be made of the residual left hemiparesis, the pinned fracture of the right femoral neck, the chronic constipation, the bilateral cataracts, and the obesity. Treatment can now be planned and an estimate formed of the likely prognosis.

3 Functional capacity

The interplay of all these factors, and their cumulative effect upon the subject, will dictate her functional capacity—in other words, her disabilities, and more important, her abilities. Of these, the most vital are mobility, and continence, and the ability to dress, wash and feed herself (Fig. 5.2).

4 The social background

A knowledge of the patient's functional capacity will indicate what sort of things will need to be done for her by other people. A knowledge of her social background will indicate whether those people exist, and how much they are able and willing to do for her. The geriatric team is now in a position to decide whether it is realistic to aim for complete

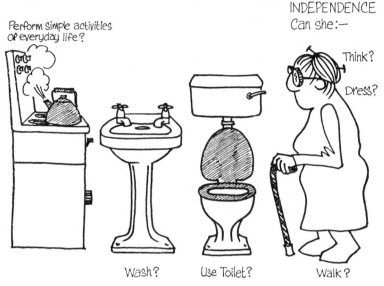

Fig. 5.2

independence, or independence with a degree of support, or whether some kind of institutional care will be required, and if so what.

It should be possible for any doctor, possessed of common sense, patience and the modicum of professional skill which carried him through his finals, to make this kind of complete assessment. It can therefore be made:

(a) IN THE WARD

In the ward—by the admitting doctor.

(b) IN THE OUT-PATIENT CLINIC

Different units differ widely in the importance which they attach to holding regular out-patient clinics. The advantage of clinics lies in allowing a complete examination, in favourable conditions, accompanied by adequate investigations, without the necessity of admitting the patient.

(c) BY DOMICILIARY CONSULTATION

These can only be carried out by the consultant, and they attract a small fee; he only visits at the general practitioner's request. The purpose of such a visit is to enable him to obtain the consultant's advice when the patient is too unwell for it to be practical for her to travel to the out-patient department or is frightened to do so. Here again, the facility is used much more extensively in some departments than in others, but does have the advantage that the consultant can see for himself the housing situation and meet the family or friends and stress to them that the hospital expects to discharge patients as well as to admit them!

(d) BY ASSESSMENT VISIT

This is usually carried out by a more junior member of the medical staff, often accompanied by a health visitor or remedial therapist, and usually at the request of the family doctor. (Many geriatric units also make considerable use of reports submitted by their geriatric liaison health visitor, who visits alone and may provide invaluable information.)

What action can be taken

There are many ways in which the geriatric physician may be able to help other than merely by offering a bed. Sometimes he will shed fresh light on the diagnosis and thus the likely prognosis. He may suggest alterations in drug therapy or emphasize that the family doctor is doing all that can reasonably be done. Sometimes he will merely try to offer some support and reassurance to the relatives, or advise them concerning life with granny and the mutual preservation of sanity. Occasionally he will act as a signpost, directing the patient towards some kind of social care, or towards the psychiatrist or another specialist colleague. And sometimes he will make use of another facility of his department, of which mention must be made.

The geriatric day hospital

The use of the geriatric day hospital has been increasing steadily in this country since the late 1950s, and now a unit without this facility is gravely handicapped by comparison with its neighbours. The day hospital exists for the treatment of the elderly sick, just as the geriatric wards do: and indeed, it serves as an 'office-hours' ward where patients can be examined and receive medical and nursing treatments including injections, enemata, and dressings. It serves as a surgery where minor ailments can be treated and where other services such as chiropody are

available. It serves as a rehabilitation unit for occupational and physiotherapy. Finally, the social aspects of a patient's attendance greatly
improve her outlook and morale. The advantages to the rest of the
department can be enumerated as follows:

1 Earlier discharge of in-patients because they will be able to continue
their therapy whilst living at home.
2 The commencement of treatment for out-patients who may be
awaiting admission.
3 The avoidance of certain admissions altogether: the entire programme of investigation and treatment can often be carried out on a day
hospital basis provided that the distance involved is not too great.
4 The prevention of relapse on discharge after in-patient rehabilitation.
5 The relief that may be afforded to relatives.
6 The day hospital will supplement the facilities of the wards, and
in-patients will benefit from attending because of the high level of
activity and the daily influx of patients from their own homes. In this
way, the transition from in-patient to out-patient care is less sharp,
and patients can be groomed for their return home.

It is not appropriate here to describe in detail the *modus operandi* of a
day hospital, but it receives its patients either after discharge from the
ward, or following assessment in one of the ways outlined above. A
specific objective has been set for each patient, who will usually attend
once, twice, or thrice weekly for a couple of months or so before being
reviewed at a multidisciplinary case conference, to see how nearly the
objective has been achieved. Because of its convenience, nine to five
routine, its stream of new patients, and often its new buildings, the day
hospital is comparatively easy to staff with a team of high quality and
good morale.

In-patient facilities: progressive patient care

1 The assessment ward

The vast majority of patients are admitted to an acute assessment ward
whose main function is diagnosis. This ward consists of beds which
have access to resident junior medical staff as well as full X-ray and
laboratory facilities and good physiotherapy and occupational therapy
departments. There is no reason to suppose that the acutely ill elderly
patient requires, or deserves, any less sophisticated medicine than her
younger counterpart. Most of these patients will be very feeble at
first and will require turning in bed, or at least lifting out of bed and
dressing and washing, and lifting on and off the commode. But in
addition, many will need intravenous infusions and transfusions and

blood pressure and fluid balance charts as well as the usual special medical procedures. These wards will therefore need to have more skilled nurses (technically speaking) than the continuing-care wards. In terms of numbers similar levels are required as on the general medical wards. The practice of geriatrics demands nurses with special skills and attitudes.

An adequate intensity of nurse staffing is very seldom available, and the nurses are perpetually overworked. It should not be forgotten that nurses play a major part in rehabilitation, so short-staffing is not only dangerous but also militates against successful re-ablement. When under pressure, the geriatric unit should therefore resist the temptation to put up extra beds, which will jeopardize the treatment of the patients already in the wards, and will tax still further the overstretched staff. A smaller number of better staffed beds is generally more efficient. Shortages of staff lead to poor morale, and under these circumstances it may be advisable temporarily to close a proportion of the beds.

It is one of the crucial duties of the geriatrician to engineer sufficient throughput to meet the demands for new admissions. This duty is the cross he has to bear; contrary to popular belief, the main difficulty facing the geriatric department is not in admitting patients, but discharging them. We can investigate, treat and rehabilitate our patients until, having survived this onslaught of therapeutic zeal, we can state that they are fit to be discharged from hospital. What is so much more difficult is to ensure that conditions at home are such that the patient can be received back into the community. It is much easier to admit an

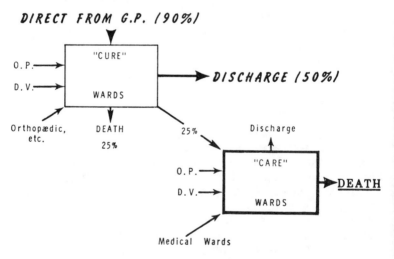

Fig. 5.3. Flow pattern of a geriatric department

old lady than it is to discharge her, and once she is in hospital, the delicate fabric of relationships that previously enabled her to maintain a precarious independence is all too often torn, never to be rewoven.

Although there is a great deal of variation, it is common to find that some 80 to 90 per cent of the admissions come directly from the general practitioner and the remainder are transfers from other hospitals or departments. Under these circumstances, it should be possible to discharge from the geriatric department more than half of the patients admitted. In this age group, it is to be expected that there will be a heavy toll from serious diseases such as bronchopneumonia, strokes, and malignant disease, and almost a quarter of the admissions will die within a few weeks. And the remaining quarter, or slightly under, are those who neither die nor get better because they have irreversible but non-fatal conditions, often with mental impairment. Such patients cannot be quickly rehabilitated up to a state of personal independence, and therefore require prolonged hospital care. Some of them will make unexpected late recoveries, and will leave hospital (Fig. 5.3).

2 The rehabilitation ward

It is common practice to set aside one or two wards for slower stream rehabilitation, for instance for hemiplegic patients who are expected to take a couple of months to recover skills such as walking. They will not be transferred during the initial phase of the illness when a great deal of nursing and medical attention is required, but will be kept in the admissions ward until they are no longer critically ill and investigations have been completed. The purpose of the rehabilitation ward, as the name implies, is to provide physio- and occupational therapy in a setting of increasing self-reliance where the emphasis is always on grooming the patient for her ultimate discharge. This involves the planned, progressive withdrawal of help—particularly by the nurses.

3 The continuing-care wards

It has already been emphasized that for those for whom rehabilitation has proved impossible, care, rather than cure, becomes the realistic aim. The function of the continuing-care ward is to relieve pain and discomfort as far as possible and to make life as worthwhile as lies within the power of the nursing staff, rather than to set the scene for intensive or sophisticated treatment. The day-to-day medical management of the patients is generally in the hands of a local general practitioner (whose wisdom and experience frequently makes him better suited to this role than his junior hospital colleague), but the beds remain under the overall control of the consultant in geriatrics, who makes regular visits.

The most important person in the patient's life is the nurse, and if she is cheerful, kind and enthusiastic, this will outweigh to some degree, the old person's handicap. Voluntary workers can also be of inestimable value in brightening the patients' lives in numerous and often unorthodox ways.

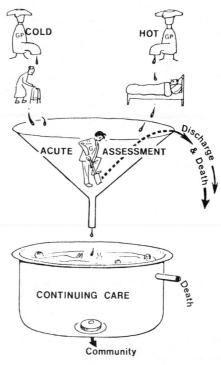

Fig. 5.4. The geriatrician is striving to discharge as many patients as he can from the assessment ward, and acts as the final common path to continuing care, whence the outflow back to the community is firmly plugged!

Medical investigation and intensive remedial therapy play a correspondingly lesser part in the activities of the ward. This decreasing scale of complexity and cost is best illustrated by a patient transferred from a very high technology service such as neurosurgery, where the cost of care is probably well in excess of £300 a week, through the geriatric department to the continuing-care ward at somewhere near a third the price. Where economies should *not* be made is in the standard of amenity of such a ward, which should be made as bright and pleasant as possible. In many ways, the long-stay patient to whom the ward is going to be her home for months or even years, deserves more in the way of creature comforts than her granddaughter who is rushed into hospital for a few days to have her appendix out.

One final point concerning continuing care. It has been said that one of the most crucial functions of the geriatrician is to be the final common pathway to long-stay hospital care. He must ration this resource so that no patient is admitted to such a bed until every possible avenue of discharge has been explored. If he allowed his colleagues in other specialties freedom of access to these beds, they would become blocked within a few weeks with patients who did not really need them. The temptation to transfer a hemiplegic patient out of an acute bed after a couple of weeks might not always be resisted (Fig. 5.4).

In our own practice in Cambridge, the segregation of patients is much less rigid, and our wards can be better divided into 'fast' and 'slow'. The fast wards are used for purposes of admission, investigation, and rapid rehabilitation, and the slow wards for slower stream rehabilitation and continuing care. The latter wards also accommodate a few patients whose treatment has been satisfactorily completed but whose discharge is fraught with difficulty, and whose functional level must be maintained while they are waiting. They also admit selected cases who have been previously assessed by the consultant.

The catchment area

The geriatric physician's responsibility does not start and end with the patient whom he happens to be examining. His duty also lies with those whose family doctors are seeking his help on their behalf. He has an important duty to make the maximum overall use of the facilities available to him, within a specified catchment area. These catchment zones have defied official definition even within the reorganized health service and often bear little relationship to either local authority or health service boundaries. They have evolved through practice and usage and a series of historical accidents in order to try to match the available facilities to the population served. There can be conflict between the provision of a high standard of care, which entails restricting beds to the number that can be adequately spaced and staffed, and meeting the commitment to the catchment area, which involves running as many beds as are required.

The beds—how many and where?

It has been proposed by the DHSS that the number of geriatric beds should be ten beds per thousand elderly (over 65 years of age) to allow for regional differences in age structure. Higher figures have been suggested, notably in Scotland. It would be more realistic to base the guideline on the population aged over 75, and 28 beds per thousand would probably be about right. What is much less clear is how these beds should be divided among the three categories mentioned above, but in practice probably between one-third and one-fifth of the total number will be actively turning over. There is general agreement that the acute assessment (and fast stream rehabilitation) beds should be sited in the district general hospital, but still much less general achievement of this aim. Many geriatric beds of all categories are still to be found in purely geriatric hospitals which are mainly old workhouses thinly disguised. It seems likely that in the future, most of the longer-stay beds will be situated in the new community hospitals which, at the time of going to press, are still very much at the drawing-board stage.

The acute admitting wards for geriatric patients must be located in the District General Hospital for a number of reasons.

1 Aged patients often have numerous problems requiring full investigation so that those susceptible to treatment can be treated and those inevitably soon to die can be spared further discomfort as far as possible. The sophisticated diagnostic tools available today often protect frail elderly subjects from unpleasant invasive procedures. The advent of computerized axial tomography of the head has been followed by a sharp reduction in the number of lumbar punctures, air encephalograms and carotid angiograms performed. A liver scan is often so strongly suggestive of metastatic disease that biopsy is quite unnecessary. Indeed, the geriatric department is a major user of the nuclear medicine service. It is also a major user of advice from other specialties, and needs to be on the same site as ophthalmic, vascular, orthopaedic, and genitourinary surgery.

2 The converse side of the coin is the help that these same departments, and others, increasingly need from the geriatrician. When he is on site, his expertise becomes available to all elderly patients and those looking after them, in whatever specialty.

3 The close relationship which should exist between the discipline of geriatric medicine and the other medical specialties can only thrive when both are under the same roof. This facilitates the rotation of medical staff in the training grades and the creation of posts with duties shared between general and geriatric medicine. Other grades of staff (nursing and rehabilitation) also benefit from rotation through the department and are more enthusiastic to do so when it is on site.

It is becoming increasingly apparent that numbers of beds are not the be-all and end-all of geriatric practice, but that the quality of the beds is at least as important as the quantity. The non-bedded facilities of the geriatric department may well be more important still.

The progress of a patient through the geriatric department can therefore be represented as a series of stages which may follow each other, or which may all start immediately after admission. The first of these stages is the medical one; examination, investigation, the establishment of a problem-orientated diagnosis, and the institution of appropriate treatment. This is very much the doctor's province, and failure is likely to culminate in death or permanent disability. The second stage is rehabilitation from the presenting disabilities and is the function primarily of the remedial therapists but includes the whole team. If they fail to realize their goal, the patient will probably require continuing hospital care. The final stage is that of the return home, and is the concern of the social worker and geriatric health visitor. If the rest of the team have fulfilled their tasks, but she is unable to reinstate the patient in the community, the outcome will be eventual placement in residential care. (Fig. 5.5.).

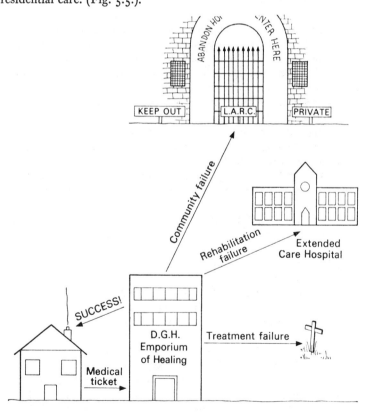

Fig. 5.5

Admissions policy

Geriatric medicine only works if patients can be admitted without significant delay. Many authors have commented on the disastrous results when a waiting-list is allowed to build up. A sick elderly person has to receive effective sensible treatment *now*, and has to be got up and out of bed and back on her feet *now*, if the opportunity is not to be missed for ever. If she is left at home, in bed, for a week or so, she will either die, or recover only to be permanently bedridden with contractures and pressure sores.

One other point that should be made is that just over a half of elderly hospital patients are in geriatric beds, the remainder being in general medical or surgical, or orthopaedic, gynaecological, or radiotherapy beds. In 1975, 23 per cent of all admissions to general hospitals were aged over 65. But they stay longer than the young and it has been forecast that by the end of the century 80 per cent of all hospital beds will be occupied by this age group. At the last count, 50 per cent of general medical beds contained elderly patients, so that geriatric physicians cannot possibly claim a monopoly of medicine in the elderly.

Some requests for admission have a purely medical content. Many, however, involve less tangible factors such as the social background, local knowledge, and ethical considerations. Furthermore, a bed once offered to a geriatric patient may be occupied by her for many months or even years, unlike the surgical bed offered to a patient suspected of having developed acute appendicitis.

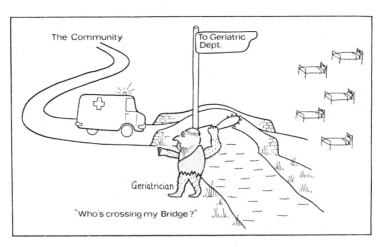

Fig. 5.6. 'Under the bridge lived a big, ugly troll'

For all these reasons, the decision to accept a patient is a difficult and responsible one, and is perhaps ordinarily best undertaken by an experienced member of the medical staff (Fig. 5.6). Requests for admission fall into four main categories.

1 'Hot'

Medical emergencies, e.g.
Acute stroke
Pulmonary oedema
Diabetic keto-acidosis

Here the decision is simple and will often be made by a house officer in the middle of the night—the patient must be admitted forthwith if there is a bed available, and if not, a bed will have to be found elsewhere.

2 'Very warm'

Cure and care

Typified by the old lady who has developed an eminently treatable condition such as a chest infection or heart failure, but who meanwhile has no one to look after her. Such an admission will normally be arranged during 'office hours' rather than at midnight, but may well not be able to wait over the weekend. In theory, discharge should be rapid but in practice it often takes old people a long while to recover their former level of activity after illness.

3 'Warm'

Specific therapeutic objective, e.g.
Rehabilitation following a stroke where the patient is not critically ill.
Investigation and treatment of anaemia.
Mobilization of an arthritic who has 'gone off her feet' after a fall.
Effective treatment must be provided as soon as possible. Otherwise the patient will succumb to bronchopneumonia, or at best, the resulting state of disability and dependency will become irreversible. Equally, prompt discharge must be assured when (and if) the objective has been achieved, so it is important to be aware in advance of possible adverse factors, either in the patient (notably dementia), or in her circumstances (notably hostile relatives, unsuitable accommodation, or isolation and lack of support). Too often, it is the new but treatable problem that precipitates admission, and the long-standing but untreatable problem that blocks discharge.

It may be possible to suggest an alternative to admission, such as day-hospital treatment, particularly if there are supporting relatives at home. In order to make the right decision, the geriatric physician will need as much information as possible. For this reason he may propose an early out-patient consultation, or domiciliary assessment by a doctor or health visitor.

4 'Cool'

Provision of care—this may be temporary (if the daughter will take over again after her own illness) or permanent. In order to be an NHS responsibility, the requirement must be for nursing, as opposed to hotel type care such as the local authority is obliged to provide. It is very seldom justifiable to ask for this type of admission as a matter of urgency because in most instances the need for care will have been predictable for the past several weeks or months.

Reasons for avoiding unnecessary admission

1 PATIENT'S WELLBEING

(a) 'Institutionalization' leads to apathy and deterioration of intellect and personality.
(b) Unfamiliar surroundings and faces tend to induce confusion.
(c) Professional competence cannot compete with filial self-sacrifice, and pressure sores may develop or a virulent organism cause a fulminating chest infection.
(d) The various home supports may crumble, once the keystone—the patient—has been withdrawn, so that discharge prospects become steadily more remote with each passing day.
(e) Repeated moves are likely to ensue, and these are bad for old people.
(f) Once the patient has been tidied away into a warm comfortable hospital bed, any pressure to provide the *right* sort of care ceases.

2 WIDER CONSIDERATIONS

(a) If pressure is exerted to have a patient admitted, that pressure will prevent subsequent discharge. One more hospital bed is unavailable to the seriously sick.
(b) Willingness to accept patients not properly a geriatric responsibility merely masks deficiencies elsewhere and encourages repeated inappropriate demands. As there is usually great difficulty in discharging these patients, the department will become constipated, so that it cannot offer a proper service to general practitioners and

their patients. The morale of the department suffers, further impairing the service.

(c) A patient who really needs psychiatric care on account of noisy, restless, antisocial behaviour, is difficult to tolerate in a ward where she will disturb seriously ill patients and distract the staff from their task of nursing the sick and helpless, without having recourse to excessive sedation. It has been well said that the lack of a psychiatric bed does not make a 'psychiatric' patient into a 'geriatric' patient.

Death Certification

By the very nature of the work of the department, it is inevitable that the house physician in geriatric medicine will frequently be called upon to complete death certificates. He should perform this final duty to his deceased patient with the utmost promptitude in order to spare the bereaved relatives the additional distress of uncertainty and delay. A common error is to specify the pathophysiological manifestation of disease rather than the disease entity. Terms such as 'congestive cardiac failure,' 'left ventricular failure', or 'atrial fibrillation' are too non-specific. It is the underlying heart disease (usually ischaemic), which is the cause of death, which must be stated on the certificate. The certifying practitioner must have been in attendance during the final illness, but need not have seen the body after death.

Notifying the Coroner

It may be obvious that the coroner should be informed, for example when death is the result of a road traffic accident or suicide. But in geriatric practice it is often very difficult to decide whether or not death is due to 'natural causes'. For example, an old lady who suffers from dizzy spells has a particularly nasty fall in her own home and factures her femur. Some months postoperatively she contracts bronchopneumonia and dies. Foul play is not suspected, but the accident may well have been a contributory factor. Here, common sense might indicate that involvement of the coroner is inappropriate, though had the chest infection supervened during the acute phase of the admission he should certainly have been informed. If the fall had occurred in hospital, or during employment, or if the relatives appear in some way dissatisfied, he should be notified. If there is the slightest doubt, a discussion with the coroner or his officer will clear things up. The following are guidelines to the sort of case to be referred to the coroner.

1 No certificate can be given, either because there has been no doctor

in attendance, or because the doctor does not know the cause of death.

2 Violence, suspected foul play, poisoning, drug addiction, and neglect (e.g. hypothermia). Alcohol is among the drugs and poisons included.

3 Accidents which have materially contributed to death—especially road accidents. Also cases where an operation or anaesthetic has materially contributed, or has been necessitated by injury.

4 Prisoners.

5 Death due to industrial disease.

6 Service pensioners whose pensionable disability may have predisposed to the death.

7 Where relatives have criticized the medical or nursing care.

The coroner will order a post mortem examination, and in cases of sudden death where there has been no attending physician during the fourteen days preceding death, this may well enable him to issue a coroner's certificate. Where he is still not satisfied, and in all cases where death is from other than natural causes, he will hold an inquest.

It occasionally happens that a patient is admitted to hospital in a moribund state and expires almost immediately of some cause, probably natural, such as myocardial infarction or a stroke. Under these circumstances, it may be possible to procure certification from the general practitioner.

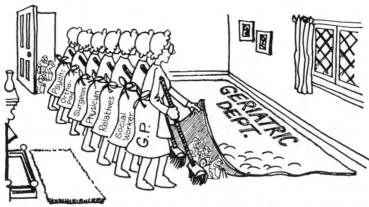

Misuse of the Department

Fig. 5.7

CHAPTER 6 · REHABILITATION

Forty years on, growing older and older,
Shorter in wind, as in memory long,
Feeble of foot, and rheumatic of shoulder,
What will it help you that once you were strong?

(Harrow School Song: E. E. BOWEN, 1872)

Rehabilitation is a concept which even today commands little more
than lip service from many members of the medical profession. To the
orthopaedic surgeon and the rheumatologist it is a part of his daily
bread and butter. To the geriatric physician, it is an essential part of his
service to his patient, and a matter of life or death to his department.
But to many other doctors, it represents an area of apathy, ignorance,
and inadequacy, and their participation is often limited to making
vague encouraging noises in the background. A very large proportion
of this work falls to the nurses, and the art of geriatric nursing has been
defined as 'the enlightened withdrawal of support'. The experts in the
field are the remedial therapists, whose techniques often appear to
doctors to lack the seal of scientific respectability. Drugs can be evaluated against a placebo by means of a double blind cross-over trial, but
no one has devised a convincing placebo physiotherapist let alone a
patient so blind that she is unaware whether she is having exercises or
not. The mysteries of short-wave diathermy remain closed to the
medical student, and not many consultants know one end of a wheel-
chair from the other.

Fortunately, physical methods of treatment were evolved and became
accepted before the current passion for statistical evidence of efficacy.
Some of the difficulties inherent in analysing the results of treatment
were emphasized in a recent study of stroke patients. This showed that
those who received most treatment improved the least—because they
were the most disabled. Those receiving occupational therapy were more
depressed than those not receiving it—because they were selected for
treatment on the grounds of having the worst strokes. Just as a patient
with a perforated peptic ulcer needs surgery, so does a patient with
a stroke need rehabilitating, and few would be prepared to defend
the ethics of a trial designed to prove it. The technical details of the
methods employed are outside the scope of this book, but a few general
principles can be described.

77

Rehabilitation consists in enabling the patient to achieve the maximum recovery of function, and thereby to lead as active, full and independent a life as possible. Sometimes this means that the patient makes a complete or almost complete recovery from the effects of the illness. Failing that, it means that she is taught to cope despite the persistent residual effects of her illness. Rehabilitation, or re-ablement, implies that the patient is disabled, so it is necessary to consider the types of disability which occur in geriatric practice.

Disability after acute systemic illness

An acute illness such as pneumonia or a myocardial infarct is likely to induce a state of profound physical weakness rendering the sufferer quite incapable of getting herself out of bed and onto the lavatory seat, let alone down to the kitchen to make the breakfast. During this period, someone will have to minister to the patient, and unless there is a devoted relative to do so, she will need to be admitted to hospital. In either event, once the imminent danger is past, most patients can get out of bed, and, after a brief convalescence, gradually feel their way back into full activity. This does not apply to the old and the feeble, who are likely to find that they have entirely lost their confidence and who may take some weeks of expert tuition before they can take to their feet again. This is occasionally true after an operation, and the elderly man who has undergone elective prostatic surgery may require prolonged post-operative rehabilitation. When the pre-operative condition is good, however, and the mind is alert, there is often surprisingly little difficulty in recovering mobility.

A useful distinction can thus be drawn between rehabilitation from an illness, and rehabilitation from its treatment. And of all the forms of treatment known to modern medical science, the worst offender in this respect is bed rest. It is very much easier to prescribe a period in bed for an elderly patient than it is to dig her out again afterwards. Although a spell in bed may be necessitated by debility, it is doubtful whether it should ever be enforced as a therapeutic measure in elderly subjects, who should be sat up in a chair and mobilized as soon as their general condition permits.

Disability after an acute illness is probably increasing. Before the advent of antibiotics and diuretics, an old lady was very likely to succumb to an episode of pneumonia or heart failure. Nowadays she receives technically expert treatment, but all too often it is not until several weeks have elapsed that it is apparent that she will never walk again. Ideally, she should receive comprehensive treatment from the outset, not only with drugs but also with physical measures to restore her to full activity. The objective is that she should remain active and independent until, months or years later, her final illness carries her off with merciful speed. She thereby avoids the prolonged twilight phase of pre-death dependency, and it is this phase which leads to informed lay criticism of the profession for 'keeping all those poor old things alive'.

Disability due to chronic locomotor disease

In the young, this type of damage usually occurs acutely, particularly as a consequence of traffic accidents, and a typical example would be paraplegia due to injury to the spinal cord. Even the young are not spared the ravages of chronic disease, and in this age group disseminated sclerosis must rank high among the disabling diseases seen in this country. Among the old, pride of place must be accorded to cerebro-vascular disease, with degenerative joint disease, Parkinson's disease and rheumatoid arthritis also occurring commonly and causing a great deal of suffering and immobility. Rehabilitation may be required as a result of the gradual progress of the underlying disease, or because of a more sudden deterioration—for instance, an old person may take to her bed for a few days simply in order to keep warm during a cold snap.

Rehabilitation is likely to take much longer than it does after an acute illness, and the aim is often more modest. It may be unrealistic to try to restore the patient to her previous functional level and the objective will then be the more limited one of teaching her to overcome her disabilities and still cope somehow with the simple activities of everyday life.

Disability due to irreversible damage of acute onset

The patient who sustains a fracture of the neck of the femur usually requires a nailing or plating procedure, or even replacement of the femoral head by a prosthesis. These are fairly major operations, and, in the elderly, are likely to be complicated by post-operative respiratory infections and leg vein thrombosis, so that a considerable amount of expert re-ablement is going to be necessary. The original fall which caused the injury may well have been one of many, in a frail old body who was becoming progressively unsteady on her feet. And in addition to these adverse factors, she is now left with various anatomical changes —she has a piece of metal in her femur, there is probably some residual shortening and rotation of the affected leg, and the hip joint is likely to undergo degenerative changes even when the initial post-operative pain has subsided. A more glaring example, because of the greater post-operative anatomical deficit, is the amputee.

Another example of an illness which may be critical in the early stages, and which also leaves a lasting defect in its wake, is a stroke. Sometimes the onset is not particularly dramatic, but it is often attended by impairment or loss of consciousness, by difficulties with swallowing leading to dehydration, and by incontinence which will predispose towards the development of pressure sores. The survivors of this phase of the illness are left with a neurological deficit which can be expected to diminish somewhat over the course of the next couple of months or so, but to an unpredictable extent, and only a very few are left with a hand as good as it was before. The process of rehabilitation, and the roles of the various professionals concerned is best illustrated by an account of the progress of these victims.

Rehabilitation of the stroke patient

The pathology, investigation, and treatment of the various types of stroke illness is discussed elsewhere, but an outline of the programme of re-ablement is appropriate at this point. The consequences of failure, in terms of human suffering and hospital-bed occupancy, will be appreciated when the incidence of the disease is considered. There are estimated to be over 100,000 new episodes of stroke annually in England

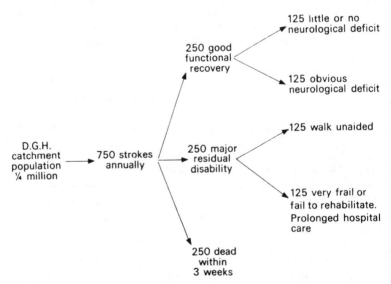

Fig. 6.1. Incidence and effects of stroke (approximate only)

and Wales—in other words, the population of a city the size of Cambridge. About 50 per cent of these die within the first month, and of the survivors, half make a good recovery and become personally independent while the remainder do much less well and some 20 per cent of the total require continuing hospital care. A district hospital serving a population of a quarter of a million could thus expect 500 to 750 episodes of cerebrovascular accident to occur within its catchment area each year, and it has been suggested that the quality of the management offered may dictate whether 50 or 150 of these patients are eventually transferred to longer-stay beds. Seventy-five per cent of the stricken are over 65 years old. In one British study of recovery after strokes in the elderly, it was found that 20 per cent recovered almost fully except for a clumsy hand. Forty per cent remained somewhat handicapped and continued to use a tripod or other aid in order to get about. Thirty per cent became long-stay patients, and 10 per cent died during the ensuing four months. Other authors have described their results in groups of younger patients, in whom the outcome, not surprisingly, is better. However, there are probably some 100,000 severely disabled stroke survivors in the Kingdom (Fig. 6.1).

WHO AND WHERE?

The most important person in the rehabilitative process is the patient herself, and it is her own determination and intellect and fortitude which will in the last resort decide the outcome. Those who look after her, whether relatives or nurses, are almost as important, for their expectations can engender an attitude of invalidism or one of increasing independence. The professional expertise of the re-ablists is essential if the best possible result is to be achieved, and it falls to the doctor to co-ordinate the overall programme.

In all but the mildest cases it is thus to the patient's advantage to be assessed and treated in hospital, where the activities of all these experts can be focussed upon her. But if she can be sat up out of bed at once, and if there are willing daughters to exercise her as well as to provide basic care, and if she is within easy travelling distance from a day hospital or at least a physiotherapy department then it may not be necessary to resort to admission.

THE TIMETABLE TO RECOVERY

The rate, and degree, of recovery, are so variable that even the most expert are frequently confounded. Having said that, it is useful to consider the process as comprising three phases. The first two weeks are spent in recovering from the acute illness. The ensuing two months are devoted to relearning the basic skills such as walking; and it will probably take most of the following two years to achieve the maximum re-integration of the patient into society.

1   *Initial stage*

The medical management of the seriously ill or unconscious stroke patient is discussed elsewhere, but there are many who do not fall within this group but who are nevertheless initially unwell and bedfast. Such patients need two hourly turning to prevent the development of pressure sores, and a cradle to support blankets and reduce the risk of contractures. The use of splints may be required if contractures seem to be imminent, but may lead to pressure sores and occasionally to increased spasticity. Difficulty with swallowing will necessitate feeding by naso-gastric tube to ensure adequate hydration, and severe incontinence at this stage can only be managed by catheterization.

In the fully conscious patient, profound aphasia is probably the single most frustrating symptom and great care must be taken not to treat her as a child nor to speak over her as if she were unconscious: indeed, even in the presence of marked receptive dysphasia, she should be reassured that recovery will shortly begin, and that the present state of helpless and undignified dependency will be a transient one. All four limbs are passively put through their full range of movement several times a day, and the patient is encouraged to try to resist at the first signs of returning muscle power. Passive movements can now be replaced by active movements of both affected and unaffected limbs. As soon as she is well enough, the patient is sat out of bed: this may reduce cerebral oedema and certainly permits a better view of what is going on around her. It also reduces the impression of being an invalid, and this boost to the morale is reinforced by substituting her own clothes for the nightdress or pyjamas so symbolic of sickness. It is essential to see that she has a pair of sensible, supportive shoes instead of loose, down-at-heel slippers, for she is now ready to be coaxed onto her feet.

2   *Increasing activity*

The first stage may have taken two days or two weeks, but as soon as is possible without undue strain and fatigue, a programme of increasing activity is introduced. The patient is taught to lift and adduct her bad arm with the good one, to prevent the development of a frozen shoulder. When the paralysed arm is not being exercised, it should be supported in a sling to prevent painful limitation of shoulder movement. An object held in the hand will help to restore tone and position sense and assist flexion of the fingers while discouraging contracture formation. Standing with support is encouraged as soon as possible because even a weak leg can weight-bear if the knee is extended. Bed-end exercises against a plank at the foot of the bed enable the patient to stand with the support of the bed-rail. Walking practice, initially with the physiotherapist bracing the patient's leg with her own, is the next advance. Parallel bars may be extremely useful, but the hand is often too weak to hold on firmly enough. A tripod or similar support, held in the good hand, is often the most successful aid to independent walking. The patient is instructed in simple techniques such as how to turn over in bed and how to get up if she falls. The provision of suitable beds and chairs is important as the chair will need to be higher than normal and the bed lower than normal (preferably adjustable, for the sake of the nurses) for most patients to learn to get up from them with ease and safety. As soon as possible she is left to take herself to meals and to the lavatory, and if necessary, is given practice in climbing stairs. Those who are handicapped by persistent foot-drop with inversion can be helped by means of a caliper which may perhaps be discarded later. Occasionally it is helpful to splint a flaccid limb with a plaster back slab to provide additional support.

Other problems may include incontinence (q.v.), and regular toiletting opportunities are often successful. Otherwise a catheter can be introduced as a (hopefully) temporary measure. Enemata may be necessary to clear up obstinate constipation. The patient who persistently stumbles into obstructions on the paretic side may have to have it pointed out that she has a visual field defect, and that she will have to make a conscious effort to turn her head in that direction to avoid such obstacles. This must also be explained to the relatives in order to avoid misunderstandings.

The patient is encouraged to undertake the routine necessities of everyday life for herself as soon as she can, and one of the most fundamental of such activities is dressing. Many of these functions require the use of the hands, and it is helpful to support the affected arm in a sling suspended from the ceiling to enable it to undertake purposeful active movements. Treadle machines and hand looms also provide stimulating outlets for activity by weakened muscle groups and basic skills can be re-learned in the assessment kitchen and bedroom.

Brief mention must be made of two techniques sometimes employed by physiotherapists in the treatment of hemiplegics, including those of advanced years. Proprioceptive neuromuscular facilitation ('P.N.F.') is a method of promoting the response of the neuromuscular mechanism through bombarding the proprioceptors with stimuli. Patterns of stimulation used are based on mass movements of muscle groups, and multiple joint movements.

Proponents of the Bobath technique see the hemiplegic's main difficulty as the abnormal co-ordination of posture and movement. The aim is to inhibit abnormal postural reflex activity and to facilitate more normal reaction patterns. Undue effort is avoided as this may increase spasticity and lead to widespread abnormal reactions. Use is made of key points of control, mainly proximal, to suppress patterns of activity—e.g. extension of neck and spine, external rotation at shoulder with extended elbow, and abduction and external rotation at the hip with extension of hip and knee.

3 Discharge and after

The successful outcome of rehabilitation is discharge from hospital, but the process does not stop there. Further hospital attendance as a day patient may be beneficial: and at home, the occupational therapist may be able to advise concerning the use of the many gadgets (Fig. 6.2)

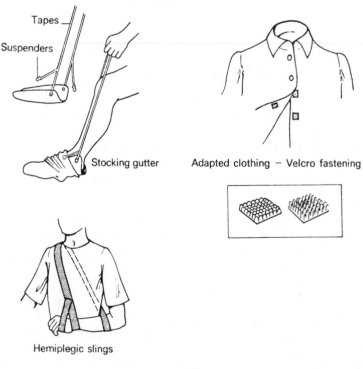

Tapes

Suspenders

Stocking gutter

Adapted clothing — Velcro fastening

Hemiplegic slings

Fig. 6.2

Aids to daily living

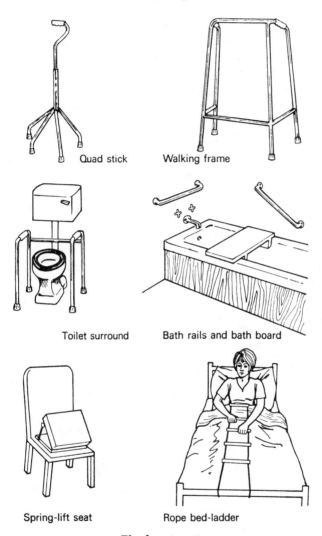

Quad stick   Walking frame

Toilet surround   Bath rails and bath board

Spring-lift seat   Rope bed-ladder

Fig. 6.2—*(contd.)*

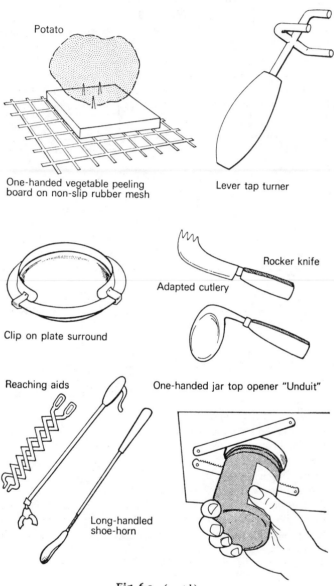

Potato

One-handed vegetable peeling
board on non-slip rubber mesh

Lever tap turner

Clip on plate surround

Adapted cutlery

Rocker knife

Reaching aids

One-handed jar top opener "Unduit"

Long-handled
shoe-horn

Fig. 6.2—(*contd.*)

now available to enable the patient to cope with her residual disabilities. It may also be necessary to suggest various modifications to the house, or even to arrange rehousing in more suitable accommodation. For those who live with their children it is often necessary to educate the family out of an over-protective attitude. It is psychologically and physically helpful if the patient is involved in household chores such as washing up, even if her harassed daughter could do it unaided in half the time! Psychological support outside the home is now available at well over fifty *stroke clubs*, a laudable exercise in self-help where the emphasis is generally on social aspects rather than on therapy.

Finally, it should again be stressed that the rate of recovery varies tremendously, and that its degree is unpredictable. One is often disappointed by a poor outcome when every feature had appeared to be favourable. Equally, one is frequently gratified by the late recovery of a patient when all hope of achieving independence has long evaporated. However, the harsh realities of economics make it essential to use scarce skills in the most effective way possible—in other words, to focus them where they are most likely to achieve results. This entails a certain amount of streaming. All stroke victims are given a fair crack of the rehabilitation whip, but it is important to be selective so that the more promising candidates can receive more intensive treatment. Our efforts at rehabilitation are more effective if they are not spread too widely and thinly, and for this reason it is useful to have some guidelines to the results which can be realistically anticipated.

Some general rules concerning strokes

1 Persistent unconsciousness is a bad sign—good recovery rarely follows.
2 Conjugate deviation of the eyes is a bad prognostic sign.
3 Legs do better than arms—less fine movements are involved.
4 Proximal muscles do better than distal ones—less fine movements are involved.
5 Spasticity is better than flaccidity, provided contractures are avoided—tone is necessary for weight-bearing.
6 Sensory loss is worse than motor loss—especially position sense.
7 It is better to damage the dominant hemisphere—probably because of the disastrous loss of body image which often complicates infarction of the non-dominant hemisphere.
8 The patient who has not made good progress at six months is unlikely ever to do so.

Factors adversely influencing recovery

THE HOSPITAL

It is sad, but true, that almost as many elderly patients are made worse by our hospitals as are benefited by them. We like to think that our patients come into hospital unable to walk, and are discharged able to get about unaided. Unfortunately, in some hospitals, almost as many are ambulant on admission but become immobile during their stay. In other words, the hospital helps to create its own long-stay patients. Sometimes this is unavoidable, when for instance a patient becomes infected by a virulent organism currently resident in the wards. Sometimes it is entirely avoidable when for example an aged patient is thoughtlessly confined to bed because this is the rule for the particular disease concerned. Most often, it is simply due to inadequate staffing—the staff is too thinly spread, and the quantity of beds is preserved at the cost of their quality. The effects may be obvious—there is an increasing number of pressure sores. They may be much less obvious: it is quicker to dress and bath a patient than it is to supervise her early, tentative attempts to dress and bath herself. Every time these simple services are performed for a patient, it acts as a reinforcement of the habit training whereby she learns to accept the rewards of passive submission to a role of complete dependence. Every activity is a therapeutic opportunity.

THE PATIENT

1 *Dementia*

It has been repeatedly shown that dementia is the single most potent factor preventing discharge from hospital. However much power returns to the limbs affected by a stroke, significant dementia will render the victim unable to co-operate fully with the remedial therapists. On the other hand, we have all encountered patients whose intellect has remained intact and who have been enabled thereby to overcome formidable neurological deficits. Exactly the same applies to other types of illness such as arthritis and fractures of the hip, as well as acute illnesses such as pneumonia. Preservation of mental function will allow sufficient re-learning to take place to permit the patient to cope with her residual disability: dementia interferes with this process.

2 *Motivation*

Not all our patients are cast in an heroic mould, stoically determined to live a full and active life against overwhelming odds. Apparent poor motivation may be due to an underlying depressive illness. Real lack of motivation exists when the patient enjoys receiving attention and being waited on. Furthermore patients might be trained by the hospital that unquestioning acceptance of all this attention is the hall-mark of the 'good' patient. Sometimes it is quite unreasonable to expect a frail old lady to struggle to return to the cold, lonely cottage with no bath or indoor w.c. from the warm cheerful hospital where she has experienced comfort and care beyond her dreams. Or to aspire to local authority care with its means-tested scale of charges when the hospital is free (except for loss of pension).

It may seem obvious that it is impossible to make someone well if she does not want to get better, and among younger patients this has been demonstrated. In one study it was found that those who were eligible for compensation for their back injuries fared very much worse than another group with similar injuries who were not eligible, and another showed that injuries sustained on the sports field have a far better outlook than similar injuries sustained at work.

3 Age

All our patients are elderly, but the very very old not surprisingly rehabilitate less well. This may be due to that vague, but none the less real clinical condition known as 'frailty': or it may be due to the greater likelihood of other concomitant diseases as well as the one currently being treated. In extreme old age, the will to survive in the face of illness may give way to a detached acceptance of approaching death.

4 Communication and sensory deprivation

Motor dysphasia renders the patient incapable of expressing her difficulties. Receptive dysphasia makes her unable to comprehend the instructions she receives and the reassurance and encouragement she should be getting. The hard of hearing are in a similar predicament. Vision is used in posture and balance, especially when position sense is defective, and the unsighted have an additional formidable disability to overcome.

5 Neurological deficits

Mention has already been made of the unfavourable effects of sensory loss and neglect of the affected side when predicting the outcome of a hemiplegia.

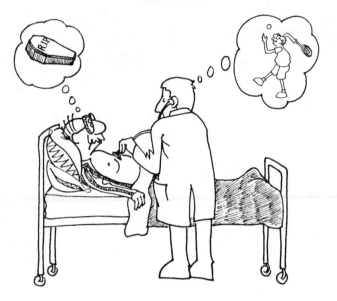

SOME AGREEMENT SHOULD BE REACHED CONCERNING THE LIKELY OUTCOME.

Fig. 6.3

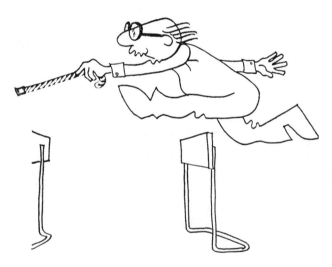

THE AIM SHOULD BE A REALISTIC ONE

Fig. 6.4

6 *Associated diseases*

Unrelated disorders such as obesity, arthritis or a previous amputation are clearly likely to militate against successful rehabilitation. The same applies to complications arising during the phase of severe illness, notably pressure sores and contractures.

7 *Pathological*

Account must be taken of the cause of the patient's disability, and whether the disease process is still active. Evidence of widespread atherosclerosis will adversely affect the prospects of rehabilitating a stroke patient: similarly, severe uncontrolled hypertension in slightly younger patients carries a poor prognosis and the possibility of a recurrence of the stroke.

Based on these principles, it should be possible to plan a reasonable programme for each patient. Two final points should be stressed: the outlook should be discussed, in fairly optimistic terms, with the patient, so that she and her therapists are aiming towards the same goal: and that goal should be realistic (Figs. 6.3, 6.4).

CHAPTER 7 · SPECIAL FEATURES OF GERIATRIC MEDICINE

'Are you in pain, dear mother?'
'I think there is a pain somewhere in the room'—said Mrs Gradgrind—'but I could not positively say that I have got it!'

from *Hard Times*, by CHARLES DICKENS

Illness, in this country, is more and more something that happens to you when you grow old. Thanks to affluence, public health measures, and immunization, we are spared the frightful infections which afflicted the children and the youth of previous centuries. Currently, we are even spared the incessant warfare which has, within living memory, decimated our young men. Unless you succumb to the effects of self-induced disease (deliberate self-poisoning, over indulgence in alcohol or tobacco, mis-use of the car, motor cycle or hang-glider, participation in criminal, terrorist or urban guerilla activities—either voluntarily or as an innocent victim), the chances are that you are going to enter old age. Because everyone dies, it follows that everyone experiences a period of ill-health, even if mercifully brief. Most people, in the affluent nations of this enlightened era, avoid ill-health throughout childhood, adolescence and middle age. For these reasons, the main burden of serious ill-health encountered by those in the healing professions falls on the old.

Most young people are well, and most ill people are old

This is why it is essential to become familiar with the special features of disease in the elderly, and the special approach required for the successful practice of medicine in this age group.

Whole person medicine

The disease cannot be considered in isolation from the rest of the patient. From her point of view, perhaps the most important thing about being unwell is the effect that this will have on her capabilities and functional capacity. This can only be assessed in the light of some knowledge of her premorbid functional state, and her response to rehabilitation is likely to depend on her mental function and motivation more than anything else. Once more, we need to know what she was like before she became ill. The close interdependence of disease, disability, and intellectual function cannot be sufficiently emphasized. Finally, some familiarity with the family situation and surroundings will enable us to help our patients to plan realistically for the future.

The ageing physiology

One of the fundamental physiological aspects of the ageing process is the impairment of homoeostatic mechanisms so that the *milieu interieur* cannot be maintained in the face of environmental hostility. This renders old people vulnerable to various stresses.

One example of this is their liability to dehydration. The fit young adult, liberated in the Sahara desert, will conserve his fluid by concentrating his urine maximally. When, because of his obligatory urine production, he does start to lose water and electrolytes, he will preserve his vital plasma volume at the expense of his interstitial fluid. The aged kidney is unable to respond to water deprivation by concentrating the urine to the same degree, and the distribution of the body fluids among the various compartments may not be to the best advantage. The kidney's role in the regulation of the ions in the plasma, and in the maintenance of acid-base balance, also becomes impaired: these mechanisms continue to function adequately under normal circumstances, but lose their reserve to meet unusual challenges.

Defective homoeostasis makes it more difficult to maintain a constant body temperature, and the main cause of hypothermia is a cold house. Chemical insults are also handled less effectively and more than 50 per cent of people aged over 70 have abnormal glucose tolerance tests. Drugs tend to be metabolized and eliminated more slowly, so that the old are at special risk of developing drug toxicity.

Immunological responses tend to become reduced, and this lowers resistance to infection. They may also become altered and there is a high incidence of auto-antibodies in old age.

Pathology

Degenerative changes, particularly in the arteries and joints, are an almost universal accompaniment of ageing, and lead to a heavy burden of disease in old age. Malignant disease also becomes increasingly common with advancing years and the majority of deaths from this cause occur after the age of 65. Infections play a large part in terms of both mortality and morbidity, and affect particularly the respiratory and urinary tracts. The effects of trauma are also frequently encountered, mainly due to falls and other accidents in the home, and include fractures in the region of the hip, fat embolism, subdural haematoma, collapse of vertebral bodies, and other fractures.

Pathologists sometimes express surprise when they perform a post-mortem examination on a patient who has died in her nineties, and find the major vessels almost free from disease. They should not be surprised because to survive to such an age, vascular disease must have been either late in onset or slow in progression. But it is misleading to regard those who are spared the ravages of atherosclerosis until an advanced age as a 'biological elite'. They probably do not represent a separate population from the rest of us, but simply one extreme of a continuous distribution curve of health. A recent series of necropsies performed on nonagenarians showed that coronary atheroma was moderate to severe in 75 per cent, and cerebral atheroma, in 58 per cent (but only 22 per cent in a series of subjects aged 70–90 years).

Multiple pathology

When dealing with younger patients, it is customary to try to explain every symptom, sign, and abnormal laboratory finding in terms of a single pathological process. This approach is completely inappropriate in the old. Once people are in their eighties, they commonly show evidence of several different pathological processes—some active, others inactive, but nevertheless contributing to the total disability. Inactive conditions may include the scars of battles fought long ago against serious disease, such as a withered leg from childhood poliomyelitis. They may include more recent calamities—strokes or pinned femora. Cataracts, deafness, degenerative joint disease and atherosclerosis are all conditions which are likely to develop slowly and to progress. Disorders such as anaemia and cardiac failure which have been diagnosed earlier, can be kept under control by continued medication. Others, like an hiatal hernia or diverticular disease, will probably whisper of their continued presence down the years. And in addition to some, or all, of these pathologies, the latest symptoms may suggest that the unfortunate patient has now developed a gastro-intestinal neoplasm, a urinary tract infection, or some other unrelated disease. A complete diagnosis must take all these problems into account, and must also make some attempt to allocate to each its priority and its activity. A problem-orientated approach is essential.

Special diseases of the elderly

Some disorders are by their nature almost peculiar to this age group, and others have been forced by circumstances to concentrate their efforts on the old in this country during the present half-century.

Some of the diseases with an inherent predilection for the aged are among the commonest afflictions of our time. These include strokes, Parkinson's disease, dementia, and prostatic disease. Among the less common may be mentioned the plasma cell dyscrasias, chondrocalcinosis, and giant cell arteritis and polymyalgia rheumatica. Other conditions have always been liable to attack those past middle life and are now being seen more frequently in extreme age, and these include hypothyroidism, pernicious anaemia, and motor neurone disease. Herpes zoster, erysipelas and ischaemic colitis are also traditional scourges of the old and frail.

The diseases which have changed their habits and now flourish among the old, are mainly those associated with deprivation. Tuberculosis is one of them, and is now chiefly encountered among immigrants and the aged. The others are the deficiency diseases—scurvy, osteomalacia, and folate deficiency.

Certain disorders, notably leukaemia and bronchopneumonia, have a bimodal age incidence which favours the very young and the very old. Others, though often commonly affecting those of middle age or over, present special syndromes almost confined to the old. Among these may be mentioned masked thyrotoxicosis, hyperosmolar non-ketotic diabetic crisis, and thrombotic non-bacterial endocarditis.

Altered presentation of disease

Diseases often present in a less florid and dramatic way in elderly subjects: the organs, it has been said 'suffer in silence'. An acute abdominal catastrophe is easy to recognize, if not to identify with any certainty, in the young. But in the old it is rare to find the same unmistakable picture of board-like rigidity and agonizing pain and profound shock. Myocardial infarction is often comparatively painless, and may cause the victim to feel a bit off colour, or to lose consciousness briefly, or to become confused: it may be completely 'silent', or it may present calamitously with a cerebral vascular accident. It is common to find an almost complete lack of the physical signs usually associated with pneumonia, and old people, like children, generally swallow their sputum; evidence of this disease may only be recognizable radiologically. The staring eyes and the hot, sweating, shaking hands and the irritable fidgeting of the young woman with Graves' disease are conspicuously absent in her grandmother with thyrotoxicosis.

The violent responses of youth become subdued by senescence. Pain, fever, and leucocytosis all tend to be damped down. Vague, non-specific terms are common in geriatric case histories—'collapse', 'falling about', and 'gone off her feet' are common presenting symptoms. In fact, geriatric medicine is dominated by the 'four Is':

Intellectual failure
Instability
Immobility
Incontinence.

These are the four great symptoms of disability which inevitably seem to lead to pleas for hospital admission. These pleas for action are often made by agencies other than the patient herself. It is frequently the relatives, or the neighbours, or a social worker who seeks medical advice on her behalf—the patient neither seeking nor welcoming it. There is commonly a lack of self-referral, particularly in regard to the following symptoms.

1   Intellectual failure

Intellectual failure may be due to a transient toxic confusional state or to a chronic dementing process. The first of these is usually reversible,

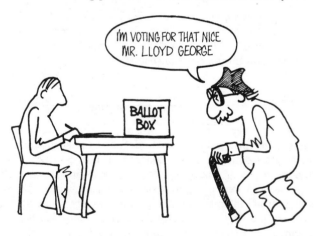

Intellectual Failure.

Fig. 7.1

but the second is most often progressive and renders the patient unrehabilitable. It is therefore incumbent upon the physician to differentiate them. It is also his duty to help the relatives by means of advice and encouragement. Both conditions are often intolerable to the family or other supporting persons on account of wandering, restlessness and anti-social behaviour.

2 Instability and immobility

Instability and immobility are the likely outcome whenever an old person has to take to her bed for a few days because she has developed a mild chest infection and is too weak to do for herself. The bronchitis does not require admission, but the ensuing disability may do so. Instability, or falling about, may easily have serious consequences. It may be due to anything from Stokes–Adams attacks, through postural hypotension, to hip disease or subacute combined degeneration. Falls

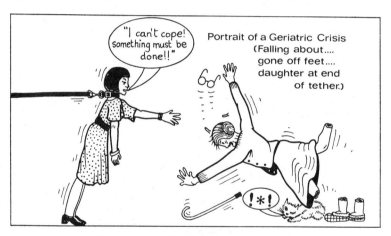

Fig. 7.2. Instability leading to acute acopia

lead in turn to loss of confidence and a reluctance to walk at all, and the final result is immobility. Early rehabilitation may restore mobility, but otherwise fixed flexion deformities and contractures will develop and the opportunity for successful treatment will be lost. Immobility can also be due to a variety of other factors, some of them psychological. The cold, the bereaved, the isolated and the depressed sometimes take to their beds through apathy—and are then unable to leave them again. The bored and the demented sometimes become immobile simply by disuse of their walking skills. The meek can be bullied into immobility by well-meaning but overworked attendants who find it quicker to do everything for them. And sometimes walking is painful due to arthritis, so life seems to be better in bed.

3 Incontinence

Incontinence, like the preceding disabilities, makes life difficult and unpleasant for those at home. It is also exceedingly demoralizing for the sufferer. 'Accidents' may occur because of difficulty in getting to the toilet in time because of reduced mobility or because of urgency.

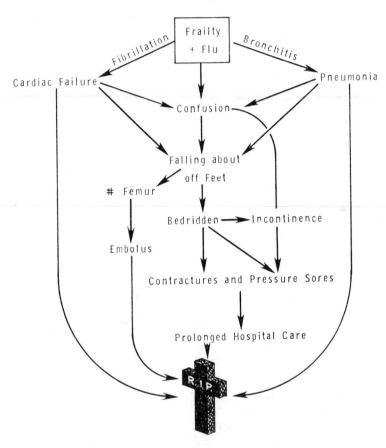

Fig. 7.3. Cascade of disasters triggered by minor illness

There may be total unawareness of the need to empty the bladder or rectum, or even of the act of doing so. And occasionally there may be apparently deliberate defaecation in inappropriate places, such as the waste-paper basket or the living-room carpet. From the social point of view, these distinctions are fine ones, but they are important when

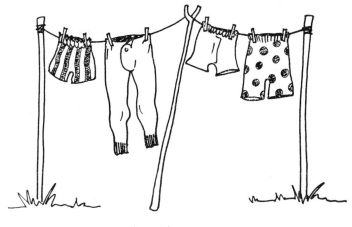

Incontinence

Fig. 7.4

trying to decide the most hopeful avenues of investigation and management.

Examining the aged patient

There are a number of practical points to bear in mind.

1   The history may be discursive, the process of disrobing, laborious, and the examination, exhaustive, so that by the time the crucial part of the consultation is reached, the patient (and perhaps the doctor) is too fatigued to co-operate. It is essential to amass as much information as possible as you proceed. For example:

(a) The gait. This should be studiously observed as the patient enters the consulting room or makes her way to the examination couch. It may yield clinical information such as foot-drop, festination, or the 'stammering' pattern of cerebrovascular disease. It will be very likely to yield practical information concerning the patient's ability to look after herself.

(b) A few simple preliminary enquiries (age, name of G.P., how did you get here?), together with the history, will indicate the patient's orientation and grasp of her circumstances, and give a good idea of her mental function.

(c) Are clothes, hair, nails unkempt? Dirt often indicates neglect and will alert the examiner to the possibilities of malnutrition, dementia, and hypothermia.

(d) History-taking provides an opportunity for circumspect observation, and the initial overall impression offers the best chance of spotting myxoedema, Parkinson's disease, or Paget's disease of the skull.

(e) Abrasions and bruises mean she has been falling about, whether she mentions it or not, and injuries are sometimes of non-accidental origin.

(f) Fidgeting and inability to sit still are features of anxiety and of the generally hyperkinetic thyrotoxic patient—unless, on closer inspection, the movements are choreiform in character. Oro-facial dyskinesia and other involuntary movements can be quietly analysed during the interview.

2   The general inspection always embraces an assessment of the state of hydration. Because of the impaired homoeostasis already referred to, the aged are especially liable to become dehydrated or oedematous. A common finding, and one of serious portent, is the 'top and bottom syndrome' of dehydration of the upper part of the body and oedema of the legs. The 'dry skin wet lungs syndrome' is another familiar paradox which makes assessment of overall fluid balance very difficult.

3   Can she see? Not such a banal question as it may appear. The answer is often neither yes or no, but 'a bit'. It is then necessary to answer some further questions: how much? why? would new (or clean!) glasses help? can she see enough for her needs, or is she debarred from activities she would greatly enjoy—sewing, reading, television?

4   Can she hear? If she keeps asking 'What did you say?' is she really deaf, or is she covering up a failure of comprehension? Check the ears for wax.

5   The chest. Look for kyphoscoliosis, a very common finding which may betray metabolic bone disease. Displacement of the apex beat may be due to skeletal deformity, although it generally indicates cardiac enlargement. However, this in itself is very common, and is not necessarily of gloomy prognostic import. In particular, it correlates poorly with ECG evidence of severe ischaemia or hypertrophy.

6   The abdomen. Always consciously ask yourself if the bladder is palpable. The enormously distended bladder picked up on routine examination is a recurring source of surprise in the geriatric out-patient clinic.

Always examine the rectum—not only for tumours, but for constipation (which may have been denied ten minutes previously), for black stools, and for enlargement or irregularity of the prostate.

7   The nervous system. The chief difficulty lies in securing full co-operation. The command 'relax' immediately throws all muscle groups

into spasm (this is by no means confined to the old), but the desired result is sometimes achieved by asking the subject to rest his head back against the pillow, gaze at the ceiling, and think about winning the football pools.

A good catch-all test is 'clap your hands'. Everyone co-operates, and if it is done with reasonable elan, it excludes gross weakness, loss of body image, ataxia or bradykinesia.

Absent ankle jerks are exceedingly common in persons over 75 and are not evidence of any specific neurological deficit. Distal impairment of vibration and position sense again seems to be a part of the ageing process rather than a hallmark of disease. It may contribute to the unsteadiness of gait often found in extreme old age. While examining the legs, check that passive movement of the hips is full and look for inequality of limb length and rotation. Severe hip disease and even fractures are sometimes picked up in this way.

8   The blood pressure—see Chapter 14. Of limited significance if high, of potential significance if low, of considerable significance if showing a marked drop on standing accompanied by pallor and distress.

Limitations

It is not always justifiable to pursue the diagnosis as far as one might in a younger patient. Limitations may be imposed on investigations by the frailty of the subject and the increased risk that many procedures therefore carry, and this risk must be balanced against the therapeutic possibilities and the long-term prognosis. In the field of radiology, for example, much can be learned from plain films of the chest, abdomen, and bones, without any danger or discomfort. Barium meals are well tolerated, on the whole, and often give useful information. The discovery of a carcinoma of the stomach may well influence the overall management of the patient and her family even if surgery is not contemplated. A barium enema, on the other hand, is an uncomfortable procedure which calls for considerable co-operation from the patient, and which carries some risk of perforation of the bowel. Nevertheless, if the simpler procedure of sigmoidoscopy is unrevealing, a barium enema is the proper next step provided that the general condition of the patient will allow. Quite apart from carcinoma of colon the barium enema is helpful in the medical assessment of patients with suspected diverticular disease, ulcerative colitis and Crohn's disease. Intravenous urography is usually well tolerated and provides valuable information about the anatomy of the kidneys, ureters and bladder. Other special procedures in the X-ray department are only occasionally called for.

There are often limitations on the treatment which can be offered, and in particular the pros and cons of surgery may be difficult to weigh up. The aim of treatment may have to be more modest than in the young, and the extended care of the disease is often a more realistic goal than its cure.

When not to treat

To diagnose, in the very old, is not invariably to treat. A localized breast carcinoma, picked up on routine examination, may well cause no interference with the patient's general well-being within her foreseeable life span. To advise resection would be meddlesome and pointless.

Medicine can easily be practised by reflex action—bronchopneumonia equals a course of ampicillin. This kind of practice leaves the profession open to the criticism of 'keeping all those poor old things going when their lives are a burden to themselves as well as everybody else'. Bronchopneumonia is rightly regarded as the old man's friend, and it is often inappropriate to salvage someone who will only have to die less peacefully a few weeks or months later. Geriatricians are not committed to the pointless prolongation of meaningless lives. The main objectives of geriatric medicine are concerned with the quality rather than the quantity of life. If the potential quality of life can reasonably be judged to be unworthwhile, due to dementia or suffering or severe disability, it is the belief of the authors that positive steps should not be taken to prolong it. If these factors are not known to the house physician admitting the patient in the middle of the night, she must of course be given the benefit of the doubt and treated. All too often there is inade-quate communication between the family doctor and the hospital, and energetic therapy may cause distress to the relatives as well as the patient. The family, on these occasions, sometimes show a better sense of proportion than the medical attendants. When in doubt, their feelings should be solicited without unfairly placing them in the position of having to make the final decision. To withhold treatment is not to practise euthanasia, and indeed is not always to the patient's detriment. To intervene may prolong dying rather than prolonging life. The legitimate aim of medicine is to extend well-being, not to extend disease: to delay decline, rather than to delay death. Too many old people accept their aches and pains as the inevitable accompaniments of advancing years. Too often, this stoical resignation is reinforced by the family and even by the general practitioner. It is one of the rich rewards of geriatric practice to be able to alleviate much of this suffering through accurate diagnosis and judicious treatment.*

* For non-specific 'Failure to thrive' or 'Going-off' syndrome see Appendix, p. 356.

CHAPTER 8 · MENTAL ILLNESS

He taketh away the understanding of the aged.
(Job XII, 20)

Because mental illness makes an incalculable impact on every aspect of the care of the elderly, the importance of a simple psychiatric assessment is a recurring theme throughout this book. The major mental disorders encountered among old people are brain failure and depression.

Brain failure

The advantage of this term lies in its deliberate vagueness. Although difficult to define, it is easy to understand because it implies impairment of the higher cortical activities such as cognitive function, intellect, concentration, memory, personality, affect and orientation. Like failure of the heart, kidney or liver, it may be acute and reversible, or chronic and progressive. Like failure of these other organs, it may be compensated and compatible with a reasonable degree of activity, but if it is decompensated the overall function of the organism is threatened. And like failure of these other organs, its cause may be intrinsic brain disease or some extrinsic factor. Its very presence may be difficult to establish. A classification of brain failure is given in Table 8.1.

Acute brain failure—the toxic confusional state or delirium

This is an important and common presentation of physical disease in an old person, and is almost as non-specific as vomiting in a child.

Clinical features

1 The onset is abrupt. As this information will not be volunteered by the patient, the duration of confusion is the most crucial information to be sought from a relative or neighbour. Patients with underlying dementia are particularly vulnerable, and sudden confusion often represents acute-on-chronic brain failure, so these enquiries must embrace the previous mental state. Other predisposing factors include anaemia and malnutrition; sensory deprivation through deafness or

Table 8.1. Brain failure in the elderly

	Acute—Toxic Confusional State	a. Secondary	*Chronic*—Dementia b. Senile (Alzheimer type)	c. Atherosclerotic
History	Hours/days/weeks	Rapidly progressive 3–18/12	>6/12	>6/12 Hypertension, strokes, fits
Pathology	Underlying disease	Underlying disease	Senile plaques Neurofibrillary tangles	Multiple infarcts
Cause	Drugs Infections Cardiac failure/infarction Stroke Metabolic	Drugs Space-occupying lesions N.P. Hydrocephalus B12 deficiency Myxoedema Syphilis	Neuronal fall-out Slow Virus Auto-immune Aluminium (?significance) Choline acetyl transferase deficiency	Hypertension Vascular disease
Course	Lucid intervals common	Variable	Progressive—no lucid intervals	Stepwise—lucid intervals and intercurrent delirious states
Activity	Mentally active Fear & other emotions	Usually vegetative	Initial depression or agitation Emotional flattening Mental vegetation	Emotional incontinence
Hallucinations Delusions	Frequent	±	Rare	Occasional
Personality	Preserved	Sometimes destroyed	Early disintegration	Preserved until late
Focal signs	±	±	o	Common

blindness; social isolation; and sudden removal to strange surroundings and people.

2 The condition is potentially reversible with appropriate treatment of the underlying cause and hence the importance of its recognition.

3 Symptoms and signs of the underlying disease may be detected—or they may be entirely lacking.

4 The patient is confused and is inclined to misidentify persons.

5 She is likely to be disorientated in time and place.

6 She may be deluded in her interpretation of external events and surroundings.

7 She may also be hallucinated, and become disturbed by the sight of imaginary people or things. Anxiety is commonly a prominent feature.

8 The overall impression is usually one of noisy restlessness, referred to as delirium. The degree of delirium often fluctuates, possibly with lucid intervals. There may be periods when the patient becomes obtunded with clouding of the sensorium.

Causes

1 DRUGS

It seems logical to mention alcohol first, because it is widely used, socially acceptable and readily available on self-prescription. Confusion can be induced through acute over-indulgence, and more notoriously through sudden withdrawal when the well-known syndrome of delirium tremens may result. Geriatricians are by nature an unsuspicious lot, because their patients suffer more commonly through the deprivations imposed by society than through the self-induced ills of affluence. Nevertheless, it is not uncommon for elderly persons of greater financial than social resources to seek solace in the gin bottle. When this is accompanied by dietary self-neglect, the ill effects are likely to be potentiated.

The dangers of medically prescribed drugs in this age group are emphasized elsewhere. Certain drugs which are widely prescribed with impunity for younger patients are very likely to induce a confusional state when given to the old. The barbiturates are infamous in this respect and are no longer used in geriatric medicine. However, levodopa and benzhexol are worthy of especial mention as they are so often given to the aged, as are corticosteroids.

2 INFECTIONS

Localizing signs of acute infections may be absent or minimal among geriatric patients, and even general disturbances such as fever may be conspicuously absent. Infections of the respiratory and urinary tracts are particularly likely to present with confusion of sudden onset.

3 STROKES

Minor episodes of cerebral infarction can present in the same way. Sometimes they involve the so-called 'silent' areas of the cortex, so that it is almost impossible to detect any specific neurological deficit, except by those refined techniques of neurological examination which require complete co-operation and an above average I.Q. on the part of the subject!

4 HEART DISEASE

As with most degenerative disorders, the pathological changes which lead to heart disease may take a life-time to develop, but their clinical manifestations may occur suddenly and out of the blue. Once again, in old age the classical presenting features are often conspicuous by their absence, and acute confusion due to a dramatic reduction in cerebral perfusion may be the only clue to a painless myocardial infarct. A change in cardiac rhythm—usually the advent of atrial fibrillation with a rapid ventricular rate, but sometimes the onset of bradyarrhythmia such as complete heart block—can have the same effect, and so can heart failure and hypotension due to cardiac or extra-cardiac causes.

5 METABOLIC AND ENDOCRINE

Diabetes in the elderly is often mild, but infections can exacerbate it and lead to water and electrolyte depletion and cause confusion; its treatment can easily induce hypoglycaemia which can be even more dangerous. Acidosis, fluid imbalance, uraemia, jaundice and anaesthesia are other conditions which are likely to cause confusional states.

Management

The most important step is the identification, and if possible, correction of the underlying cause. Sedation is undesirable but sometimes un-avoidable and is discussed later under the dementing diseases.

Chronic brain failure—the dementias

Incidence and importance

It is no exaggeration to say that the Health and Social Services are reeling under the onslaught of these disorders, which have reached epidemic proportions. There are three main reasons for their staggering impact.

1 INCIDENCE

It is estimated that 10 to 15 per cent of those over 65 have significant impairment of the intellect, and that half of these are severely affected. The incidence increases linearly with advancing years. There are thus around three-quarters of a million sufferers in the United Kingdom, and they comprise $1\frac{1}{2}$ to 2 per cent of the total population. A considerable increase in their number during the next decade can be reliably anticipated, as one in five persons over the age of eighty has the condition.

2 EFFECT

Progressive failure of the intellect and disintegration of the personality is more completely destructive of the quality of life than any purely physical disability. Social competence and continued independence are impossible. Co-operation with remedial therapy is minimal, and it has been repeatedly shown that brain failure is the greatest single determinant of continued hospital care.

3 ALIENATION

Dementia is more difficult to tolerate than most physical diseases and is more likely to alienate the affections of even the most devoted family. After the first flush of youth, it is the intellect and personality that we love, rather than the body, and to have a demented spouse is to be bereaved without being widowed.

Diagnosis

This terrain abounds with pitfalls for the unwary. They include:

1 AGE ITSELF

For some medical students and nurses, hospital provides their first encounter with persons in their eighties. How can they be expected to distinguish between the normal and the abnormal?

2 INTELLIGENCE TESTING IN THE ELDERLY

Old people perform poorly in intelligence tests, partly due to disinterest and partly no doubt to the poorer educational opportunities available during their youth. A true decline appears to start at 50 to 55, but tasks requiring speed show an earlier decline and the elderly are more easily "thrown" by the inclusion of irrelevant material. There is evidence that the fall off in performance starts later with each succeeding generation. A physiological decline in intelligence is a different phenomenon from the onset of dementing disease.

3 COMMUNICATION

Blindness is bound to interfere with orientation. Deafness and dysphasia make communication very difficult even though the mind remains perfectly alert.

4 BARRIERS

There are often socio-economic and cultural barriers between a young professional helper and the patient, whose standards and expectations may be very different.

5 MOTIVATION

Some assessment of intellectual function is a mandatory part—perhaps the most important part—of the assessment of the elderly patient. This does not mean that she is immediately subjected to a barrage of questions concerning current political figures, which may both cause offence and lead to justifiable speculation by the patient as to whose sanity is open to doubt! Perhaps more pertinently, such questions do not reveal the extent of the subject's grasp of her own circumstances, which is more closely related to her social competence. The same objections apply to the numerous psychometric questionnaires which have been described, although mental test scores are of value in research and in following progress. Ideally, any test used should be quick and easy, and should fit naturally into the interview. It should test recent rather than distant memory, and should, as far as possible, overcome cultural barriers. A little tactful probing will reveal whether the patient can give a good account of herself (it will require corroboration because some become expert at filling in gaps in a plausible manner!), whether she is familiar with the nature of the interview, whether she has a realistic grasp of how she copes at home, and whether she can recall where she lives, what she has had for her last meal, and how she has been conveyed to the surgery/clinic/day hospital. At this stage, she can be invited to specify the month and year. Other more formal tests include the recall of addresses, numbers or sentences: simple mental arithmetic such as 'serial sevens': categories (towns, colours, domestic animals): and, for in-patients, 'ward orientation'—the identification of places and people in the environment. In hospital, apparent reluctance to identify the place may be because of illness and fatigue, or it may be because the patient was bundled into an ambulance without being told where she was going.

6 DEPRESSION AND NEUROSIS

Depression is common in the early stages of dementia. Conversely, depression often leads to a state of withdrawal and inanition which closely mimics dementia. There is a group of elderly females of low intelligence and socio-economic status who show neurotic traits and who become so unable to cope with life that they acquire a label of dementia (neurotic pseudo-dementia).

7 ECCENTRICITY

It is often very hard to draw the line between increasing eccentricity and mental disease. One example of pseudo-dementia is the Diogenes syndrome*, a variation on the senile squalor theme. It is typified by an old person living in a state of extreme self-neglect and filth and with a tendency to hoard rubbish. When protests by the neighbours lead to professional intervention, such people are completely unrepentant, and found to be of perfectly sound mind although somewhat suspicious, and tend to be from a high socio-economic group: the degradation of life-style seems often to follow bereavement.

8 PLAUSIBILITY

In in-patients, ask the ward sister! She will have been able to observe the patient's behaviour and will not be deceived by a plausible veneer.

Clinical features

Dementia is to the cerebral cortex what congestive failure is to the myocardium. It is the clinical syndrome which is the likely outcome of any pathological process affecting the organ concerned, without telling us much about the nature of that pathological process. There is a diffuse impairment of the intellect and personality. It is usually, but not always, of insidious onset, when the relatives will testify to a gradual failure of the intellect over many months or years. It is usually, but not always, progressive, though the rate varies enormously.

* Diogenes—Greek philosopher noted for his contempt of social niceties.

Initially, awareness of failing mental powers often leads to profound depression. There is commonly a stage of nocturnal restlessness, and during this trying phase, the patient will get dressed to go to work at 2.00 a.m. or 3.00 a.m. or she will indulge in such quasipurposeful activities as incessant rummaging in the drawers. This mindless restlessness is frequently accompanied by anxiety. At a later stage, the clinical features are those of apathy and lethargy rather than noisiness and activity.

Other faculties which decline early in the disease include concentration and short-term memory, although the long-term memory is often surprisingly intact. Personal hygiene deteriorates and the behaviour may be disinhibited, antisocial or aggressive. Conversation is at first appropriate although often erroneous, later it is quite inappropriate, and eventually, cannot be sustained at all. The patient becomes incontinent, disorientated and then unable to obey the simplest instruction. It may become difficult even to engage her attention as she sits fidgeting and plucking at her clothes. Finally, dementia is a fatal disease and it is claimed that the life expectancy at diagnosis is reduced to 25 per cent of the normal for that age, but that it is longer in the atherosclerotic than the senile variety. Demented patients become susceptible to self-neglect (malnutrition, dehydration and hypothermia), bronchopneumonia, falls, and strokes.

The main features can be summarized as follows, in approximate order of progress:

Depression—early, before loss of insight
Concentration↓
Memory loss—short term→long term
Cognitive function↓→Misidentification: grasp of circumstances↓
Capacity for self care↓→self neglect
Restlessness, wandering
Personality↓→personal habits and hygiene↓
Behaviour disinhibited, noisy, antisocial, dirty, aggressive
Hallucinations, delusions (not typical)
Disorientation
Incontinence
Eventually—unable to answer simple questions appropriately, difficult to engage attention, immobile, plucks at clothing etc.

Classification

THE SECONDARY DEMENTIAS

There is a large number of organic diseases which may lead to chronic brain failure, which may be reversible if the appropriate treatment is given in the early stages. Although none of them is very common, the possibility of such a dramatic improvement in the patient's welfare makes it important to bear them in mind. Having said that, it is often difficult to decide which patients should be investigated. Clearly, those with other features suggestive of a remediable condition should be subjected to the relevant tests. Of the others, those under 75, in good physical condition, with rapid deterioration over a few months, should be selected for investigation. The examination of choice is computerized axial tomography (CAT), unless the subject is too demented to co-operate, in which case a radioisotope scan should be performed. One or two of these diseases may be singled out for mention with relevant features.

Myxoedema

'Myxoedema madness' was one of the many diagnostic triumphs recorded in 'Dr. Finlay's Casebook'.* Although the other features of hypothyroidism will normally be apparent, they develop so insidiously that they are likely to escape observation by the family or even by the general practitioner because of their frequent contact with the patient. Early replacement therapy with thyroxine should restore complete physical and mental health.

Vitamin B_{12} Deficiency

'Megaloblastic madness' is the name given to the dementia which may result from vitamin B_{12} deficiency, because the marrow will show a megaloblastic picture even if the patient has not yet developed overt anaemia. Sometimes there are other features due to damage to the spinal cord and peripheral nerves. The commonest cause of this deficiency is pernicious anaemia in which auto-immune gastric atrophy results in a failure to produce both gastric acid and intrinsic factor. Without the latter, the terminal ileum is unable to absorb ingested vitamin B_{12}, but the response to injections of the vitamin is occasionally very gratifying. Even more rarely, dementia in association with folate deficiency may respond to folic acid.

Drugs

Drugs can cause chronic dementia as well as acute confusion. Old age is usually, but by no means invariably, accompanied by such dire financial straits as to deny regular access to alcohol. Other forms of

* Dr. Finlay—beloved early twentieth-century Scottish village G.P. created by the novelist A. J. Cronin and subsequently popularized on television.

chronic toxicity can produce mental changes and one which is perhaps worthy of special mention is bromism. This was formerly a common condition, because various compounds of bromine used to be popular ingredients in pharmaceutical preparations. The elderly may be very faithful to their proprietary remedies, and five cases of bromism were described in 1971, all showing neurological signs in addition to their mental changes. Long-term barbiturate usage can also result in dementia, often associated with ataxia.

Trauma

The results of trauma of the brain may be catastrophic and obvious, as in the 'lame brain syndrome' after a severe head injury. They may be delayed and irreversible, as in the punch-drunk boxer, or they may be deceptive and insidious as in the old person who develops a subdural haematoma many days or weeks after a fairly trivial blow on the head, perhaps received in a fall. A history of trauma is obtained in 50 to 70 per cent of patients: symptoms have seldom been present for more than three months. The collection of blood effectively forms an intracranial tumour, and its manifestations depend on its exact location, but are often simply a change in intellect or personality (See Chapter 13). Impaired or fluctuating consciousness and hemiparesis occur in a quarter to a third of cases, and headache less frequently. Plain skull films should be done to try to locate the pineal: radioisotope scanning may yield a positive result, but the CAT scan is the definitive investigation in a co-operative patient.

Tumour

Exactly the same applies to tumours, which may grow rapidly and cause headaches and epilepsy and pressure on vital parts of the nervous system, but which may be very slow growing—commonly the case with a meningioma. A subdural haematoma or a meningioma compressing the relatively silent frontal lobes can result in a clinical picture indistinguishable from atherosclerotic dementia, although the CAT scan, or brain scan may yield the diagnosis and may lead to surgical intervention with a happy outcome.

Normal Pressure Hydrocephalus

It was initially thought that this rare condition was easy to diagnose and satisfactory to treat, but these early hopes have not been entirely fulfilled. The hydrocephalus is usually idiopathic and, as the name implies, the CSF pressure is normal. A CAT scan demonstrates gross enlargement of the lateral ventricles. Fluctuating, but progressive mental changes are usually associated with signs of a spastic paraparesis. CSF shunting operations sometimes bring dramatic benefit, but there is also an appreciable morbidity.

IRREVERSIBLE DEMENTIA—THE CHRONIC BRAIN SYNDROME

It is usual to distinguish between the senile and atherosclerotic forms, but the two varieties co-exist in about 20 per cent of patients.

SENILE, PARENCHYMATOUS, OR PRIMARY NEURONAL DEMENTIA

The majority of sufferers are women. It has therefore been claimed that the greatest problem facing the profession today is the fact that old women's bodies outlive their brains. The course is progressively downhill, with destruction of the personality and flattening of the emotions. Parietal lobe symptomatology is common, and upward gaze may be defective. The pathological findings include cortical atrophy, widening of the sulci, and dilatation of the ventricles. There are senile plaques in the cortex measuring five to 100 microns in diameter, and, more specifically, neurofibrillary tangles within nerve cell bodies. Neuronal loss is most marked in the posterior hippocampal cortex. Aetiological theories include the following:

1 *Neuronal fallout*

It was long held that the loss of nerve cells from the cerebral cortex at a rate of 100,000 a day was an aspect of the ageing process which was responsible for this condition. It remains unclear whether the cell population falls more rapidly in these patients than in agematched controls.

2 *Auto-immunity*

An auto-immune mechanism has been suggested on the basis of the occurrence of amyloid deposits rich in IgG within the plaques, but direct evidence is lacking.

3 *Viruses*

The uncommon dementing disorder, Creutzfeld-Jakob disease, has been transmitted from man to primates, and a case has occurred in the recipient of a corneal graft from a donor found to have the disease.

This raises the possibility that senile dementia is one of the transmissible slow virus encephalopathies.

4 *Aluminium*

Aluminium is known to be neurotoxic and to produce neurofibrillary tangles. An increase in the aluminium content of the brain in senile dementia has been reported. The significance of this finding is uncertain, and it may be a phenomenon of normal ageing.

5 *Neurotransmitter deficiency*

Acetyl choline is one of the main excitatory neurotransmitters within the brain, and seems to be particularly concerned with memory. The acetylation of choline is dependent upon the enzyme choline acetyl transferase. The discovery of abnormally low concentrations of this enzyme in the amygdala, hippocampus and cerebral cortex of patients with Alzheimer's disease and, more recently, senile dementia, is an extremely promising development. Another enzyme which may be deficient in senile dementia is glutamate decarboxylase which catalyses the synthesis of the neurotransmitter gamma aminobutyric acid (GABA).

ATHEROSCLEROTIC, OR MULTI-INFARCT DEMENTIA:
ISCHAEMIC BRAIN DISEASE

Men are more frequently afflicted, and a history of hypertension, minor strokes, or focal epilepsy is common. Residual neurological signs should be sought, and emotional lability may be a clue to pseudobulbar palsy. Deterioration typically occurs in a stepwise manner, with confusional episodes and comparatively lucid intervals. The personality remains recognizably that of the patient in his younger days.

The pathology is as the name implies—disseminated softenings due to multiple infarcts. When their volume totals over 50 ml, brain failure is likely. Causative factors are those of arterial disease in general.

Management

The role of the doctor in the management of the elderly demented patient is threefold.

1 To establish the diagnosis, to treat the treatable, and to offer some sort of prognosis for the untreatable majority.

2 To support patients in their own homes or those of their relatives.

This entails counselling and encouragement as well as symptomatic drug therapy.

3 To advise concerning the provision, rationing and management of institutional care when maintenance at home has become impossible.

SUPPORT

In some ways the near relatives are even more important than the patient herself, and a frank discussion of the situation with them can in itself be therapeutic. In this way, the conflicting emotions of affection and rejection, guilt and resentment, can be brought out into the open, and the nature of the disease explained. Home support can be arranged, and in particular, some form of day care may liberate a daughter for two or three days each week and thus preserve HER sanity!

MEDICATION—SPECIFIC

It has been said that to diagnose the chronic brain syndrome is to switch off. This highlights not only the importance of excluding treatable conditions, but also the lack of specific treatment for the condition. It is difficult to believe that drug therapy might be capable of influencing what is basically a degenerative process, but the same would have been said about Parkinson's disease prior to the advent of levodopa. It is stretching credulity even further to claim that the rigid calcified atheromatous vessels of the circle of Willis so familiar in the postmortem room could possibly respond to vasodilators. Furthermore, the difficulties involved in mounting a scientific trial of a new preparation in a condition with so few measurable parameters and with such inherent variability are formidable, and, even if a statistical effect could be demonstrated, in the individual patient it would have to be quite a large one to be clinically worthwhile. The discovery of a really effective agent would rank as the most important advance since penicillin, and none of the drugs currently marketed has been greeted with the fanfare of enthusiasm from the scientific press that this would justify.

The drugs which have been claimed to enhance mental function in these patients fall into two groups. The vasodilators, it is hoped, will increase cerebral perfusion, and in view of the theoretical risk of a 'steal' phenomenon arising, it is probably just as well that they appear to be ineffective. The cerebral activators increase cerebral metabolism as indicated by utilization of oxygen or glucose, or enhance metabolism by improving enzyme systems. Some of the newer drugs do all this, and reduce platelet stickiness and blood viscosity besides (Table 8.2).

Hyperbaric oxygen has been claimed to produce lasting benefit, but its administration is too formidable an undertaking for routine use.

Table 8.2. Drugs purporting to improve mental performance

Proper name	Trade name	Comments
Cyclandelate	Cyclospasmol	Vasodilator
Isoxsuprine	Duvadilan	Vasodilator
Inositol nicotinate	Hexopal	Vasodilator
Naftidrofuryl	Praxilene	Increases ATP levels, oxygen-sparing effect
		Used in peripheral vascular disease
Meclofenoxate	Lucidril	Shown to disperse lipofuscin granules
Dihydroergotoxine mesylate	Hydergine	Effect on astrocytes
		May cause bradycardia
Pyritinol	Encephabol	Increases glucose utilization. Not UK

Vasopressin is thought to play a part in the process of memory consolidation, and is undergoing trails in chronic brain failure.

It seems probable that a greater contribution can be made to the preservation of the intellect and personality by purposeful activity and social integration. Attention to the general health, and particularly the correction of vitamin deficiency, anaemia, and cardiac failure, are also important measures.

MEDICATION—SYMPTOMATIC

In both acute and chronic brain syndromes it may be necessary to resort to drugs to control such manifestations as anxiety, agitation, restlessness, hallucinations, and seriously disturbed behaviour. The relief of distressing symptoms is humane, and is also likely to be appreciated by others. It is very important, however, to avoid constraining the patient within a 'chemical straitjacket' and so over-sedate her as to render her a drowsy, withdrawn, immobile vegetable. Thus in general small doses are given initially and increased to obtain control of symptoms. Table 8.3 shows the drugs recommended by the authors.

Sedatives and tranquillizers

Among these drugs the best known and most effective are the phenothiazines. They are all liable to cause excessive drowsiness in large doses, and they may lead to the side effects of hypotension, impaired temperature control, Parkinsonism, tardive and oro-facial dyskinesia, and obstructive jaundice.

Chlorpromazine (Largactil) was the first of these drugs to be widely

Table 8.3. Medication for elderly confused

	Proper name	Trade name	Suggested dose
Night sedation	Chlormethiazole *or*	Heminevrin	0·5–1 gm
	Dichloralphenazone	Welldorm	0·65–1·3 gm
Daytime restlessness or irritability	Haloperidol	Serenace	0·5–5 mg thrice daily
	±Lorazepam *or*	Ativan	1 mg thrice daily
	Thioridazine	Melleril	10–50 mg thrice daily
	or Chlormethiazole syrup	Heminevrin	5–10 ml (250–500 mg) thrice daily
Paranoid symptoms in delirium	Trifluoperazine	Stelazine	1–5 mg thrice daily
Severe delirium	Haloperidol		10 mg i.m.
	Paraldehyde		5 ml each buttock (GLASS syringe)
	or Chlormethiazole 0·8%		i.v. infusion 60→10 drops/minute (CARE)

N.B. It is commonly recommended that procyclidine 5 mg thrice daily should be given with haloperidol and the phenothiazines to prevent Parkinsonism.

used, and is as effective as any of its successors. A small starting dose would be 10 mg three times a day, but it is occasionally necessary to use doses as high as 150 mg thrice daily. It is sometimes given in a combined regime with chloral or haloperidol. Trifluoperazine (Stelazine) is equally effective in doses of up to 30 mg daily. Thioridazine (Melleril) 30 to 300 mg daily is slightly less potent, and promazine (Sparine), in the same quantities as chlorpromazine is considerably milder in its effect and less toxic. Perphenazine (Fentazin) is effective given intramuscularly in a dose of 2.5 to 5 mg and fluphenazine (Moditen) is available in a long-acting injectable form.

Among the so-called minor tranquillizers, the benzodiazepines now have pride of place. The most popular is diazepam (Valium) which can be given in doses of from 2 to 5 mg three or four times daily. Other drugs which may be very useful are chlormethiazole (Heminevrin) 250 to 500 mg thrice daily, and haloperidol (Serenace) 0.5 to 5 mg thrice daily. Haloperidol is also particularly liable to cause involuntary movements and a Parkinsonian syndrome. It is a butyrophenone derivative.

Hypnotics

Nocturnal restlessness may be largely due to the discomfort caused by a full bladder or rectum, and attention should be directed to these possibilities. Difficulties with sleeping are also common among the depressed and the anxious, and are prominent in the early stages of intellectual failure. For those who find insomnia a problem, it is worth trying a warm milky drink or a cold alcoholic one as a nightcap. It is commonly necessary to use an hypnotic, and chloral is one of the safest for use in elderly subjects. It is now available rather more acceptably in tablet form as dichloral phenazone (Welldorm). Another useful drug which has a short half-life and does not interfere with psychomotor function the following day is chlormethiazole.

CUSTODIAL CARE

Institutional care is considered in Chapter 4. Some local authorities tolerate confused, wandering and incontinent residents in their ordinary residential homes, while others make separate provision in homes for the 'elderly mentally infirm'. It appears inevitable that in the future, the great majority of applicants accepted for local authority care will fall into this category. Ambulant, demented persons with violent and antisocial behaviour require supervision by nurses trained in mental illness. When the family can no longer shoulder the burden, these patients come under the care of the mental hospital. It may be possible to arrange institutional care on a 'relief' basis, with admission for a few weeks several times a year tailored to the family's needs. All too often, however, it is permanent. Accommodation is very scarce, and there are at least five demented patients in the community for every one in hospital. Within the institution, much can be achieved by occupational therapy and simple aids to orientation, to make the most of remaining brain function.

Legal aspects of intellectual failure

The legal implications of incapacity to handle financial affairs are discussed in Chapter 19.

The question of compulsory admission to mental hospital occasionally arises, although the vast majority of elderly in-patients are admitted on an informal basis. Provision for compulsory admission is contained in several sections of the 1959 Mental Health Act (currently under scrutiny), but the one most frequently used is Section 25. Following application by the next of kin or a social worker, it is necessary to obtain two medical recommendations, one by a doctor with knowledge of the patient (usually her family doctor) and one by a psychiatrist, the two doctors not to be on the staff of the same hospital. The patient is then admitted for observation for a period of 28 days, but may be discharged during this time by the consultant psychiatrist responsible for her. If, in an emergency, only one doctor can be contacted, Section 29 provides for emergency admission for three days.

As a last resort, Section 47 of the National Assistance Act (as amended in 1951) entitles the general practitioner to apply to the District Community Physician for the compulsory removal to hospital or a residential home of a person who, on account of grave disease, is in a serious state of self neglect and whose health would be endangered by remaining at home. This requires the support of a magistrate and is valid for three weeks unless it is possible to give a week's notice, when it may be valid for three months.

In general, however eccentric the patient and however appalling her living conditions, if she wishes to remain in her own home, she must be allowed to do so, provided that she is not a danger to others. If she is a danger to herself but understands and accepts the danger, her wishes must once again be respected. It is wrong to try to insist on institutional incarceration simply because a scene of squalor and neglect offends the eye. One does not have to be socially competent to remain free. But if the patient is at risk through mental illness, but is unwilling to accept advice, then it may be necessary to have recourse to the Mental Health Act.

Depression

Depressive illness in the aged is common and causes a great deal of suffering and death. Community surveys have suggested an incidence of up to 15 per cent for moderate to severe depression. Contrary to popular belief, suicide is a real risk and the oldest $14\frac{1}{2}$ per cent of the population account for 25 to 30 per cent of cases. It is probable that the success rate is higher among suicide attempts by older people because many live alone and are found too late and because resuscitation is more difficult. As with dementia, disease must be distinguished from non-disease. By this, it is meant that there are certain circumstances in which it would be abnormal NOT to feel unhappy. Bereavement, loneliness, poverty, pain, and the knowledge of one's dwindling powers and imminent dissolution are the lot of many of the old. A state of helpless dependence combined with a total inability to communicate natural anxieties and fears commonly follows a stroke. In these situations, it may be questioned whether it is more appropriate to prescribe antidepressants, or to try to influence favourably the underlying misfortunes of the afflicted by means of counselling or social engineering.

True depression in the aged is the master of disguise of geriatric medicine—it is the great imitator of other diseases. It frequently leads to a state of withdrawal and inanition which mimics dementia. It may result in lethargy and sluggishness and thus masquerade as hypothyroidism. It can induce a state of akinetic mutism closely resembling brainstem infarction. And it can reveal itself less floridly in the exaggeration of symptoms only too readily attributed to concomitant disorders such as osteoporosis or degenerative joint disease. The opposite side of the coin is the presentation of other diseases with the symptom of depression. Serious organic diseases such as occult carcinoma may make their presence felt by a vague loss of well-being, sometimes vocalized by the sufferer as feeling 'low' or 'off colour'. Dementia, too, can first manifest itself in the same way.

Depression is perhaps above all the disease which must be treated irrespective of the general health of the sufferer. In medicine it is essential to preserve a sense of proportion, and what is the value of prolonging life, if life itself has no meaning? In younger patients, if life can be maintained, the disease can be expected eventually to go into remission. In the old, it will so undermine the general strength that the remission, when it comes, will probably be too late. If the illness is at all severe, treatment is therefore mandatory. Fortunately there are now a number of effective drugs available which can modify the disease and accelerate remission.

The morbidity of this dreadful disease—the anorexia and weight loss, the insomnia, the self-neglect—is seldom relieved significantly by purely symptomatic measures. The symptoms and the causes of depression without disease, however, may often be assuaged by fairly simple measures: loneliness, for example, may respond to regular contact with the relatives, or visits to an over sixties club.

The endogenous type of depressive illness in particular seems to be associated with depletion of biogenic amines, particularly 5-hydroxy tryptamine and the catecholamines. The tricyclic and related group of antidepressants appear to act by inhibiting the re-uptake of released noradrenaline and other amines via binding sites into cellular stores in the presynaptic neurones and thereby potentiating their action.

Factors pointing to a favourable prognosis include previous attacks in earlier life, and a severe degree of depression.

Drug treatment

THE TRICYCLIC AND TETRACYCLIC COMPOUNDS

This group of drugs is the most popular and successful treatment available for depression of moderate severity. Imipramine (Tofranil), and its derivatives (trimipramine, desipramine), is more suitable for the retarded, withdrawn type of depressive, and it can be given in a starting dose of 10 mg three times a day. Elderly patients often respond satisfactorily to smaller doses than are customary for the young and middle-aged. If this dose is ineffective, it should be increased to 25 mg as soon as it appears to be well tolerated. Amitriptyline (Tryptizol), on the other hand, has a sedative effect (unlike its derivatives, nortriptyline and protriptyline—both with a stimulant effect), and is thus indicated when depression is accompanied by anxiety, agitation and restlessness. Many patients will respond to a dose of less than 25 mg three times a day, but twice this amount may well be required. If nocturnal restlessness is a problem, a large proportion or the entire dose (50 to 100 mg) can be given on retiring. This is a drug in which the quantity given seems to be critical, so it is worth adjusting the dose before abandoning it as ineffective.

None of these preparations has any significant effect on the mood of the normal subject, and most of them tend to take at least two weeks to exert any beneficial effect on the patient with a depressive illness. They have anticholinergic properties, and are thus prone to lead to tachycardia, dryness of the mouth, constipation, hypotension, and hesitancy of micturition: they can also produce confusional states. The newer products are claimed to be more effective with fewer side-effects but these claims await substantiation.

OTHER DRUGS

The monoamine oxidase inhibitors have largely fallen into disuse before the advancing tide of newer agents (Table 8.4). Of those mentioned, L-tryptophan has the soundest rationale and appears to be very safe.

There is a small group of elderly patients who remain unaccountably drowsy, withdrawn, apathetic, and poorly motivated. It is justifiable in this situation to resort to an amphetamine analogue, which may produce an excellent response. Caution should be exercised, and a suggested starting dose would be dextroamphetamine 2.5 mg at breakfast and lunch.

Other forms of treatment

Many old people develop an agitated type of depressive illness, and a combination of a tranquillizer together with an antidepressant is then required. Finally, no old person who is severely depressed and who shows little response to medication in adequate doses should be denied

Table 8.4. Anti depressant drugs for the elderly

Proper name	Trade name	Suggested starting dose	Comments
Amitriptyline	Tryptizol	10 mg thrice daily	Tricyclic. Sedative effect
	Lentizol	25 mg at night	
Imipramine	Tofranil	10 mg thrice daily	Tricyclic
Clomipramine	Anafranil	10 mg thrice daily	Tricyclic. Injectable for rapid effect
Dothiepin	Prothiaden	25 mg thrice daily	Tricyclic. Well tolerated by the frail
Maprotiline	Ludiomil	10 mg thrice daily or 25 mg at night	Tetracyclic. Rapid action. Side effects rare
Mianserin	Bolvidon	10 mg thrice daily	Tetracyclic. Few side effects. Drowsiness
Viloxazine	Vivalan	50 mg thrice daily	Bicyclic. Few side effects. Nausea, vomiting.
L-tryptophan	Optimax	1 gm thrice daily	Precursor of 5-HT. Non-toxic. (? effectiveness)
Flupenthixol	Fluanxol	0·5 mg thrice daily	Rapid effect claimed
Doxepin	Sinequan	10 mg thrice daily	Anticholinergic and cardiotoxic side-effects infrequent
Nomifensine	Merital	25 mg daily	Well tolerated. Dopamine agonist

N.B. It is important to become familiar with just one or two.

the benefit of electro-convulsive therapy. Even the frail often tolerate ECT very well, and it may prove life-saving.

Schizophrenia

Schizophrenics, like the rest of us, grow old, and sometimes the disease tends to burn itself out. 'Late paraphrenia' is regarded by many people as a form of schizophrenia which manifests itself for the first time late in life. It is less florid than the usual form of the illness, and takes the form of paranoid delusions which may be difficult to differentiate from the suspicions and fears which may be perfectly normal in an isolated and somewhat eccentric old person. It is usual to try the phenothiazines in such cases, but the response is often disappointing. It is important to be sure that the hallucinations and delusions are not iatrogenic, because certain drugs, such as those used in the treatment of Parkinson's disease, not uncommonly induce them without the other manifestations of delirium.

Neurosis

Anxiety neurosis is probably the commonest psychiatric disorder encountered in geriatric practice and represents a vast sum total of human suffering. It may be a recrudescence of a lifetime of neurotic symptoms, or it may arise *de novo* in late life. Anxiety is a frequent accompaniment of depression, of the early stages of dementia, and of physical illness. On the other hand, patients with anxiety neurosis are often depressed and often experience physical symptoms. These physical symptoms (palpitations, breathlessness, giddiness, abdominal discomfort, bowel fixation) may be so predominant as to amount to hypochondriasis. Other common features include isolation and a poor marital track record.

The treatment is symptomatic, and firm reassurance following a full physical examination may be very helpful. Minor tranquillizers (diazepam 2 mg thrice daily) are occasionally useful, and depression is treated along the lines already described. A gentle sedative may be required at night; and the various day-care facilities can do much to relieve loneliness, if the patient can be persuaded to attend.

Institutional neurosis must also be mentioned since its importance lies in the fact that it is invariably iatrogenic and that it is therefore preventable—at least in theory. Regrettably it is still true that a visit to an institution for the care of the elderly is likely to reveal considerable numbers of persons sitting around the periphery of the day room in silent and apathetic immobility. This attitude of passive acceptance is by no means invariably a hallmark of dementia or depression, and represents a powerful argument for delaying custodial care as long as possible or, better still, avoiding it altogether. Within the institutional environment, the organization of activities involving meaningful participation offers the best means of avoiding this 'mental bedsore'.

CHAPTER 9 · IMMOBILITY

Teach us to live that we may dread
Unnecessary time in bed.
Get people up and we may save
Our patients from an early grave

RICHARD ASHER, 1947

Introduction

About 20 per cent of patients admitted to a geriatric unit will have a history of being house bound for more than two years. Over half (53 per cent) of our population over the age of 65 years report having difficulty in getting about their house. It should therefore not be surprising to discover that a complaint of 'gone off her legs' is a frequent presenting symptom when a request is made for admission to a department of geriatric medicine.

The possible causes for such immobility, whether long standing, recent or progressive, are many. Some of these conditions are reversible if correctly diagnosed and treated. The remainder can nearly all be improved or made tolerable if correctly managed.

Table 9.1. Causes of immobility

Pain — in bones	— osteomalacia, osteoporosis, Paget's disease, malignant disease and trauma
— in joints	— osteoarthritis, rheumatoid arthritis, gout and pseudogout
— in muscles and soft tissues	— polymyalgia rheumatica, ischaemia, polymyositis
Weakness	— endocrine, metabolic, haematological, haemodynamic, neurological
Psychological	— inertia, anxiety and fear, depression and dementia.
Iatrogenic	— over-sedation, parkinsonism, postural hypotension, metabolic disturbances

Pain

Pain is likely to cause immobility but great variation is found in patients' responses. Many patients will remain mobile in spite of severe pain—

others will give up more readily. The patient's personality traits will therefore be as important as the site, severity and cause of her pain.

The main sites of pain which reduce mobility

1   Bones
2   Joints
3   Muscles and soft tissues

Bone pain

Pain in bones is noted for its persistence and severity. Although often worsened by movement and weight bearing, it will also in many instances continue at rest, thus interfering with sleep.

Causes of bone pain

1   TRAUMA
2   OSTEOPOROSIS
3   OSTEOMALACIA
4   PAGET'S DISEASE
5   MALIGNANT DISEASE

1   TRAUMA

Relatively minor trauma resulting in bruising will not sufficiently impress a casualty officer to make him take the situation seriously. No fracture having been seen, the elderly patient may be sent home, but because of the pain, retire to bed and hence start her career of immobility.

Pathological fractures may occur in bones affected by any of the conditions to be mentioned. This possibility should be considered as an explanation for the development or worsening of pain and immobility in a patient known to have abnormal bones. The precipitating trauma may be so slight as to go un-noticed. In these cases the degree of pain is sometimes less than in traumatic fractures as total tissue damage at the site may be less.

In scurvy subperiosteal haematoma can occur and, although rare, this condition is more likely to appear in the elderly than in any other group. In addition, it is eminently treatable and extra effort should therefore be made to keep it in mind.

One should be wary of missing a fracture in patients with other painful conditions affecting mobility—such as rheumatoid arthritis. The hemiplegic patient, especially with aphasia, is particularly at risk in this respect. Impacted fractures without deformity are very easy to miss.

2 OSTEOPOROSIS

Osteoporosis is common and is frequently confused with osteomalacia. The bone structure in osteoporosis is normal but the amount of bone present is reduced. It is such a common phenomenon in geriatric medicine that the view is often held that it is part of the natural ageing process, although it is still accepted that more accelerated forms are pathological.

Twenty-five per cent of women over the age of 65 are said to have osteoporosis, but only 6 per cent of men. Because of this sex difference a hormonal cause is often postulated, but there is no real evidence that the menopause has a lasting effect on bone. Women are thought to

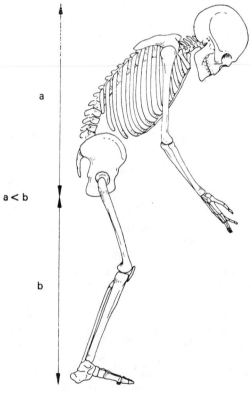

Fig. 9.1 (a)

achieve a smaller maximum bone mass in their prime—they therefore get off to a worse start. If bone loss is a normal ageing process, this would help to account for the sex difference, as women have a longer life expectancy.

There are some known causes such as:

1 Bed rest
2 Steroid therapy
3 Thyrotoxicosis
4 Cushing's syndrome

these should all be sought and corrected if possible.

No simple diagnostic test is available to confirm the diagnosis of osteoporosis. The calcium, phosphorous and alkaline phosphatase levels of these patients are normal unless there has been a recent fracture. X-rays of affected bone will show generalized rarefaction and changes in the trabecular pattern in the femoral neck have been said to be of value in diagnosing the condition. Vertebral changes are often seen particularly biconcave (cod-fish) vertebrae and more seriously partial or complete collapse of vertebrae. These vertebral changes might be suspected after measuring the patient. Vertebral collapse will reduce

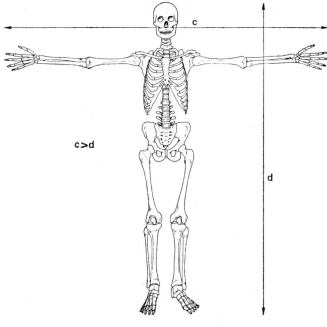

Fig. 9.1 (b)

crown to pubis distance and span will exceed overall height. Other clinical features which may be present are a marked transverse abdominal crease and actual contact between the rib cage and the pelvic brim (Figs. 9.1a & b). It should be remembered that these changes may also occur in kyphosis due to other causes (see Table 9.2).

Table 9.2. Causes of kyphosis

Bone collapse	secondary to osteoporosis
	secondary to osteomalacia
	secondary to trauma
Bone destruction	secondary to neoplastic disease
	secondary to infection
	secondary to Paget's disease
Neuro-muscular causes	Parkinson's disease
	old Polio
Joint disease	ankylosing spondylitis
	rheumatoid arthritis

The treatment of osteoporosis also presents many problems. It is generally accepted that once it has occurred, the osteoporosis is irreversible. Although some clinicians advocate the use of hormones—both female and anabolic—there is no convincing evidence of their effectiveness. Others advocate the use of fluoride and some give both vitamin D and calcium. This combination may well be justified if the theory that osteoporosis and osteomalacia often occur in combination can be confirmed.

The use of analgesics is also debated, as some observers feel that pain only occurs when fractures happen and analgesics should not therefore be required between crises. Nevertheless, many patients complain bitterly of continuous pain—usually in the back. Rarefaction may be the only abnormality seen on their X-rays. The variability of pain in Paget's disease is well recognized and possibly the same variation occurs in osteoporosis. If the patient complains of back pain and no more serious cause can be demonstrated, then analgesics are justified and should be given regularly. This is a more acceptable policy than the use of rigid supporting corsets with their effects on respiration and the possibility that the resulting immobility of spinal movements will worsen osteoporosis. However, after acute vertebral collapse, strict and firm bed-rest together with potent analgesia may be unavoidable. The patient should be mobilised as soon as pain permits.

3 OSTEOMALACIA

This is very easily treated and the results can be very dramatic although it is relatively uncommon. The true incidence of osteomalacia in old age is not definitely known—amongst admissions to geriatric departments, it is thought to occur at the rate of 4 per cent. Such a frequency will mean that a unit with a turnover of 1,000 patients annually will have the opportunity of correcting this disorder 40 times each year.

Osteomalacia means softening of the bones—the bones are soft because they are inadequately calcified. Calcification is impaired because of lack of vitamin D or its metabolites. Like all deficiency diseases it can be treated by simple replacement therapy, although where possible, the cause of the deficiency should be corrected. In old age, however, the cause of the lack of vitamin D may not be precisely detected because of difficulties in performing extensive and exhaustive tests in old and disabled patients. The following causes should be considered.

1 dietary deficiency
2 malabsorption (including gastrectomy)
3 impaired metabolism of vitamin D due to liver or renal disease
4 the effect of drugs (especially anti-convulsants) on vitamin D absorption and metabolism
5 the lack of endogenous vitamin D production secondary to sunlight exposure, especially in the housebound

Often evidence will be found to suggest that osteomalacia in old age is due to a combination of many of the above factors.

Osteomalacia is a diagnosis which should be considered in all patients with painful immobility. Suspicion should become greater if the pain is mainly proximal—in hips, thighs and shoulders and sometimes in the back. If hip movements are weak as well as painful—leading to a 'waddling gait' and difficulty in climbing stairs, clinical suspicion should mount. The next step in confirmation should be the estimation of serum calcium, phosphorus and alkaline phosphatase levels. The complete positive biochemical picture is a low calcium and phosphorus, giving a product of less than 1·6, together with a raised alkaline phosphatase. Care in interpretation is needed when the serum albumin is low, as this will artificially reduce the calcium level. Not all the parameters need to be abnormal for the condition to be present—but a raised alkaline phosphatase level is probably the most suggestive (it can of course also be raised for many other reasons). X-rays are usually unhelpful—the bones simply showing the non-specific changes of rarefaction, but pseudofractures seen in the cortex of a bone are diagnostic. Radioisotope bone scanning may prove to be a useful investigative procedure. Bone biopsy is the only sure way of confirming the diagnosis —a 0·5 cm core of bone may readily be removed from the anterior iliac crest under local anaesthesia. Cases with osteomalacia will demonstrate wide uncalcified seams of osteoid tissue.

Treatment is by regular administration of combined calcium and vitamin D tablets BPC, each containing 500 units of vitamin D. Some authorities recommend starting with a parenteral injection of 600,000 units of calciferol. The only known danger of treatment is the production of hypercalcaemia and response has therefore to be monitored by regular serum calcium estimations. The use of ultraviolet light is devoid of this danger. If a dietary or gut cause is found, efforts should be made to bring about any necessary correction. See Chapters 3 and 15. 1 αcholecalciferol (a metabolite of vitamin D) is indicated where there is a definite hepatic or renal cause.

If no other significant disabilities are present, the response to treatment should be very satisfying, with a return to normal mobility.

4 PAGET'S DISEASE

This is a combination of excessive bone breakdown associated with rapid replacement, resulting in deformity and increased fragility. Any bone can be affected but those of the pelvic girdle and the tibia and the skull are most frequently involved. In many instances, the condition is completely asymptomatic and is revealed by routine X-ray or biochemical screening. Paget's disease seems most common in people of Anglo-Saxon descent, and is rare in Asia and Scandinavia.

On X-ray, an affected bone is often thickened and bowed and the normal trabecular pattern is distorted and there are patches of rarefaction and sclerosis. The characteristic biochemical change is a raised bone alkaline phosphatase, but usually with normal calcium and phosphorous levels. The serum calcium level can, however, be raised when an affected bone is immobilized. The finding of raised hydroxyproline excretion in the urine (the product of collagen degradation) is further evidence for activity of the disease.

Many patients are severely disabled by the severity and persistence of bone pain. Although affected bones are often large, they fracture easily and this causes yet more pain. The distortion of the bones may give rise to symptoms due to pressure on other structures—especially where parts of the nervous system pass through bony canals. High output cardiac failure is a rare complication of the condition resulting from the increased vascularity of the bone. However, the heart failure found in most of these patients is more commonly due to associated cardiac pathology. The most serious complication of all is the development of sarcomatous change in an affected bone but this is very rare.

Until recent years, treatment for Paget's disease has been purely symptomatic, consisting of analgesics and orthopaedic measures. The discovery of the hormone calcitonin has, however, considerably altered the situation. When given intramuscularly, it can reduce bone resorption.

The main indication is to relieve pain but in the long term it may prevent bone deformities and the subsequent liability to fracture. The treatment is, unfortunately, expensive and inconvenient, and should not yet be used routinely, but only when simpler measures have failed. The long-term effects have yet to be evaluated. Similarly the effectiveness of other forms of treatment such as mithramycin, glucagon and diphosphonates is still to be assessed. Treatment with fluoride is no longer popular.

5 MALIGNANT DISEASE

The commonest form of malignant bone disease is that due to secondary spread. The metastases are usually from primary lesions in the prostate, lung, breast, thyroid and kidneys. The majority of secondary deposits in bone are osteolytic (areas of bone appearing as if eaten away) but the lesions secondary to carcinoma of the prostate are sclerotic (areas of increased density). Familiar sites for any of these lesions are the vertebral bodies, ribs, pelvis and upper ends of the femur and humerus —all places where the marrow is particularly vascular.

Secondary deposits are often painful and demand symptomatic relief by potent analgesia or radiotherapy. Palliation is usually all that can be hoped for in most cases. Painful bone secondaries from a carcinoma of the prostate may justify treatment with oestrogens (see Chapter 19). In elderly women, hormone replacement therapy may also be justified in carcinoma of the breast with bone lesions. Bone metastasis from a primary in the thyroid (if well differentiated) might respond to treatment with radioactive iodine.

The onset of paraplegia due to spinal secondaries constitutes a radiotherapeutic emergency. Immediate treatment is essential to offer any hope of avoiding complete paralysis and an indwelling catheter.

Elderly patients with multiple myeloma need careful assessment before specific treatment with cyclophosphamide or melphalan is commenced. These forms of therapy are dangerous and should be used only when likely to be beneficial.

Although steroid treatment has many complications in the elderly, worthwhile benefits may be obtained from its use in the presence of hypercalcaemia due to bony secondaries.

Painful joints

As painful joints are frequently made more uncomfortable by weight bearing and movement, they are likely to lead to immobility. It may be difficult to differentiate between pain in the joint and pain arising from adjacent bones and muscles.

The main types of arthritis in old age.

1   OSTEOARTHRITIS
2   RHEUMATOID ARTHRITIS
3   GOUT AND PSEUDOGOUT
4   OTHERS AND MIXED FORMS

1   OSTEOARTHRITIS (OR DEGENERATIVE JOINT DISEASE)

This is a chronic destructive arthropathy most commonly found in the
elderly. X-ray surveys have indicated an incidence in old age in excess
of 80 per cent; giving support to the concept that osteoarthritis is only
an exaggeration of the normal ageing process. However, only about a
quarter of those with X-ray changes also complain of joint pains.
Although osteoarthritis affects all parts of the spine, and less frequently,
joints of the upper limbs, it is involvement of the hips and knees which
most frequently leads to immobility.

Osteoarthritis is classically not symmetrical but often both hips or
both knees or sometimes all four joints are damaged, but not equally.
Obese people are particularly vulnerable to osteoarthritis and arthritics
are particularly likely to put on weight because of their immobility.

It is not only walking which becomes impaired because of pain and
limitation of joint movement. Loss of the ability to get out of bed or to
rise from a chair will mean the end of independence. If no relative or
helper is available to assist with these movements or to use a hoist, life
at home will be impossible.

The skilled use of analgesics initially on demand, but later given
regularly and in effective dosage, can help to maintain mobility. If
mobility has been lost, it may be regained in some instances by the
combination of analgesics and physiotherapy. The aims of the therapist
will be to increase the range of limited joint movements, and to stabilize
joints by strengthening the surrounding muscles which are commonly
wasted. Instruction in the use of a walking frame will also help, the
frame sharing in the weight-bearing and making movement less painful
and more steady. The occupational therapist will also be of assistance.
Advice about seating, particularly height, stability and type of arms,
will be of value; spring-assisted seats adjusted to the patient's weight
will also be beneficial in some cases. Special aids for picking up articles
from the floor—'lazy tongs'—aids for putting on socks and stockings
and elastic shoe-laces, are simple measures, but of great value and will
help to maintain the independence of a disabled person.

Surgical advice should be sought if drugs and physiotherapy do not
bring about sufficient relief and improvement. Hip replacement provides
rapid and lasting results. Severe uncontrolled pain which interferes
with normal activities is the major indication for operation. The patient

must be otherwise fit and well motivated and in particular must be without any evidence of intellectual impairment.

2 RHEUMATOID ARTHRITIS

This is usually thought of as a symmetrical polyarthritis due to synovial proliferation, predominantly affecting young or early middle-aged women. As it is a chronic disorder which rarely kills its victims, they will often survive into old age, most will have no major disabilities. In others although the disorder might be quiescent considerable joint destruction will have occurred. The sufferers may have to give up their long-fought battle to maintain their independence and mobility, not necessarily because of their joint deformities but due to the acquisition of other disabilities in other systems. Some of these additional burdens may be secondary to the rheumatoid disease or its treatment—iron and folic acid deficiency anaemia and osteomalacia also have a high incidence in chronic rheumatoid patients. Once detected, such problems are reversible and great gains may be made in functional capacity.

Rheumatoid arthritis arising in old age for the first time is not uncommon. Unfortunately the exact incidence in this age group is not known, but out of a group of geriatric patients with acute onset arthritis, about one-third were diagnosed as having rheumatoid arthritis. The disease is essentially the same in young and old but in the latter men are equally at risk and a rapid onset is more common.

The management of active rheumatoid arthritis is, however, different in older patients. In young sufferers, prolonged bed rest is sometimes advocated, and may be a good investment in the avoidance of later damage. The situation in the elderly is quite different—bed rest itself becomes more dangerous, and the time for investment to show a profit much shorter. The usual aims are therefore to maintain mobility with physiotherapy, to prevent deformities with splints, and to minimize symptoms with drugs. Anti-inflammatory drugs, especially aspirin, remain the first choice. If gastro-intestinal side effects are troublesome then enteric coated preparations or benorylate should be used. A potent, long acting anti-inflammatory drug, such as indomethacin, taken at night will help with early morning stiffness. Patients who cannot tolerate these preparations should be tried with propionic acid derivatives. Although gut side effects are less frequent they may still arise—there is considerable variation in patient preferences.

A short, sharp course of steroids may sometimes be justified in order to obtain rapid results so that the period of immobility can be kept to a minimum.

Gold and penicillamine should only be used under the direction of a rheumatologist.

3   GOUT AND PSEUDOGOUT

The mechanism of pain in both of these conditions is an inflammatory reaction provoked by the presence of crystals in the synovial fluid. In gout, the chemical substance is uric acid, and in pseudogout, pyrophosphate salts.

Classically gout affects the metatarsophalangeal joint of the great toe, and is easily diagnosed. Confirmation may be obtained on X-ray and a serum uric acid estimation. In old age, women are also victims to this arthropathy.

Pseudogout most commonly affects the knees. The radiological finding of chondrocalcinosis is not sufficient to make the diagnosis, but fluid from the affected joint must be examined for leucocytes and crystals. Because of the gross joint swelling, there is usually no difficulty in obtaining the necessary synovial fluid.

The onset of both forms of gout is usually sudden, and together they account for about 12 per cent of cases of acute arthropathy in old age and are equally common. In patients with true gout, there will sometimes be a family history, and the attack may have been precipitated by diuretic therapy. Gout secondary to a blood dyscrasia (leukaemia or polycythaemia) is three times more common in the elderly than in other groups.

Treatment of the acute attack of either form, is with potent anti-inflammatory drugs such as phenylbutazone. If there is evidence of renal damage, in true gout, then allopurinol should be started in order to modify uric acid metabolism and prevent further damage.

4   OTHER ARTHROPATHIES

It should always be remembered that the elderly can suffer from any joint disorder. Psoriatic and septic arthritis do deserve a separate mention as they are not uncommon. In dealing with elderly patients, it is always wise to consider the possibility of mixed forms of arthritis especially osteoarthritis with rheumatoid arthritis, and the latter with septic arthritis. Effusions may arise in joints after trauma and they may be bloodstained.

Muscular pain

Muscular pain and weakness may be the cause of immobility. The patient may complain of 'arthritis' or 'rheumaticks' but on direct questioning and clinical examination it becomes clear that the main problem is in the muscles.

Causes of muscle pain

1 POLYMYALGIA RHEUMATICA
2 ISCHAEMIA
3 POLYMYOSITIS
4 MISCELLANEOUS

1 POLYMYALGIA RHEUMATICA

This is a variety of collagen disorder found mainly in the elderly. The symptoms and signs are widespread, and it is generally regarded as part of the spectrum of disease which includes temporal arteritis. In polymyalgia rheumatica, the muscle symptoms are most marked, the patient complaining of pains—stiffness and 'rheumatism'—especially in the early morning. In temporal arteritis, headache and scalp tenderness are most pronounced. The second name does at least concentrate attention on the arteries, where the characteristic giant cell granulomata will frequently be found.

Other findings which, if present, will help to suggest the diagnosis, are a mild pyrexia or normochromic anaemia and a very high ESR.

It is the risk of sudden occlusion of a vital artery, such as one of the cerebral or coronary vessels which makes the diagnosis and treatment of this condition urgent. The ophthalmic artery appears to be especially at risk. Biopsy confirmation of the diagnosis is highly desirable. Anti-inflammatory drugs will relieve the muscle symptoms, but steroids are required to prevent the more serious complications. The maintenance dose will be decided by monitoring the patient's ESR and symptoms but a high starting dose such as Prednisone 20 mgs three times daily will be required.

2 MUSCLE ISCHAEMIA

Ischaemia of muscles on exercise (intermittent claudication) will limit the range of mobility. When sufficiently severe to cause rest pain complete immobility is likely. In old patients with severe arterial narrowing, it is unlikely to be restricted to a single vessel, and by-pass surgery is seldom a practical possibility. The use of vasodilators is also disappointing, but sympathectomy will sometimes bring about sufficient improvement to avoid amputation.

In mentally alert patients with severe peripheral ischaemia causing rest pain, amputation may be the only answer. If properly prepared, physically and psychologically, the results can be extremely good, and an independent life regained after a period of intensive rehabilitation.

In patients with severe cerebrovascular disease causing dementia or strokes, the decision concerning treatment of an ischaemic limb is much more difficult. If the prospect of regaining any independence is not good, then symptomatic pain relief is the kindest course to take (see Chapter 14).

3 POLYMYOSITIS

This is a rare non-specific inflammatory disorder mainly affecting the proximal limb girdle muscles. The affected muscles are weak and tender and there may also be an associated dermatitis. The skin is frequently oedematous, of violaceous hue and the face and upper limbs are mainly affected.

Although the condition is usually due to collagen disorders in younger patients, it is more often a manifestation of neoplastic disease in the elderly.

Treatment is removal of an identifiable tumour if practicable, or symptomatic treatment with steroids. The prognosis in old age is usually poor.

4 MISCELLANEOUS

Pressure sores on heels are unfortunately frequent in disabled elderly patients. They are often extremely painful and a real obstacle when remobilization is being attempted.

Painful feet due to corns, bunions and toe-nail deformities play a very significant role in making old people immobile (see Chapter 18).

Weakness

Weakness is a prominent symptom of any serious systemic disease. It is a very difficult symptom for patients to describe and equally difficult for doctors to assess. Full examination of the patient may localize the weakness to certain muscle groups and elicit the necessary clues for making a correct diagnosis. Simple laboratory investigations can then be performed to confirm the clinical suspicions.

Causes of weakness

1 ENDOCRINE
2 METABOLIC
3 HAEMATOLOGICAL
4 HAEMODYNAMIC
5 NEUROLOGICAL

1 ENDOCRINE CAUSES OF WEAKNESS

Although rare, these causes are important, as most are reversible. Disorders of the endocrine system are, however, often difficult to detect in old age, the classical pictures rarely occurring and the familiar clinical symptoms and signs are frequently absent or modified.

After diabetes mellitus, thyroid disorders are the most frequent endocrine abnormalities in the elderly. These amount to about 5 per cent of all geriatric unit admissions, and about half will be suffering from hyperactivity. In a small proportion of these patients, proximal muscle weakness will be the only clinical abnormality, the more florid symptoms and signs of younger patients being absent. In these cases laboratory support will be required to substantiate the diagnosis. Altogether, about half of geriatric patients with thyrotoxicosis have some evidence of myopathy.

In myxoedema, immobility is most likely to be secondary to the general slowing down and loss of initiative that is part of thyroid deficiency. The description of apathetic thyrotoxicosis in old age is a splendid example of the difficulties and confusion that can arise in the practice of geriatric medicine (see Chapter 16).

Both hyper and hypo activity of the adrenals can result in decreasing mobility. In Cushing's syndrome whether primary, secondary or as a non-metastatic complication of a malignancy, the weakness can often be seen to be associated with proximal muscle wasting and hypokalaemia. The weakness of Addison's disease is more vague and more generalized.

2 METABOLIC CAUSES OF WEAKNESS

Osteomalacia has already been mentioned as a cause of immobility through the mechanism of bone pain. However, the situation is often complicated, as proximal muscle weakness is also a frequent part of the clinical picture. Vitamin D replacement is fortunately successful in treating both of these aspects of osteomalacia.

Reduced body potassium causes muscle weakness and should always be sought as a possible precipitating factor for immobility. The potassium changes of Cushing's syndrome have already been mentioned;

other significant causes are dietary deficiency, excess loss in diarrhoea or
vomiting, or renal loss through diuresis or impaired tubular function.

The dehydration which so rapidly complicates many acute illnesses
in old age will often delay recovery. It is due to a combination of water
and electrolyte loss and impairment of the thirst mechanism. The
resulting prolonged immobility may then become self-perpetuating (see
Chapter 16).

3 HAEMATOLOGICAL CAUSES OF WEAKNESS

Anaemia is dealt with in Chapter 17. Because of the slow onset of
anaemia in many elderly patients, due to chronic blood loss, it can be an
insidious cause of decreasing mobility. In the megaloblastic anaemias,
this is often even more pronounced, due to the widespread cellular
changes which are not restricted to the haemopoietic system.

4 HAEMODYNAMIC CAUSES OF WEAKNESS

The best example of this mechanism is the reduced effort tolerance
which frequently follows in the early stages after a myocardial infarction.
It should be remembered that such attacks in old age are often silent
and therefore easily overlooked. The patient will simply complain of
weakness and tiredness, possibly with increased dyspnoea on effort, and
will, if allowed, retire to bed. A brief period of rest is obviously justified
in this situation, but as soon as possible, the patient should be persuaded
and encouraged to become mobile again. If the attendants are overprotective and too sympathetic, the patient may rapidly become
permanently immobile.

5 NEUROLOGICAL CAUSES OF WEAKNESS

A stroke producing paralysis of a leg will obviously reduce mobility.
However, predominant sensory loss will cause just as severe difficulties
in walking. The sensory problems will need careful evaluation to ensure
proper management. Otherwise the inability to walk, in the absence of
paralysis, might be attributed to lack of motivation.

Parkinson's disease with either marked increased extra-pyramidal
tone or akinesia, or both, will also present many mobility problems (see
Chapter 13).

Peripheral neuropathies will also hamper mobility, as will paraplegia
and cerebellar disorders. As complete a diagnosis as is possible will be
required before the correct course of treatment and rehabilitation is
commenced. These topics are discussed in a little more detail in
Chapter 13.

Psychological disorders

In Chapter 8 psychological disorders of the elderly are described. They play an important role in reducing the patient's mobility.

Psychological causes of immobility

1 INERTIA
2 FEAR AND ANXIETY

1 INERTIA

This may feature in the clinical picture of both dementia and depression. In the early stages of dementia, it frequently takes the form of passive dependence. These patients have no insight into their problems and will simply decide that their walking days are over. No amount of persuasion will change their opinion. In those patients in whom dementia takes a prolonged course, the terminal phase is frequently one of complete immobility. The patient becomes bed-fast and curled into a foetal position, in spite of the efforts of enthusiastic nurses and physiotherapists.

In depression there is a general slowing down of bodily functions manifest as inertia. Recognition of the depression is of the utmost importance, since it can be reversed in many cases by appropriate treatment.

2 FEAR AND ANXIETY

Fear and anxiety, especially of falling, are common causes of reluctance to walk in geriatric practice. Chapter 10 documents the many causes of falls in old age. The consequences may be so serious that these fears are fully justified. The stoical members of the elderly population will be able to cope with the anxiety caused by the many risks encountered in old age. Others will not be so successful. Correction of the possible causes of falls will obviously be beneficial. Other useful measures, are instruction in how to get up off the floor after a fall, and how to use a walking frame and other aids. Easy access to an alarm-call system is also reassuring; this might take the form of a telephone, for which financial assistance can be available, or a portable system such as a whistle or an aerosol alarm. Tranquillizing drugs in small doses will also be helpful in some cases, but in others, the side effects will be more troublesome than the original symptoms.

Iatrogenic causes of immobility

There is a high frequency of drug-induced disease in old age, amounting to about 10 per cent of all admissions and out-patient referrals.

Over-sedation will result in an inert withdrawn and immobile patient. The drugs may simply have been given as night sedation, but the hangover effect may continue into the next day. Sedation, necessary during an acute toxic state, may be continued unnecessarily after the precipitating crisis has been resolved, and thus hinder the patient's recovery.

Many of the tranquillizers used in modern medicine will induce parkinsonian features in old patients and thus impair mobility. Postural hypotension is also often caused by drugs, and symptoms that the patient experiences on standing will encourage her to remain in bed or seated. Hypokalaemia, secondary to diuretic therapy and laxative administration, will be associated with weakness and reluctance to move. Osteomalacia can be due to long-term treatment with barbiturates and other anticonvulsants and the resulting weakness and bone pains may lead to immobility. There may also be an associated megaloblastic anaemia due to the same drug.

Bed rest itself is used as a therapeutic tool, but if used to excess in old age, rapidly leads to self-perpetuating immobility. Periods in bed should therefore be kept to a minimum.

The complications of immobility

Although one of the aims of geriatric medicine is rapid and full remobilization after periods of illness, there will remain certain occasions when bed rest is needed, or is the only humane way of managing a patient. During this period of confinement to bed or chair, continuous efforts should be made to limit the risks associated with immobility.

The avoidable complications of immobility

1 DEHYDRATION AND ELECTROLYTE IMBALANCE
2 VENOUS THROMBOSIS
3 CONTRACTURES
4 SPHINCTER DISTURBANCES
5 PRESSURE SORES

1 DEHYDRATION AND ELECTROLYTE IMBALANCE

The bedfast patient depends on her nursing attendants for an adequate supply of fluids. The scale of supply must be related to her physiological needs and not simply to expressed demand.

2 VENOUS THROMBOSIS

Venous thrombosis of the pelvic and leg veins is a problem of immobility. It is therefore commoner in the elderly and its management is more difficult. Special efforts are therefore needed to prevent the onset of this complication. In most instances, this means the avoidance of dehydration and the encouragement of active and passive movements. Even with an enthusiastic and devoted staff, the risks of developing a thrombosis in a completely paralysed leg is very great (60 per cent). Anticoagulant therapy in geriatric patients carries special risks (see Chapter 19) but should not be withheld on the grounds of age alone.

3 CONTRACTURES

The prevention of contractures is yet another reason for stressing the importance of frequent active or passive movements of limbs. During a period of enforced immobility each joint should be passed through its full range of movements, as many times as possible during the 24 hours. This can be done by the patient in some instances or by her relatives, the nursing and medical staff, and where special skill is required by the physiotherapists. It is only by such attention that the muscles can be protected from permanent shortening with fibrosis. Pain may trigger off flexion contractures and must therefore be adequately treated. Resultant flexion deformities of the hips and knees preclude walking. The judicious use of splints will ensure that should fixity occur the final position will permit maximum function of the limb. Splints must be carefully and individually made so that they perform their tasks efficiently and do not cause pressure sores.

Where contractures have developed, they can sometimes be corrected. Gradual extension, assisted by warmth and analgesia, can eventually correct some of the less severe deformities. Surgical correction by tenotomy will be justified in many patients to relieve discomfort and to facilitate rehabilitation.

4 SPHINCTER DISTURBANCES

It should always be remembered that the most rational and socially competent person, if confined to bed and lacking adequate attention will, on occasions, be forced to be incontinent.

Prolonged periods of inactivity, often together with a reduced appetite, will lead to slowing of gut motility. Constipation is then likely, and if not corrected will worsen day by day, until faecal impaction occurs. The faecal mass will then be too large to be passed. This large faecal mass lying in the pelvis will impair bladder control and urinary incontinence is likely. As the situation worsens, spurious uncontrollable diarrhoea will occur, as liquid faeces trickle past the obstructing mass. The patient will then have the indignity of being both incontinent of urine and faeces, although still mentally alert and fully orientated. If such a patient is aphasic, the distress and embarrassment she experiences but cannot express, is enormous.

Those caring for the elderly therefore need to be aware of these complications and prevent their occurrence and rapidly correct them if they arise. Attention to these basic functions is properly the concern of both doctor and nurse. (See Chapter 11.)

5 PRESSURE SORES

These can be divided into superficial and deep varieties. The superficial type is the more frequent and consists of a break in skin continuity. And as its name suggests, it does not ulcerate deeply. The deep type is less common, but carries a much more sinister prognosis. It arises in the subcutaneous tissues and then extends superficially to and through the skin. In addition it may progress inwardly to affect muscle and even bone.

Pressure sores are very liable to occur in ill old people. The actual frequency will depend on the quality and quantity of the nursing staff and their equipment. Unfortunately 2·5 per cent of patients in general hospitals develop pressure sores. Many factors play a role in the aetiology of pressure sores. As the name suggests pressure is of great importance, particularly if it is prolonged. This will especially apply to the unconscious, the paralysed, those with impaired sensation and those in whom movement and position change are excessively painful. When an area of tissue is compressed between a bony prominence and a firm surface, it becomes ischaemic as blood is prevented from flowing through the vessels. Not only is the magnitude and direction of the pressure important, but also the efficiency of the patient's cardio-vascular system in forcing blood through the threatened area, and the amount of oxygen carried by the blood. Therefore, patients with reduced blood pressure, widespread vascular disease, anoxia and anaemia are all at increased risk.

Local and persistent irritation and trauma to the skin are other important contributing factors. Examples are friction from rough sheering movements of skin across bedding, and maceration due to prolonged contact with urine or sweat.

By paying attention to the known risk factors, a great deal can be achieved in the prevention of pressure sores. A scoring system has been designed to ease the recognition of the likely victims (see Table 9.3). Scores of less than 14 are closely associated with the development of pressure sores; a falling score is also a serious warning signal.

Table 9.3. Method of scoring for vulnerability of developing pressure sores (after Exton-Smith, Norton and McLaren)

Score	General physical condition	Mental state	Activity	Mobility	Incontinence
4	Good	Alert	Ambulant	Full	Not
3	Fair	Apathetic	Walks with help	Slightly limited	Occasionally
2	Poor	Confused	Chair-bound	Very limited	Usually/Urine
1	Very bad	Stupor	Bed	Immobile	Doubly

Maximum score 20. Score of 14 or less indicates severe risk

Patients at high risk should be turned at two hourly intervals as this is the best way of preventing trouble. Extra aids which can be utilized are special foam or sheep-skin pads for pressure points. A large cell ripple mattress (with cells of 11–15 cms) can be usefully employed. It must, however, be in perfect working order, and must not be used as a substitute for detailed nursing care. The use of a water bed is also beneficial, especially for those patients at very great risk and in whom frequent turning is painful and causes distress. Net suspension beds are a cheap and convenient method of nursing vulnerable patients'.

Although the nursing staff is traditionally blamed if a patient develops a pressure sore, the medical staff must accept some of the responsibility. If a rapid and accurate diagnosis is made on admission, some of the precipitating factors can often be reduced or reversed. If treatment is effective, more rapid mobilization can be achieved. Over-sedation should be avoided as it can itself be a significant contributing factor.

Pressure sores cause considerable distress to the patient, and extra work for the nursing staff. The patient's recovery will be delayed by weeks or months or even prevented altogether. The development of a severe pressure sore will increase the cost of a patient's hospital care by £2,000 or more.

Table 9.4. Areas for attention

Relief of pressure
Improvement of general condition
Avoidance of skin irritation
Applications and local measures, e.g. debridment and cleansing

CHAPTER 10 · INSTABILITY

Falling my love again
What shall I do?
Never wanted to
I can't help it.

After the 'Blue Angel'

Falls are certainly very common in old age, their causes being many and their outcome often serious. The frequency of a patient's falls may become so great that an independent life in her own home becomes impossible. The trauma suffered during falls may directly or indirectly precipitate an elderly person's death. Fear of falling may so demoralize a victim that she gives up the struggle to live.

Quite often the causes of the falls will be clear from the history but sometimes details are very sparse. Loss of consciousness, lack of witnesses or poor short-term memory may all limit the amount of available information. When the clinical history is incomplete or absent it becomes especially important to obtain clues from a careful and detailed physical examination supplemented by relevant investigations. The causes of falls will therefore be described under the headings of the systems which are at fault. Little more than a list can be provided in this chapter but details of all the conditions mentioned can be found elsewhere in this book. These conditions variously cause falls as a result of syncope, giddiness, weakness, clumsiness or tripping.

Environmental causes

The poor housing of the elderly and the frequent state of disrepair of their accommodation was described in Chapter 3. Defects such as uneven floors, worn carpeting and badly lit steps and stairs are frequently the underlying cause for a fall or trip. Additional domestic hazards are unseen pets, and trailing electric wires (Fig. 10.1).

Neurological causes

CONFUSION

In any confusional state, the subject may become exposed to increased

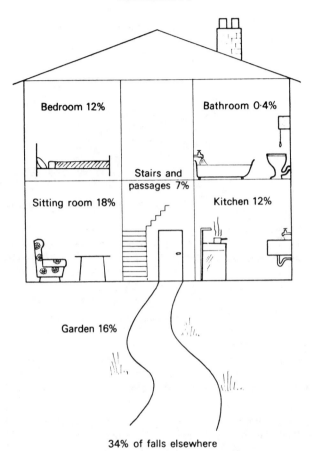

Fig. 10.1. Location of domestic falls resulting in a fracture

dangers by entering unfamiliar surroundings inappropriately dressed and with a clouded level of consciousness. For example untied shoe laces and knickers round ankles are dangerous, especially at the top of a steep staircase.

POOR VISION

The presence of visual field defects such as hemianopia following a stroke, or a central scotoma in glaucoma increase the risk of obstacles being overlooked. Lens opacities and retinal degeneration can give rise to similar risks. Visual defects in the elderly are often made worse by poor lighting frequently found in homes.

Table 10.1. Neurological causes for falls

(I)	Turns		fits
			TIAs
			drop attacks

(II) Spasticity — pyramidal — diffuse cerebrovascular disease / paraparesis of lower origin ; extra pyramidal

(III) Weakness (one or both legs) — upper motor e.g. mild or recovered stroke DS., MND. / lower motor e.g. old polio, peripheral neuropathy

(IV) Sensory—esp position — cord (post column) / peripheral nerves

(V) Special senses — poor vision / labyrinthine disorders

(VI) Cerebellar atoaxia

DAMAGE TO THE VIII NERVE AND ITS CONNECTIONS

Vertigo, whether due to changes in the labyrinth as in Ménière's syndrome or damage to the auditory nerve, for example by streptomycin, exposes the patient to the increased possibility of falls (see Chapter 18).

POOR RIGHTING REFLEXES

It has been clearly demonstrated that 'body sway' is greater in the elderly. When an elderly person stands still, considerable body movements occur as she tends to fall, and then corrects herself. The same happens in the young but the correcting systems are so efficient that hardly any movements are detectable. Many old people, in their own way, are aware of their own difficulties, and realize that once they are starting to fall they have little chance of regaining equilibrium. Dizziness, giddiness and light-headedness all require careful evaluation.

FITS

Anyone who has a grand mal seizure whilst standing up will fall to the ground. People who suffer from epilepsy in youth may well continue to have attacks throughout life.

The onset of genuine epileptic fits in old age will raise the possibility of a space occupying lesion, but often none is found. In most cases, the aetiology is thought to be vascular and supporting evidence of vascular disease in other systems can usually be found.

The diagnosis of epilepsy is based on the same criteria in old age as in youth. Because of the added dangers of anticonvulsants in geriatric practice, extra care should be taken in their prescription. Not all elderly epileptics require anticonvulsant therapy as in some cases it will cause symptoms worse than the illness.

TRANSIENT ISCHAEMIC ATTACKS (TIAS)

This refers to episodes of cerebral ischaemia which can affect either the carotid or vertebral circulations. Their duration is variable, usually only a few minutes or hours, but must be less than 24 hours to justify the title. If the area of ischaemia is situated in the carotid territory, the attack is likely to take the form of a disturbance of visual field, speech disorder or a sensory or motor defect in one or both limbs on one side. When located in the vertebral region, diplopia, vertigo and dysarthria usually occur. Falling can accompany either variety of TIA. Difficulties will sometimes be experienced in differentiating these attacks from epilepsy, but involuntary movements and incontinence are not features of transient cerebral ischaemia (see Chapter 12).

DROP ATTACKS

These are aptly named attacks as the victim just drops to the ground, much to her own surprise. There is no warning, no loss of consciousness and no neurological deficit. The victim's embarrassment is prolonged by her inability to rise without help in the absence of any obvious weakness. Sometimes pressure against the soles of the feet may reactivate the lost reflexes and the patient may then be able to stand without help. As the cause of these attacks is not clear it is not surprising that there is no known effective treatment or method of prevention. It has been suggested that these attacks are due to vertebral ischaemia with loss of postural reflexes.

CERVICAL SPONDYLOSIS

Osteo-arthritic and osteoporotic changes in the cervical vertebrae are usually responsible for the deformities which can lead to compression of the vertebral arteries. Interference with the vertebral blood flow is most likely during neck movements. The wearing of a cervical collar may prevent attacks, but to be effective, it needs to be tight and closely fitting and is therefore unacceptable to many patients.

It will probably have been realized that there is considerable overlap between the four causes of falls just described, cerebral ischaemia being most frequently implicated. As a result clinical differentiation is often difficult and sometimes impossible except in the case of witnessed classical epilepsy.

PARKINSON'S DISEASE

The characteristic festinant gait of Parkinson's disease is a cause for falls. The rapid shuffling steps associated with a flexed posture and extra-pyramidal rigidity expose the patient to the increased risks of accidents and loss of balance.

In addition, some patients with this disease also have an associated tendency to postural hypotension. In marked cases, this is described as the Shy-Drager syndrome.

PERIPHERAL NEUROPATHY

When position sense is lost, the risks of falling due to loss of balance are great. Even the loss of other modalities will lead to difficulty in walking and increase the possibility of accidents. There may also be an associated autonomic neuropathy, making postural hypotension a further hazard.

Cardio vascular causes

MYOCARDIAL INFARCTION

In view of the known high frequency of vascular disease in old age, it will not be unexpected that myocardial infarction is common. However, the classical clinical picture with characteristic chest pain is rare in geriatric practice, affecting only about 20 per cent of myocardial infarction victims. Almost 10 per cent of the remainder will present as a syncopal attack.

HYPOTENSION

This will often be the cause of the patient's fall during a myocardial infarction. The sudden drop in blood pressure may result in inadequate

Table 10.2. Cardio vascular causes for falls

(I)	Hypotension	Postural following silent myocardial infarction following pulmonary embolus following sudden bleed
(II)	Dysrhythmia	sudden bradycardia sudden tachycardia Stokes-Adams attacks
(III)	Effort syncope	due to postural hypotension due to aortic stenosis
(IV)	Carotid sinus syncope	

cerebral blood flow, with resulting syncope. Other causes of a sudden reduction in blood pressure include concealed bleeding, especially in the gastro-intestinal tract and pulmonary emboli. The latter are common in the elderly because of the high incidence of venous thrombosis in immobile legs. Both of these last examples may occur repeatedly and lead to a series of falls.

POSTURAL HYPOTENSION

This is a common mechanism for falls. It is easily detected and can often be corrected (see Chapters 13 and 14).

CARDIAC ARRHYTHMIA

The time when an elderly person with an arrhythmia is likely to fall is when the rhythm changes, or its rate alters. The sudden onset of marked sinus bradycardia is a time of danger. The development of complete heart block is another example. Stokes-Adams attacks are certainly the most dramatic instances of falls due to a cardiac cause. The onset or change in a tachyarrhythmia, of which the commonest is atrial fibrillation, is another example. Continuous cardiac monitoring may be required to detect the relevant abnormalities.

AORTIC STENOSIS

Systolic aortic murmurs are common in the elderly and falls are also common, so it is not surprising that they sometimes both occur in the same patient. However it is difficult to confirm that effort syncope secondary to aortic sclerosis occurs in the aged as it does in younger patients with true aortic stenosis.

CAROTID SINUS SYNDROME

Sudden pressure on the carotid sinus leading to a syncopal attack may occur in all age groups. It should be reproducible but is rarely so in practice. It is probably more frequently diagnosed than it occurs.

Gastro-intestinal causes

BLEEDING

Sudden, but not necessarily prolonged, bleeding may cause a sufficient fall in blood pressure to lead to syncope. The gut in old age abounds with potential sites for such blood loss—hiatus hernia, gastric and duodenal ulcers, large bowel diverticular disease and carcinomata being the most likely underlying conditions.

DIARRHOEA

Sudden bouts of diarrhoea can lead to transient episodes of loss of consciousness. Prolonged, chronic diarrhoea can result in potassium deficiency and can lead to muscle weakness and reduced stability. Hypokalaemia has also been reported as a potential precipitant of TIAs.

DEFAECATION SYNCOPE

Loss of consciousness has been reported as occurring in constipated patients on straining at stool.

Genito-urinary causes

PROSTATISM

Old men with prostatism often experience falls at night. The reasons are multiple and frequently several are acting together. The process of straining to pass urine can in itself provoke a syncopal attack. In addition, the patient may experience postural hypotension on getting out of his warm bed—his night sedation may potentiate this risk. There are then the hazards of finding the toilet or other receptacle in the dark with the possible added difficulty of reduced visual acuity.

Musculo-skeletal causes

UNSTABLE JOINTS

The combination of degenerative joint disease associated with ligamentous changes and weak surrounding musculature is likely to result in frequent falls. Such patients are stiff and clumsy, especially when rising from a chair or on climbing stairs and it is at these times that they are most likely to fall. The joint most frequently affected is the knee, and the patient complains that it 'just gives way'.

OSTEOMALACIA

In osteomalacia, there is an associated proximal girdle muscle weakness which causes difficulty in standing and produces the characteristic waddling gait. Because of poor muscles at the hips, falls are likely, and the chances of recovering balance after tripping are greatly reduced.

CERVICAL SPONDYLOSIS

(See the neurological causes of falls.)

Metabolic causes

THYROID DISEASE

Whether over or under active, disorders of thyroid function can lead to falls. Thyrotoxicosis can be associated with a proximal muscle weakness which will reduce stability. Myxoedema may cause not only slowness of movement, but also clumsiness and ataxia, which increases the risk of accidental falls.

ADRENAL DISEASE

Addison's disease with hypotension and asthenia makes falling more likely to occur. Cushing's disease is also a possible cause for falls because of its proximal muscle weakness, and hypokalaemia.

HYPOGLYCAEMIA

Although rare, spontaneous hypoglycaemia can be the reason for a patient being found on the floor. A low blood sugar however is more likely to be secondary to treatment for diabetes.

CHRONIC ANAEMIA

When the haemoglobin level is 10 g/dl or less then risks of episodes of transient cerebral ischaemia are increased in a susceptible patient.

Iatrogenic causes

OVERSEDATION

By causing confusion, drowsiness and instability, the careless use of sedatives and anticonvulsants may expose the patient to increased risks of accidental falls.

POSTURAL HYPOTENSION

Whether due to treatment of hypertension or as a side effect of many drugs, especially the phenothiazines, l-dopa and diuretics, this is a common mechanism of iatrogenic falls.

HYPOGLYCAEMIA

See above.

ARRHYTHMIA

Drugs used in the management of cardiac arrhythmia may themselves cause disturbances of heart rate or rhythm. This is especially true for digoxin. L-dopa and the tricyclic antidepressants should be remembered as potent precipitators of various tachycardias. The adrenergic β blocker drugs may in contrast cause a bradycardia. Great care is therefore required in the use of all these drugs in geriatric medicine.

EXTRA-PYRAMIDAL RIGIDITY

When drug induced, for example by the phenothiazines, extra-pyramidal rigidity is as effective in causing falls as it is in true Parkinson's disease.

VERTIGO

This can be a side effect of the aminoglycoside group of antibiotics especially in elderly patients with renal impairment.

Complications of falls

There can be no doubt that falls in the elderly are potentially dangerous, as 5 per cent of deaths in the over-65-year-old population are due to falls. Many old people accept the risks very stoically, and consider the dangers not to be too high a price to pay for an active but hazardous old age.

It may be a much more difficult task to persuade their relatives, friends and neighbours that the risks are worth taking, and ultimately the

Table 10.3. Complications of falls

1	Loss of confidence and mobility
2	Bruising
3	Fractures
4	Subdural haematoma
5	Burns
6	Hypothermia
7	Dehydration
8	Bronchopneumonia
9	Pressure sores

major responsibility lies with the patient. Many falls will fortunately be relatively atraumatic, and the dangers are often over-emphasized by well-wishers.

Loss of confidence and mobility

Fear of falling can be a very real reason for loss of mobility in the elderly. After a few falls, some elderly people become so frightened and anxious that they will not attempt to stand even when there is plenty of help and support at hand. Terrified by their previous experiences, these people will hold themselves tightly in their chairs, and if assisted to their feet, they will slump between two helpers, pleading to be allowed to sit again. Their obvious distress is upsetting to themselves, their helpers and any on-lookers. Considerable encouragement will be needed to persuade them to regain their mobility. Aids such as parallel bars are sometimes acceptable to these patients, and tranquillizing drugs may be useful. Care must be taken to avoid such side-effects as dizziness, light-headedness or postural hypotension, which will worsen the situation.

Bruising

To the inexperienced, this might seem to be a trivial complication of falling. However, anyone who receives requests for admission to the geriatric unit will be familiar with the following story:

'Can you admit a lady of 82 who fell two days ago? She was seen in the accident department immediately afterwards but as there were no fractures, she was sent home. She is now bed-fast and incontinent.'

The above sequence of events is all too common but could easily be avoided. One cannot blame the patient, as her bed was probably the only place at home where she could be comfortable. The faults usually lie with the accident service for failing to realize that the patient's pain and discomfort require proper analgesic treatment, even if there are no broken bones. Also, proper liaison between the casualty doctor and the community nursing service could have ensured that the patient was visited frequently at home. The nurse would be able to supervise the analgesic therapy and also actively encourage the patient to get up and help restore her confidence. Unfortunately, it does not take long for a patient who is already stiff and sore following a fall to become rigid, immobile and bed-fast.

Fractures

Fractures are common in the elderly for a combination of two reasons:
1   Falls are frequent in old age.
2   Bones are fragile in old age—the nature of the bone changes is described in Chapter 9.

For a practical demonstration of these facts, one needs to look no further than a female orthopaedic ward, where approximately half of the beds will be occupied by patients over the age of 65 years. Only wards in the department of geriatric medicine have a higher proportion of elderly women.

As a complete description of all fractures and their management cannot be given here, only important points about common injuries will be discussed.

FRACTURED RIBS

With fractured ribs, it is important to take seriously the severity and persistence of the patient's pain. Effective analgesia is essential if full respiration and mobility are to be maintained. Local injections with anaesthetic are often beneficial. Tight strapping of the chest, however, should be strictly avoided as it is likely to lead to serious respiratory complications in the elderly. Many of the powerful analgesics also have a depressant effect on respiration.

COLLES FRACTURE

Although immobilization in a plaster for a fractured lower end of radius may not present much of a handicap to a middle-aged patient the situation for a frail elderly person, living alone, is much more serious. It is difficult for her to cope at home with one arm in plaster. It should be realized that, for such a patient, to be admitted to a hospital bed (or local authority residential home) is sometimes as necessary as bringing in a younger person with more extensive trauma. Such an admission should not need to be prolonged, as long as community support can be organized to provide any necessary assistance at home with personal and domestic tasks.

FRACTURED FEMUR

Fractures through the hip are far more common amongst the elderly than in any other group. It has been reported that such fractures double in frequency for each 5-year increment in age after 50. Although the fall causing the fracture may seem trivial, the complications of the trauma sustained will often be sufficient to cause death. Subsequent fatal events may be fat embolism after replacement arthroplasty or pulmonary embolus from a deep-vein thrombosis in the affected leg.

The Aims of Management should be Two-fold

1 To relieve pain.
2 To restore mobility.

Fortunately, both aims can be achieved together by modern orthopaedic surgery. Attempts to treat elderly patients with prolonged bedrest and traction are almost bound to result in disaster. Where an unstable and painful pertrochanteric fracture needs fixation, a pin and plate should be inserted. In higher fractures, the best functional results will be obtained by a replacement of the femoral head by a prosthesis. With these operations the patient should be able to weight bear on the day after operation. Speedy rehabilitation can then be encouraged and the patient happily returned to her home, independent and confident.

FRACTURED TIBIA AND FIBULA

Fractures of these bones may seem less serious than those through the femur. Unfortunately, however, the recovery rate of such patients may often be far worse. The application of a heavy walking plaster may in fact effectively prevent mobility in the frail elderly patient, because of its sheer bulk and weight. By the time the plaster is removed, the period of fixation of the knee may mean that irreversible damage with loss of free movement will have occurred.

SUBDURAL HAEMATOMA

The possibility that a fall has caused a head injury and even a subdural haematoma should frequently exercise doctors' minds (see Chapter 13).

BURNS

Half of the deaths due to burns in this country occur in the elderly.
Many of these fatalities are caused by falls onto fires or scalds caused by
hot fluid being held at the time of a fall, fit or faint. Even with skilled
care, the recovery rate for elderly burned patients is extremely poor.
Such suffering is especially unfortunate when it is realized that many
of these accidents could be avoided if proper care was paid to fire
precautions. Fire-guards and non-inflammable clothing will reduce
these risks.

HYPOTHERMIA

DEHYDRATION

BRONCHOPNEUMONIA

PRESSURE SORES

See relevant Chapters for details.

These are all possible complications of falls. The patients at risk are
those who are unable to get up once they have fallen. If they live alone,
they may remain undetected and even die. The best way of enabling a
fallen patient to summon help is a portable alarm system. Telephones
and fixed bells are of little use if one falls some distance away. In such
circumstances a loud whistle or aerosol alarm is more practical. It is,
however, important that neighbours should be able to recognize the
alarm for what it is.

CHAPTER 11 · INCONTINENCE AND CONSTIPATION

> Let me look back upon thee. O thou wall
> That girdles in those wolves, dive in the earth,
> And fence not Athens. Matrons, turn incontinent,
> Obedience fail in children . . .

WILLIAM SHAKESPEARE
Timon of Athens. Act IV, Sc. 1

From the above curse spoken by Timon as he leaves Athens, it is obvious that Shakespeare was well aware of the social implications of incontinence. To the naïve and inexperienced, the symptoms of incontinence and constipation often seem trivial and even amusing. However, to those unfortunate enough to have experienced these problems and their complications, or to have had to care for the sufferers, the devastating effects are well known.

Unfortunately, incontinence (mostly urinary) is a very common problem and one which becomes more frequent as age increases.

Table 11.1. Showing incidence of urinary incontinence

	Sex	% Incontinent
Geriatric inpatients	Male	18–40%
	Female	24–46%
Elderly at home	Male	7–25%
	Female	13–42%

In all there must be approximately 1½ million incontinent elderly people in this country, sufficient for 20 patients for each hospital bed set aside for general and geriatric medicine. It is therefore obviously unrealistic to assume that all incontinent people should be cared for in hospital. Fortunately, it is not necessary to commit all these people to hospital care as many cases of incontinence can be reversed, and those which cannot can often be easily managed at home.

Nevertheless, incontinence does remain an important reason for hospital admission. This is especially true for the elderly incontinent person living alone. When incontinent in-patients were surveyed, twice as many as would have been expected (from population patterns) had lived alone. Of those elderly people with families, the onset of incontinence is often the final straw in taxing the goodwill of the relatives. Admission to hospital is eventually precipitated in one-fifth of those who are supported by their families, when they lose sphincter control.

Incontinence

Urinary and faecal incontinence will each be discussed separately and each will be subdivided into reversible and established forms.

Mention must be made initially of forms of incontinence not really due to loss of sphincter control or other pelvic defects. It should always be remembered that in some unfavourable situations, anyone (including the author and reader) is likely to be forced into incontinence. For instance, if one cannot reach a urine bottle and in addition is unable to ask for one, incontinence will eventually occur. This predicament can torment a fully rational, but aphasic stroke patient.

A common formula for the production of incontinence in old age is:

Distant toilet + slow and painful mobility + urgency = incontinence

In many instances it will be the first two items which will be of most importance. The second two items dictate the subject's wetting distance. It has been suggested that relatively immobile people should not be further than 15 metres from a toilet or commode if accidents are to be prevented. In a domestic situation this is fairly easily achieved, but will often be impossible in many institutions which have not been purpose built.

Reversible urinary incontinence

If incontinence occurs in a mentally normal patient, it is most likely that a reversible cause will be found. With increasing mental impairment, the prospects of recovery of sphincter control diminish, but do not necessarily completely disappear. In the mentally normal, it may be very difficult to get the patient to admit to her symptoms. Such patients are sometimes so acutely embarrassed by their problem and the offence they may cause to other people that they become socially isolated. Depression and other complications will then rapidly worsen the situation, so that the quality of the patient's life is totally destroyed.

In all cases of urinary incontinence, the following list of causes should be carefully considered. Reversal of symptoms is sometimes very easy, simple and cheap, and the benefits incalculable. Neither expensive apparatus nor sophisticated investigations are needed.

Reversible causes of urinary incontinence

1 DIURESIS
2 INFECTIVE
3 MECHANICAL
4 PSYCHOLOGICAL
5 IATROGENIC

1 DIURESIS

Age changes

The power of the kidney to concentrate urine falls with age. Additional pathological insults can further reduce renal efficiency. Impaired ability to concentrate urine is a common cause of nocturia in old age, and is very likely to result in bed-wetting if the patient is confused, sedated or immobile. The avoidance of excess fluids in the evening, especially C_2H_5OH and caffeine, may help to ensure a dry night.

Hyperglycaemia

Hyperglycaemia is an exceedingly common condition in old age—see Chapter 16 and the associated osmotic diuresis will often lead to incontinence. Routine urine testing in such an incontinent patient should reveal the diagnosis and correction should be simple.

Hypercalcaemia

Hypercalcaemia is a much rarer cause for an osmotic diuresis, but if due to neoplastic disease or sarcoid (rare in the elderly), it can be reversed by the administration of steroids.

The use of diuretics can lead to incontinence in old age, but this will be dealt with much more fully later.

2 INFECTIVE

There is no doubt that urinary tract infections are common in geriatric patients. An incidence of about 20 per cent is reported. In recent onset incontinence the finding of urinary infection is significant and its treatment may lead to the regaining of bladder control. In cases of long-standing incontinence, infection may be secondary, and its treatment have no effect on the patient's sphincter control.

Atrophic senile vaginitis

Atrophic senile vaginitis is another cause of urinary incontinence, especially when the patient also suffers from restricted mobility, and is unable to cope with the urgency that results from the vaginitis. If specific organisms or fungi can be detected, they should be eradicated. In most instances, an atrophic mucosa will be found, but no pathogens isolated. Replacement hormone treatment will often be beneficial in these cases. It would seem most appropriate to give these locally as stilboestrol pessaries, but many elderly women find this an unacceptable form of treatment. They should therefore be offered small oral doses of oestrogens such as quinestradiol (500 mcg twice daily), which should avoid withdrawal bleeding at the end of the course of treament (up to six weeks).

Just as vomiting is frequently a non-specific presentation of many illnesses in children, urinary incontinence can herald distant pathology in the elderly. It is a frequent component of the acute toxic confusional state, and will clear up once the true underlying illness has been identified and corrected.

3   MECHANICAL

Retention with overflow as a mechanism for urinary incontinence has causes additional to prostatic obstruction. In all cases, the vital clue is a palpable bladder.

Faecal impaction

This is the most important cause as it is easy to prevent and simple to correct. Also detection requires nothing more complicated than the routine performance of a rectal examination. On examination, the rectum will be found to be completely filled with faeces. The hardness of the stools will depend on the length of time the bowels have been neglected. Whether hard or soft, the sheer bulk of the motions can be sufficient to obstruct the bladder outflow.

As in all things, prevention is better than cure, and the avoidance of constipation can protect the patient from considerable discomfort and embarrassment.

Prostatic obstruction

This is the most common cause of retention with overflow. The retention is usually easy to detect, as the bladder is palpable unless the patient is very obese. It is often more difficult to confirm that the obstruction is due to prostatic enlargement as a rectal examination may be normal. The part of the gland causing the obstruction may be small and internal. Serum acid phosphatase estimations are unlikely to be helpful, but an intravenous urogram may help to show the position and the cause of the blockage. If the prostate seems to be responsible, the aid of a surgeon for cystoscopy and resection will then be required. If the risks of operation seem too great, there will be no alternative but a permanent indwelling catheter. The new silastic type causes less urethral irritation and needs to be changed less often than earlier types.

Trigone and proximal urethral abnormalities

For obvious reasons, prostatic obstruction cannot occur in the female, but a similar picture can occur due to non-specific inflammatory changes in the trigone and proximal urethra, causing bladder neck obstruction. Areas of squamous cell epithelium replace the normal transitional cell type. These changes may be hormonal in origin, and it has therefore been suggested that treatment with quinestradiol might be beneficial, a trial of six weeks' duration being required (500 mcg twice daily).

Stress incontinence

Although not restricted to previously parturient women, it is certainly more common in this section of the female community. It is particularly common in those who have undergone surgical interference during a delivery. The resultant alteration in urethral alignment causes an inefficient sphincter, and any activity which increases intra-abdominal pressure is likely to precipitate the leakage of urine.

In minor and early cases, the pelvic musculature can sometimes be strengthened by physiotherapy techniques. In co-operative patients, Faradism and pelvic floor exercises can be beneficial, and are certainly worth trying. In other patients with relatively minor degrees of prolapse, a ring pessary may help. Once inserted, the ring should not be forgotten and regular review is needed. Surgical repair may be helpful in more severe cases.

Urethral abnormalities

These are very common in elderly women. About 60 per cent of female geriatric patients show evidence of urethral prolapse and a further 10 per cent have a urethral caruncle. There appears to be a direct relationship with urinary incontinence, but the exact mechanism is not clear.

In some instances, the abnormality may actually cause partial obstruction and retention of urine.

4 PSYCHOLOGICAL

Over-stressed relatives caring for a difficult old person often make the accusation that their charge deliberately causes trouble and unpleasantness. Usually the relatives are wrong, and a physical defect can be found to account for the difficulties. Nevertheless, it must not be forgotten that many old people are difficult, unco-operative and very demanding, and have usually been so throughout their lives. In old age, personality defects often become exaggerated, and incontinence may be used to manipulate relatives and increase dependency. In some instances, relatives invite over-dependency, either due to ignorance or over-protectiveness. As in all personality defects, especially long-standing ones, counselling is not likely to have a high success-rate, but sympathy for manipulated relatives can be helpful in making their burden more tolerable.

5 IATROGENIC

A toxic confusional state can be induced by a great many drugs and incontinence is often a feature.

Oversedation may produce disinhibition so that a previously well-orientated and socially acceptable patient may lapse into incontinence. Appreciation of bladder distension will be reduced. Sedation should therefore only be given when necessary, and the duration of treatment kept to an absolute minimum.

Anticholinergic drugs used in the treatment of Parkinson's disease, and also the tricyclic antidepressants may cause urinary retention and overflow incontinence may follow.

Sympathomimetic bronchodilators, such as ephedrine also carry the risk of precipitating retention, especially in patients with outflow difficulties. It is therefore important that all these drugs should be avoided in elderly men with prostatism.

Rapidly acting diuretics should only be used when quick results are essential, and not for routine treatment of congestive cardiac failure. If used in patients with reduced mobility, incontinence may result. Patients should be informed of the duration of action of the diuretic used, in order that administration can be planned to give a diuresis at a convenient time. It should then be possible to avoid nocturia and excessive micturition at other inconvenient times.

Established urinary incontinence

Although these causes of urinary incontinence are irreversible, the patient's problems and those of her attendants can often be eased. Most of the patients in this category will be suffering from an atrophic degenerative or destructive neurological condition:

1 Dementia
2 Parietal lobe lesions
3 Spinal lesions
4 Peripheral neuropathy
5 Post-prostatectomy

DEMENTIA

Intellectual failure probably leads to incontinence through two mechanisms.

Firstly, the patient becomes unable to plan ahead, and therefore does not empty her bladder prophylactically. The relevance of opportunistic micturition becomes obvious if one's own habits are studied, for example, the bladder is emptied before a lecture, not because of an overpowering desire, but because it might be the last opportunity for some time. Anyone familiar with the problems of taking young children on long journeys will also be aware of the necessity of thinking ahead as far as micturition is concerned. If such precautions cannot be taken, then micturition will eventually become unavoidable. The unfortunate demented patient might suddenly realize what is needed, but be unable to remember the location of the toilet. The problems just described can be circumvented by the attendant thinking and planning on behalf of the patient. Regular toileting may therefore avoid many, if not all episodes of incontinence; clearly labelled and easily accessible toilets are also required.

The second mechanism, is the lack of inhibition over spontaneous bladder contractions. Cystometry, in which pressure changes are measured as the bladder is gradually filled, reveals small uncontrolled contractions in demented subjects. Although the sensation of the desire to micturate can be retained, involuntary bladder emptying may occur almost without any warning. Anticholinergic drugs can be used in an attempt to control this type of incontinence. The frequent passing of small amounts of urine is sometimes an indication that these drugs might be helpful. A carefully kept incontinence chart will also provide essential information as to the most suitable time for drug administration. In some cases, regular toileting during the day controls the situation and emepronium bromide 100–200 mg at night will prevent nocturia.

THE NEUROGENIC BLADDER

The uninhibited bladder of dementia described above is a neurogenic bladder due to lack of cortical control.

In parietal lobe lesions, the subsequent loss of awareness of body image may result in loss of bladder control. It is usual, however, to restrict the term to spinal, and peripheral nerve causes.

In complete paraplegia, the victim is left with an automatic bladder, as the sacral bladder centre remains intact, but sensation will have been lost. The patient might learn to initiate bladder emptying by various tricks e.g. suprapubic pressure.

In cauda equina lesions, both motor and sensory functions are lost and any reflex control from above is also prevented. Bladder emptying becomes completely involuntary, and is usually incomplete with considerable residual urine.

In peripheral nerve lesions, it is usually the sensory loss which is of most significance. Although the ability actively to empty the bladder might remain, the patient remains ignorant of the need to do so because there is no sensation of discomfort. The bladder therefore becomes distended and atonic. In such cases, where a large resting bladder capacity can be demonstrated, but in the absence of mechanical obstruction, the use of carbachol type drugs can be justified. Regular bethanecol, initially by injection (7·5–10 mg), and then by mouth 50 mg 6 hourly is probably the best regime.

IATROGENIC

Unfortunately, some patients after prostatectomy will be completely and permanently incontinent of urine. This complication is happily rare, but unpredictable.

Management of urinary incontinence

The first step in a plan of attack in any patient with urinary incontinence is the exclusion of the reversible causes. The urine must therefore be tested for glycosuria and a specimen cultured to rule out infection. Examination of the patient, including rectal and vaginal examinations, will detect the presence of urinary retention and its possible cause. The presence or absence of vaginitis or any degree of prolapse should also be noted. A careful assessment of the patient's drug regimen is also needed to ensure that an iatrogenic cause is not overlooked.

If the incontinence proves to be irreversible, then steps should be taken to make the patient's problem manageable. Two alternatives are available. Firstly the aim can be to channel and contain the urine. Secondly, measures can be taken to absorb the overflow.

URINARY APPLIANCES

Unfortunately, none is available which is suitable for women. Several female appliances have been devised, but all either leak or cause considerable irritation, which usually results in severe soreness or even ulceration of the pudenda.

In males, the situation is better, as long as the penis is of sufficient length to remain in position in an appliance, and the patient is co-operative. A small retracted penis or a confused patient make the use of such apparatus futile. To be successful the equipment must be simple to apply and comfortable to wear. An excess of buckles, snappers and straps leads to failure. The simplest form is Paul's tubing and there are also slightly more sophisticated sheath appliances available. Both of these types may be held in place by the use of special adhesive. Bag forms (somewhat like colostomy bags) are less successful. There is no easy way of predicting which type will be most successful in any particular patient. A large variety is needed and should be kept in stock, and experimentation encouraged. It should be remembered that most appliances, even those with valves, tend to leak at night, and some absorptive device is needed in addition (see below).

CATHETERS

These are more efficient, provided that there is no leakage around the catheter. However, they can be dangerous in confused patients, who might remove them traumatically. In prolonged use, they require careful supervision, washouts if blocked, and regular changes. Recurrent infections may still be a problem. Catheters therefore offer a solution to permanent incontinence, but at a high price. However, this price can be worthwhile, if a catheter is the only way of gaining reacceptance at home or returning to a fully independent way of life. The use of modern silastic catheters reduces many of the risks and discomforts.

The catheter bag should always be concealed, e.g. in a sporran (Shepherd's sporran), or a leg-bag should be used.

PADS AND PANTS

Incontinence pads are used in the bed so as to restrict the extent of the wetness. They therefore offer some protection to the rest of the bedding and reduce laundry problems. The urine is kept away from the skin by a porous but non-absorbent layer and is then absorbed by the pad.

These pads are disposable and fairly cheap. The Kylie sheet is an absorbent sheet which keeps the skin dry. It is not disposable but should be washed and re-used.

For ambulant incontinent patients, not suitable for appliances or catheters, various absorbent pads are available. The best types not only absorb, but retain the fluid, as the collecting substance forms a gel. The collecting material is situated in a marsupial pouch and kept well away from the patient's skin. The pants themselves are reusable after washing. The patient is kept dry and odour free, both essential requirements if a full, active and social life is to be enjoyed.

Constipation

Constipation will be discussed before faecal incontinence, because it is more common and it is frequently the underlying cause for loss of anal sphincter control.

Because of considerable natural variation, it is extremely difficult to define constipation. In fact, it is much easier to say what it is not. If the patient has a regular bowel action, not necessarily daily, but with ease and without discomfort, there is no need to be concerned. Most elderly people complain of constipation as they have been indoctrinated to believe that a once a day bowel action is the only pattern consistent with good health.

Bowel transit times are greatly increased in old age. Up to three weeks is not uncommon in geriatric patients compared with 24–48 hours in fit young people. This may reflect the results of taking an unsuitable low residue diet for many years, or follow the long-term abuse of purgatives. It cannot be assumed that it is a genuine age change.

Whatever the true frequency of constipation in old age, it would seem that fear of the condition is of even greater prevalence. Although only about one-fifth of patients claim to be constipated, over half take regular laxatives prophylactically.

Causes of constipation

1 DIET.
2 PSYCHOLOGICAL, including depression and dementia and embarrassment.
3 OBSTRUCTIVE, especially scarring and neoplasms.
4 PAINFUL ANAL LESIONS.
5 INCONVENIENCE.
6 METABOLIC—myxoedema, hypokalaemia, hypercalcaemia and dehydration.
7 IATROGENIC, including environmental causes, immobility and drugs.

1 DIET

The lifelong dietary habit of taking highly refined foods with minimum bulk may be responsible for the constipation of many old people. The situation is likely to become even worse when appetite is reduced by illness. Curtailment of exercise during sickness is another aggravating factor.

2 PSYCHOLOGICAL

Unfounded concern about bowel habit in old age has already been mentioned. True constipation can, without a doubt, be a feature of depression. The mechanism can either be through a reduced appetite and dietary intake or secondary to the generalized slowing down of bodily functions which is one of the physical aspects of severe depression. As depression in old age is thought to occur at the rate of about 10 per cent, it is a significant cause of constipation. Dementia also leads to the neglect of defaecation, and constipation will have to be detected by rectal examination, as the patient will make no complaint.

3 OBSTRUCTIVE

There are many gastrointestinal pathologies affecting the elderly, which can be complicated by obstruction. Strictures can be secondary to infective, ischaemic or neoplastic conditions. In addition, long-standing herniae are common. Constipation is an early symptom of obstruction in all these examples, and is eventually followed by vomiting if not corrected.

4 PAINFUL ANAL LESIONS

The elderly are often afflicted by piles, which when thrombosed or inflamed, will make defaecation painful. Defaecation is thus discouraged and successful bowel evacuation becomes more and more unlikely. An anal fissure can lead to the same vicious circle.

5 INCONVENIENCE

A cold, dark, outside toilet situated at the end of the yard is a strong disincentive to regular defaecation. Another problem, especially prevalent among the elderly is arthritic hips, which make rising from the toilet difficult and painful, particularly when it is not at a convenient height.

6 METABOLIC

Clear-cut examples are rare, but myxoedema, hypokalaemia and hypercalcaemia can all include constipation in their symptomatology.

Dehydration is a further example, but generalized weakness due to chronic debilitating illness, together with apathy and generalized inactivity is a more frequent precipitant of constipation.

7 IATROGENIC

As always in geriatric medicine, iatrogenic disease merits inclusion. The main culprits for constipation are the codeine containing analgesics, tricyclic antidepressants, the anticholinergic, anti-parkinsonian drugs and antacids containing aluminium salts. The diuretics, by causing dehydration and hypokalaemia can also be responsible. Oversedation can remove the will to respond to a normal call to stool which, if frequently ignored, will result in constipation.

The complications of constipation

To ignore constipation can be dangerous. Its complications can not only be distressful, but also potentially serious.

1 IRRITABILITY AND CONFUSION
2 OBSTRUCTION
3 STERCORAL ULCERATION
4 MEGACOLON
5 FAECAL INCONTINENCE
6 PURGATIVE ABUSE

1 IRRITABILITY AND CONFUSION

These symptoms are likely to be most marked in demented patients. The victim will be aware of abdominal and pelvic discomfort, but be unable to express her difficulties or seek appropriate help. Patients under sedation, for example during terminal care, will be exposed to the same risks.

2 OBSTRUCTION

The abdominal distension and vomiting secondary to obstruction by hard faecal masses, may suggest a more sinister pathology, such as a neoplasm.

3 STERCORAL ULCERATION

Constant irritation of the colonic wall by hard faecal masses can lead to areas of ulceration which are liable to bleed.

4 MEGACOLON

Megacolon due to neurological defects in the colonic wall can be a rare cause for constipation. In old age, a large dilated bowel is more frequently secondary to prolonged and severe constipation, which has resulted in loss of tone of the muscle layer.

5 FAECAL INCONTINENCE

Faecal incontinence secondary to faecal impaction is dealt with below.

6 PURGATIVE ABUSE

Patients may become so obsessed about their constipation that they take purgatives in large doses so that they eventually exchange their constipation for diarrhoea. Irreversible damage may be caused to the bowel so that it becomes an inert tube. Excess fluid and potassium losses will cause severe ill-health, apathy and weakness.

The investigation and treatment of constipation

If a specific cause is suspected, the management is the same as in younger patients. The presence of other known pathologies may, however, exert great influence on decision making. A demented patient will not only be unable to comprehend the reasons for investigation, but is also unlikely to be a suitable patient for surgery and should not be exposed to the distress involved in a barium enema, and other large bowel investigations.

Where symptomatic treatment is the only acceptable possibility, the interference should be kept to a minimum. Bulk laxatives, such as Celevac, or Isogel are probably the best and safest form of treatment. Good hydration must be maintained if obstructive complications are to be avoided. The patient should be encouraged to take a diet with as high a fibre content as possible.

Senokot is a reliable and acceptable preparation, but more potent stimulants or irritants should be avoided. Lubricants such as liquid paraffin also have unacceptable side effects. Distressing rectal leakage can occur, also malabsorption of fat soluble vitamins, and inhalation pneumonia.

There is no set dosage regime for any preparation, especially in old age. The dose must be titrated against the patient's symptoms.

Whenever possible, suppositories, enemata and manual removals should be avoided. If they are needed, every effort should be made to avoid their repeated use, by employing the preparations mentioned above. Unfortunately, such efforts are not always successful (see also Chapter 15).

Faecal incontinence

As in the case of loss of control of bladder function, the topic of faecal incontinence is best considered in terms of reversible and established forms. Normal mental function will favour a reversible cause which should be carefully sought.

Reversible faecal incontinence

FAECAL IMPACTION

This is the most common reversible cause and is easy to diagnose and eminently treatable. It should never be overlooked, and never will, if routine rectal examinations are carried out on elderly patients with any bowel complaint.

To the inexperienced, faecal impaction might seem inconsistent with faecal incontinence. However, whilst the impacted mass plugs the lower end of the large bowel, the faeces above will become liquefied by bacterial action. This fluid trickles past the obstruction and runs uncontrollably through the anus. Soiling therefore tends to be continuous and the faecal matter unformed.

When incontinence due to faecal impaction occurs, immediate relief of the obstruction is required. In such instances, repeated enemata may be needed to achieve large bowel clearance. Softening preparations such as olive-oil retention enemata (150 ml) or dioctyl sodium sulphosuccinate may be required. The undignified procedure of manual removal, with unpleasantness for both patient and helper, cannot always be avoided. If very distressful, the removal can be carried out after the patient has been prepared with a small intravenous dose of diazepam.

Once dealt with, further episodes should be prevented. A high residue diet should be encouraged and supplemented with bran or a bulk laxative. In very weak and feeble patients, additional help in the form of regular simple suppositories (glycerine) may be needed, and thereby regular enemata can usually be avoided.

INTESTINAL HURRY

Most old people are unable to cope with frequent and urgent calls to stool, and incontinence is likely to occur. Rapid transit time can be secondary to gastro-enteritis, large bowel ischaemic changes, or chronic inflammatory disease. Metabolic causes, such as thyrotoxicosis, and the much rarer gastrin secreting tumours and carcinoid tumours can also increase bowel motility sufficiently to precipitate incontinence.

IATROGENIC CAUSES

First to be considered are the purgatives. These preparations are sometimes taken in great quantities by the elderly, often secretly and unnecessarily. Powerful irritating substances, such as many plant extracts (cascara and aloes) and potent osmotic salt preparations (magnesium sulphate) are to be strongly condemned as the risks of complications in old age are very high. Not only is uncontrollable diarrhoea likely, but also severe fluid and electrolyte imbalance.

Antibiotics with a wide spectrum of activity can so alter the normal gut flora, that severe enterocolitis can be caused.

Unaccustomed dietary indiscretions can also be troublesome, especially the consumption of excessive amounts of milk, fruit, and alcoholic brews.

Established faecal incontinence

Fortunately, this is less frequent than irreversible urinary incontinence.

NEUROLOGICAL

In dementia, faecal incontinence may result from lack of inhibition of the normal gastrocolic reflex. Formed motions are therefore passed involuntarily, but often at predictable times. A well-trained attendant can therefore manage the situation without too much difficulty.

Autonomic neuropathy, as sometimes occurs in diabetes mellitus and amyloid disease, will affect gut motility, and the resulting diarrhoea will be uncontrollable.

Cauda equina or spinal cord lesions may lead to faecal incontinence.

LOCAL RECTAL LESIONS

Rectal carcinoma

The tumour, by destroying the rectal sphincters, can lead to uncontrollable incontinence. Unless routine rectal examinations are carried out, these lesions will be overlooked and the possibility of treatment missed. However, even in late stages, a palliative operation with a colostomy can make a considerable improvement to the quality of the patient's life.

Rectal prolapse

By a similar mechanism, this can also lead to incontinence. Surgical correction can, however, be more successful, but not always completely so.

CHAPTER 12 · CEREBROVASCULAR DISEASE

W'en folks git ole en strucken wid de palsy, dey mus' spec
ter be laff'd at.

Nights with Uncle Remus,
JOEL CHANDLER HARRIS, 1848–1908

Cerebrovascular disease

Cerebrovascular disease is the biggest single physical cause of hospital
bed occupancy by the elderly in the United Kingdom and it is the third
commonest cause of death in the population after heart disease and
cancer. The incidence of completed stroke rises steeply in the elderly.
Despite the frequency of cerebrovascular disease, and the devastation
and human misery caused by it, this type of illness has failed to attract
the medical attention that it warrants. Clearly the modern physician
must take a much more serious view of the palsy than did Uncle Remus.

Table 12.1. Hospital bed occupancy by elderly. UK 1970

Stroke illness	18,000	20%
Diseases of heart and vessels (excluding strokes)	14,000	16%
Malignant disease	7,000	9%
Arthritis	5,000	7%

These four diagnoses account for more than 50 per cent of all bed occupancy
by the elderly (excluding mental hospitals).

Atheroma

Atheroma of the major arteries supplying the brain is the basis of
cerebrovascular disease in most cases. The lesions are patchy and the
location critical so that a small amount of atheroma in one situation
can cause more disturbance than a larger amount of atheroma elsewhere.
The earliest and most consistent location of the atheromatous plaques
or ulcers is in the extracranial vessels especially at the origins of the
great vessels from the aortic arch, and the bifurcation of the common
carotids. The basilar artery and the points where the intracranial arteries
branch are also involved. These lesions may cause stenosis of the
vessels and they are commonly the site of thrombosis.

Hypertension

In epidemiological studies hypertension is the most important risk factor predisposing to atherothrombotic cerebrovascular disease. The risk correlates with the mean blood pressure reading and adequate treatment with hypotensive drugs in middle aged patients reduces the likelihood of stroke. Other, less common, risk factors are ischaemic heart disease, peripheral vascular disease, increased blood viscosity (haemoglobin level) diabetes mellitus and previous ischaemic attacks.

Blood supply to the brain

Cerebral blood flow diminishes progressively with age from 100 ml/100 g/min in the child to 50–55 ml in the adult to a mean value of 35 ml in apparently fit elderly people. As with so many measurements

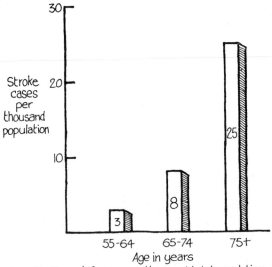

Fig. 12.1

in the elderly there is a bigger normal range of variation than in the young. The brain weight approximates to 2 per cent of the normal body weight but utilizes about 20 per cent of the total body oxygen consumption. In addition the brain requires a plentiful supply of glucose and other nutrients. A mean systolic arterial pressure of 80–90 mm Hg is required to give adequate perfusion assuming normal cerebral

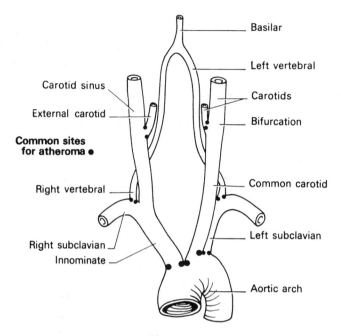

Basilar

Left vertebral

Carotid sinus

Carotids

External carotid

Bifurcation

Common sites for atheroma ●

Right vertebral

Common carotid

Right subclavian

Left subclavian

Innominate

Aortic arch

Fig. 12.2

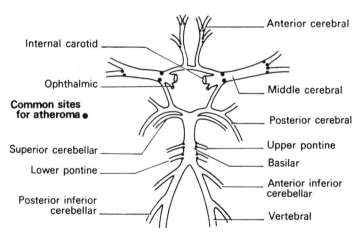

Anterior cerebral

Internal carotid

Ophthalmic

Middle cerebral

Common sites for atheroma ●

Posterior cerebral

Superior cerebellar

Upper pontine

Lower pontine

Basilar

Anterior inferior cerebellar

Posterior inferior cerebellar

Vertebral

Fig. 12.3

vascular autoregulation. Furthermore the quality of the perfusate (i.e. the blood passing through the vessels) needs to be adequate at least as regards its oxygen and glucose content. Cerebral vascular auto-regulation normally gives protection against variations in perfusion pressure, but this mechanism is impaired in the presence of vascular disease.

Four extracranial arteries conduct blood to the brain. The two internal carotids and the two vertebrals anastomose to form the circle of Willis at the base of the brain. There is another anastomotic network in the leptomeninges but after entry into the brain only capillary communication exists. The normal circle of Willis gives such a generous anastomosis that one or more of the major vessels can be blocked without cerebral damage. Unfortunately the circle is anatomically normal in only about 50 per cent of people. Multiple anomalies may be present in addition to atheromatous disease.

Atheromatous ulcers lead to stenosis, thrombosis and formation of emboli (micro or macro) destined for lodgement in the smaller vessels in the brain substance. Although the clinical presentation of cerebrovascular disease is predominantly in the elderly, the atheroma—which is the villain of the piece has been quietly building up over many years in the apparently fit and totally unsuspecting victim.

Clinical manifestations of cerebrovascular disease

The diverse clinical manifestations of cerebrovascular disease are listed in Table 12.2 and will be considered in some detail. Not uncommonly the clinical picture is a combined one or progresses from one type of presentation to another. E.g. one or two attacks of epilepsy followed by a stroke with or without an intervening phase of transient cerebral ischaemic attacks (TIAs).

Table 12.2. Clinical manifestations of cerebrovascular disease

Transient cerebral ischaemic attacks (TIAs)
Stroke—completed or ingravescent
Progressive dementia
Pseudobulbar palsy
Epilepsy

Transient cerebral ischaemic attacks or TIAs

The term transient (cerebral) ischaemic attack means a neurological disorder caused by a disturbance of blood supply to the brain in which full recovery takes place within 24 hours. These attacks usually last for just a few minutes and since full recovery occurs (by definition) they tend not to be given the attention they deserve. This is a pity because the TIA, especially in the carotid territory, may presage a full-blown stroke with permanent, gross neurological defect. Furthermore, TIAs are often eminently treatable. The patient with TIAs needs proper investigation to see what medical treatment might have to offer.

Cause of TIAs

The root cause is atheroma which with current knowledge cannot be prevented or treated. (See Chapter 14 for factors regarding aetiology.) The major additional (precipitating) causes are microemboli from platelet aggregates on an atheromatous ulcer, a lowering of systemic blood pressure below the critical systolic level of 80–90 mmHg and a poor quality perfusate. These precipitating causes of TIAs are often treatable.

Table 12.3. Causes of TIA

Atheroma of major arteries + emboli
+ fall in perfusion pressure
+ poor perfusate

Multiple emboli may produce a series of stereotyped TIAs because the emboli do not circulate in random fashion. Blood flow in the great vessels is streamed or laminar so that perfusate destined for (say) a particular branch of the middle cerebral artery is already in the appropriate stream for that part of the brain even before the blood enters the circle of Willis. Thus platelet aggregates from a lesion at the bifurcation of the common carotid artery may cause recurrent embolization in the same small area of brain because 'streaming' reduces the scatter of the emboli.

REDUCTION IN PERFUSION PRESSURE

There are innumerable causes of reduction in perfusion pressure in elderly patients. Some are listed in Table 12.4. An awareness of the factors likely to be involved together with a carefully taken history and thorough physical examination will allow the diagnosis to be made in most cases.

Postural hypotension due to drugs, peripheral neuropathy and more generalized autonomic degeneration will be dealt with in a little detail in the next chapter. The concept of being 'out of training' when applied to old people might be found difficult to accept. Yet for any level of age, disability and disease a range of fitness can be found relating more to physical and mental activity than to anything else. The person recovering from an illness (say myocardial infarction, pneumonia or surgical operation) gets fitter quicker and becomes less liable to fainting attacks if she is systematically retrained in terms of physical fitness. This positive approach to fitness is central to good geriatric practice.

Table 12.4. Fall in perfusion pressure causing TIA

Reduced cardiac output	— Myocardial infarction, dysrhythmia, heart failure.
Postural (or exercise) hypotension	— Autonomic degeneration, peripheral neuropathy, drugs, out of training (e.g. convalescent), 'steal' phenomenon.
Transient obstruction of great vessels in the neck	— Looking up (high shelf) — Looking round (reversing car) + Cervical spondylosis + Rheumatoid spondylosis + Basilar impression (Paget's disease of skull)

The fascinating but uncommon subclavian 'steal' phenomenon is seen in association with stenosis of the origin of the subclavian artery when exercise of the arm on that side causes blood to be 'stolen' from the cerebral circulation by retrograde flow down the vertebral artery. This allows the muscles of the arm to be supplied with blood at the expense of the brain and may precipitate a TIA.

Transient partial or complete occlusion of the blood vessels (especially the vertebral) due to extension or rotation of the head and neck has long been regarded as a precipitant in some cases of TIA. However in Cambridge careful vertebral angiography has failed to confirm this mechanism even in the presence of obvious cervical spondylosis. Unfortunately patency of the carotids was not assessed simultaneously. Nevertheless, the evidence suggests that clinically significant reduction in the cerebral blood flow due to movement of the head and neck is not very likely.

ABNORMAL PERFUSATE

Abnormal perfusate is often a factor in TIAs in the elderly. This compounds the problem of nutrition for a brain already threatened by lack of adequate perfusion pressure and failed vascular autoregulation. The perfusate, is of course, the blood flowing through the blood vessels. Some alterations of quality of the blood are listed in Table 12.5. Anaemia reduces the oxygen carrying capacity but needs to be moderately severe (below 10 g Hb/dl) to be significant. Polycythaemia causes

Table 12.5. Abnormal perfusate

Anaemia	— Hb below 10 g/dl
Drugs	— sedatives
	— alcohol
Hypo or hyperglycaemia (or rapid changes in level)	
Hypoxia	— cardiorespiratory failure
	— CO poisoning
Renal or hepatic failure	
Polycythaemia	

increased blood viscosity and reduced blood flow. Sudden changes in blood sugar level can precipitate focal neurological signs. Psychosedative drugs including alcohol depress cerebral function and they are also implicated in the production of postural and exercise hypotension.

Clinical features of TIAs

Two main clusters of symptoms and signs require recognition—those falling within the carotid territory and those related to the vertebrobasilar supply. With both types the onset is usually sudden, the attack

Table 12.6. Clinical features of carotid TIA

Weakness or numbness	— contralateral
Hemianopia	— contralateral
Dysphasia	— dominant hemisphere
Monocular blindness	— ipsilateral (uncommon)
Carotid artery murmur	— heard in neck

Table 12.7. Clinical features of vertebrobasilar TIA

Vertigo and nystagmus
Drop attacks
Visual loss or diplopia
Dysarthria and dysphagia
Weakness and numbness—may be bilateral
Amnesia

lasting just a few (5–20) minutes and then gradually subsiding. (A duration up to 24 hours is included in the definition of TIA.) Transient hemiparesis with variants is the usual feature in the carotid TIA whereas in vertebrobasilar TIA a more varied symptomatology develops because many different tracts and nuclei are packed close together in the hind brain. Vertigo is especially common in vertebrobasilar TIA but it carries a good prognosis with respect to the possibility of a completed stroke. Long-tract symptoms are more sinister and may herald a brain-stem infarct. Carotid TIAs seem even more likely (about a third of cases) to progress to a completed stroke at a later date.

Management of TIAs

Diagnosis is all important to allow recognition and correction of each and every treatable element in the patient's illness; for example the correction of anaemia, drug-induced hypotension or hypoglycaemia. In almost all cases the diagnosis can be made by the clinician with the help of a few investigations—e.g. plain X-rays, ECG, and blood sugar. Only in highly selected cases will specialist investigation be indicated including arteriography by direct puncture of one of the main arteries in the neck and/or arch aortography by retrograde catheterization from the femoral artery.

A few cases will have an isolated extracranial carotid artery stenosis raising the possibility of endarterectomy. Most other TIAs within the carotid territory should be considered for anticoagulant treatment. Many geriatric patients will be deemed unsuitable for both of these treatments. Furthermore these therapeutic possibilities may not be readily available even when the patient is suitable. If there is real doubt about the use of anticoagulants (see chapter on medical and surgical treatment) in a patient with suspected microemboli from an atheromatous ulcer in one of the great vessels then soluble aspirin 300–600 mg twice daily should be prescribed. Aspirin is known to reduce adenosine diphosphate (ADP) release from platelets and hence it reduces platelet stickiness and thrombus formation. Markedly raised diastolic blood pressure (something of a rarity in the elderly) requires control to bring the diastolic into the range 85–95 mmHg and the systolic to 160–180 mmHg (see Chapter 14.). Giant cell and syphilitic arteritis must also be considered in the differential diagnosis, although the latter is now rare in Britain. Episodes of cardiac dysrhythmia are treated by the appropriate drugs or the insertion of a pacemaker.

The completed stroke

The completed stroke is one of the commonest problems in geriatric practice. The neurological damage reaches its peak within six hours and results in prolonged disability. The cerebral damage can be of any grade of severity so that the residual disability ranges from minimal to maximal and the outcome often is death.

The ingravescent stroke or stroke in evolution is one which evolves over a period of more than six hours but otherwise resembles the completed stroke.

Causes of completed stroke

A major cause of cerebral infarction is failure of adequate perfusion (haemodynamic crisis) but without necessarily a block of any of the vessels. This often occurs while the patient is in bed; the blood pressure drops during sleep and the stroke becomes evident when she wakes. She may attempt to get out of bed and fall to the floor to be found by a visitor some time later. In other cases a myocardial infarct or a pulmonary embolus is the cause of the haemodynamic crisis. Thrombosis of a major artery to the brain, in the neck or in the skull, or a sizeable embolus from heart or great vessels are other less common causes.

Embolus from the heart is probably more common than hitherto suspected. It occurs classically in cases of mitral stenosis with atrial fibrillation and following myocardial infarction with mural thrombus, but also in mitral valve prolapse and in ischaemic heart disease without gross valve pathology. Intracerebral haemorrhage (often into the internal capsule but sometimes into the pons or cerebellum) and subarachnoid haemorrhage are other important causes of stroke.

Importance of blood viscosity

Red cells make an important contribution to whole blood viscosity and it has long been recognised that polycythaemic patients are prone to strokes and TIAs. More recently it has been shown that viscosity rises steeply with the haematrocrit value throughout the normal range (0·36–0·53) and also that high 'normal' haemoglobin values (e.g. 14 g/dl in females and 15 g/dl or more in males) are associated with an increased incidence of stroke. The critical effect on viscosity is the same whether due to a raised red cell mass (polycythaemia) or a lowering of the plasma volume (haemoconcentration) and the cerebral blood flow correlates inversely with the haematocrit value. Old people appear less able to compensate for the increased blood viscosity and may be put especially at risk by dehydration and the overzealous use of diuretics. Where correction of dehydration fails to lower a raised haematocrit value the possible use of repeated small venesections (200–250 ml) may be

Table 12.8. Major causes of stroke

Haemodynamic crisis
Thrombosis of artery in neck or within skull
Embolus from heart or major vessel
Intracranial haemorrhage

desirable as a prophylactic measure. Consideration should also be given to the possibility of polycythaemia rubra vera (see Chapter 17).

Clinical features in completed stroke

Cerebral infarction usually takes 1–2 hours to evolve and loss of consciousness at the onset is unusual. Embolic cases are often abrupt and with a likely source of embolus evident and perhaps a preceding history of TIA. Other cases are indistinguishable from infarction due to haemodynamic crisis. Intracerebral haemorrhage is also abrupt in onset, classically comes on during exertion and is strongly associated with hypertension (80 per cent of cases). Severe headache is characteristic and loss of consciousness occurs early in over half the cases. The general prognosis in those with deep coma is very poor. Subarachnoid haemorrhage also is often marked by sudden severe headache and impairment or loss of consciousness. There are signs of meningeal irritation (neck stiffness and positive Kernig's sign) and blood will be present in the CSF.

The patterns of symptoms and signs are as described for TIAs but are persistent and usually more severe. The carotid territory is most often involved. There may be impairment of consciousness with a flaccid paralysis of one side of the body and possibly ipsilateral sensory loss and hemianopia detectable when the level of consciousness rises. Initially the tendon reflexes may be absent because of neurogenic shock but later they are brisk on the affected side and associated with an extensor plantar response. Gross dysphasia, motor and/or sensory, is commonly an important and disastrous component of stroke involving the dominant hemisphere.

Cortical sensory loss occurs with damage to the parietal lobes and involves spatial and discriminative aspects of sensation on the side of the paralysis—especially the left. Sensory ataxia may be elicited by tests involving the appreciation of position sense in the limbs. Crude appreciation of pain, heat and cold remain intact but readily fatigue. Inability to recognize the form and shape of an object placed in the hand occurs and is called astereognosis. Disturbances of attention also occur and there may be loss of recognition of the body image and neglect of one-half of external space. These symptoms and signs—especially astereognosis, sensory inattention and failure to recognize the body image—are often referred to as the parietal lobe syndrome. In left-sided lesions there may also be disorders of visual speech functions—dyslexia, agraphia amd acalculia.

Patients with this type of disability confound the hopes of the most determined therapist. Even so recovery is possible in some cases. The patient usually pays little attention to her surroundings and fails to appreciate movement of or the actual position of the affected limbs in space. The paretic arm will be left dangling over the arm of the chair for hours on end without the patient paying the slightest attention. If able to read, the patient omits one-half of the script on the affected side. If she tries to draw a simple picture (a clock face or a house) half is left off. The patient does not appear to be aware of her disability and indeed may deny that anything is wrong.

Ischaemic lesions involving the thalamus may produce bizarre involuntary movements, severe sensory loss—especially proprioception —and distressing persistent spontaneous pain with hypersensitivity to all modalities of sensation on the side of the paralysis. This is referred to as a thalamic overreaction or the thalamic syndrome. These are most intractable symptoms but sometimes the pain responds to anticonvulsant drugs—e.g. phenytoin in an initial dose of 200 mg daily. Ordinary analgesics are ineffective.

DIAGNOSIS IN THE ACUTE PHASE

Infarction with or without thrombosis but without embolus or haemorrhage is the most common cause of the completed stroke. Embolic occlusion of a cerebral vessel is an uncommon cause in the elderly but it must be considered in a stroke of fulminant onset, without hypertension, with an obvious source of emboli and also if there is evidence of emboli elsewhere. Cerebral haemorrhage should be diagnosed in a hypertensive patient with a rapidly evolving (not fulminant) stroke and a grossly bloody CSF. Subarachnoid haemorrhage (SAH) would also be a possibility but mostly these are middle-aged patients with the maximum incidence in the 40–60 age group. Seventy-five per cent of SAH is due to rupture of an intracranial aneurysm.

Table 12.9. Cerebrovascular disease—incidence of different types Community longitudinal study. All ages

	Per cent
Cerebral infarction	53
Subarachnoid haemorrhage	14
Cerebral embolus	12
Cerebral haemorrhage	6
Lacunar stroke	2
Transient cerebral ischaemic attacks	6
Miscellaneous	5

Diagnosis from other causes of coma, such as diabetes and drug overdose, is aided by the recognition of lateralizing signs. For example with haemorrhage into the internal capsule (a common site) the head and eyes will be deviated towards the side of the lesion. The opposite cheek flaps with respiration and the plegic limbs will drop inertly to the bed after being raised by the examiner. The unaffected limbs by contrast, even in coma, fall much less abruptly.

Subdural haematoma may result from head injury but falls are so common in the elderly that the episode of trauma may be overlooked (see also Chapter 13). Cerebral tumours can present with sudden

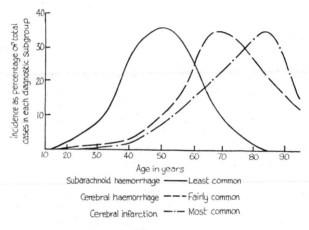

Subarachnoid haemorrhage ——— Least common

Cerebral haemorrhage — — — Fairly common

Cerebral infarction —·— Most common

Fig. 12.4

hemiplegia and may even undergo temporary remission as in a stroke. The classical triad of headache, vomiting and papilloedema is seldom seen in the elderly. Epilepsy may occur with cerebral tumour but this also happens in stroke.

CONFIRMATION OF DIAGNOSIS

In most stroke patients the diagnosis is made simply on the basis of the history, clinical examination and progress together with routine investigations including haematology profile, ECG and chest X-ray. Occasionally it is important to be more specific about the nature of the intracranial pathology. Is this a haemorrhagic or ischaemic infarct, is it a cerebral tumour or subdural haematoma? (See also Chapter 13). Non-invasive special investigations may give the answers to these questions. For example good quality plain films of the skull or echoencephalography may show a shift of mid-line structures and suggest intracerebral haemorrhage, subdural haematoma or neoplasm.

Computerized axial tomography (CAT scan) is the most valuable special investigation in selected cases of cerebrovascular disease. Provided that the head is kept still (cooperative patient, anaesthesia or coma) it will distinguish high density lesions due to haemorrhage—cerebral, subarachnoid and subdural—and also many low density lesions as in early ischaemic infarcts. Even if the infarct is not visible, the exclusion of haemorrhage and tumour is helpful. Cerebral angiography is indicated only if surgery is contemplated—i.e. mostly in younger patients with tumour or vascular malformations. However a major arterial occlusion can also be demonstrated by a dynamic radiosotope scan following an IV bolus injection. This is a much safer technique than direct angiography.

LUMBAR PUNCTURE

Lumbar puncture is not a routine procedure in the management of strokes and in many elderly patients with spinal deformity and osteoarthritis it can be very difficult to perform. Nevertheless, examination of the CSF is essential in some cases. Eighty per cent of cerebral haemorrhages have macro- or microscopic blood in the CSF but one must remember the other twenty per cent!

If anticoagulants are to be used for suspected cerebral embolus it is essential to know that there is no blood in the CSF prior to the start of treatment. Possible diagnoses of subarachnoid haemorrhage, meningitis and neurosyphilis demand an examination of the CSF.

In the case of suspected space-occupying lesions (cerebral tumour, abscess or haematoma) masquerading as stroke LP should not be performed but the opinion of the neurosurgeon should be sought. Removal of CSF in a patient with raised intracranial tension may produce a dangerous coning of the cerebral hemisphere through the tentorial opening or of the brain-stem through the foramen magnum. The absence of papilloedema is no guarantee against such an occurrence especially in elderly patients.

MANAGEMENT OF THE ACUTE STROKE

To begin with the doctor makes an overall appraisal of the patient's illness to decide the likely prognosis. To treat or not to treat that is the question. The patient suffering a first stroke against a background of previously normal physical and mental health has a good potential for survival and rehabilitation. Contrariwise the patient with established heart disease, hypertension and organic brain disease will have poor rehabilitation prospects. Coma, complete hemiplegia and conjugate gaze palsy are features which correlate with a very poor prognosis. Diagnosis of ischaemic infarction, embolus and haemorrhage respectively give an increasingly poor prognosis. Energetic treatment requires immediate hospital admission in all severe cases.

The unconscious patient must be nursed well onto her side to allow the tongue to fall forward and thus leave a clear airway. False teeth should be removed. If consciousness does not return quickly a decision regarding naso-gastric tube feeding will be required to maintain hydration and nutrition. Regular (hourly) turning of the patient is necessary to avoid pressures sores. Nursing on an alternating pressure mattress (ripple bed) or water bed is valuable in this respect. It is best to avoid catheterization immediately if the nurses can cope with the patient's incontinence. If catheterization is necessary the catheter must be removed at the earliest possible stage in recovery. Systemic illnesses must be looked for and treated e.g. anaemia, congestive heart failure and respiratory infection.

Some specific medical treatments

Cerebral oedema may increase the neurological defect well beyond the area of the infarct. Furthermore it is known that reduction of cerebral oedema in patients with head injury and cerebral tumour is beneficial. Many treatments are available for achieving this but their use in acute stroke has given disappointing results. Nevertheless, diuretics, oral and intravenous glycerol and dexamethazone all have their advocates.

Vasoconstrictors and vasodilators including stellate ganglion block have all been tried and found wanting. The normal autoregulation of cerebral blood flow is deranged in stroke, and any treatment for raised blood pressure must be cautious especially in the first few weeks. Cerebral ischaemia causes a local increase in CO_2 tension with local vasodilation, hyperaemia and oedema in the affected area. No further dilatation of these vessels is possible. Dilatation of other blood vessels elsewhere in the brain and body might result in an overall drop in perfusion pressure and make matters worse rather than better.

Anticoagulants are only indicated when it is reasonably certain that the infarct is embolic, or for the prophylaxis or treatment of deep venous thrombosis. There is disagreement as to whether treatment for cerebral embolism should be started immediately or after an interval of 1–2 weeks to allow some healing of the infarct and reduce the risk of haemorrhage. Hemiplegia is a condition with a marked predisposition to deep-vein thrombosis in the palsied lower limb with consequent risk of pulmonary embolism. The maximum advantage from anticoagulants is in the weeks and months following the stroke. Thereafter the need to continue the treatment diminishes. Special caution must be exercised in the use of anti-coagulants in geriatric practice and further information on this is to be found in Chapter 19.

Physiotherapy

Physiotherapy by whomsoever is available, should begin at once, ideally under the supervision of a trained physiotherapist. All limbs are put through full-range passive movements repeatedly each day. The paralysed limbs must be positioned to avoid damage by reason of abnormal strain on the joints. In particular, subluxation of the shoulder joint should be avoided by keeping the paralysed arm adducted and internally rotated. This can be achieved by appropriate positioning of the flaccid limb on pillows when the patient is in bed or sitting up in a chair and later by the use of a sling when the patient is ambulant. It is important that all those attending the patient are aware of the risk of subluxation (especially if the arm is pulled into abduction with external rotation) and the likely consequences of chronic pain and impaired rehabilitation.

Attention to the chest is necessary to stimulate deep breathing and coughing when consciousness returns. At this stage the patient is taught how to move the paralysed limbs with the sound limbs. Later she is taught to turn herself in bed and other techniques to reduce her dependence on others.

The longer-term rehabilitation following stroke is dealt with in Chapter 6 but it must be emphasized that the whole process is a continuum. Attention to detail is essential at all stages. The world's best team of therapists (physiotherapists, occupational therapists and speech therapists) would have their guns spiked by mismanagement of the patient at an earlier stage e.g. failure to keep a clear airway or failure to avoid pressure sores.

Recovery following completed stroke

Every patient with stroke illness presents her own peculiarities and problems for medical analysis and management. The general health, social background, personality, intellect and emotional drive are all important determinants of outcome and therefore likely to influence management decisions.

Rehabilitation (including stroke rehabilitation) is dealt with in Chapter 6 but let it be noted now that the essential foundation for stroke rehabilitation is a full assessment of the patient's disabilities and the dissemination of this information (on a need to know basis) throughout the geriatric team. Progress towards recovery is the rule but limited recovery will occur if the disability is severe. The goal is maximum independence with respect to the activities of daily living, and failure to achieve this is due often to some factor other than the paralysis of one or more limbs. These other factors—impaired intellect, impaired body awareness, disturbed sensation and failure of posture control—have been called barriers to recovery (see Chapter 6).

Mortality is high in the first few days in patients with completed stroke. Thereafter the trend is towards recovery. In one large hospital series of patients who survived the first two to three weeks, two-thirds of the patients regained personal independence and only one-quarter progressed to long-term invalidism. The remainder died within two months. In general terms the older and frailer the patient the less satisfactory the outcome but even the very old can make a good recovery. Of course a hospital series such as this cannot portray the full picture because many severe cases die at home and probably most of the mild cases would not enter hospital. Nevertheless the overall picture is more optimistic than many would have us believe.

Diffuse cerebrovascular disease

Dementia due to diffuse cerebral disease is a major cause of mental disorder in the elderly. Cerebral blood-flow studies have shown a reduction of perfusion in elderly demented subjects. It is not clear if this is the cause of the dementia or a result of the decrease in brain substance. In a minority of dementing old people the brain failure is clearly due to low cerebral blood-flow caused by cerebral arteriosclerosis. A similar picture occurs at a younger age in hypertensive patients and multiple small lacunar infarcts are the underlying pathological lesions.

Clinical picture of diffuse cerebrovascular disease

The illness takes a slowly progressive and often stepwise course of physical and mental degeneration usually associated with acute recurrent and often transient neurological upsets of various types—TIAs, little strokes, epileptic attacks. The patient dements and commonly develops unpleasant changes in personality becoming restless, wandering, cantankerous and not infrequently paranoid. Disorders of movement, posture and balance occur and sometimes there is a resemblance to Parkinson's disease. There is a generalized exaggeration of the tendon reflexes, a shuffling gait and often a tendency to fall backwards due to impaired postural fixation. Rigidity of the legs is more marked than in the arms and it gives the impression of intense active resistance to passive movement quite unlike the typical parkinsonian rigidity. The normal walking pattern disintegrates and steps are small and shuffling. These patients gradually become bedfast and lie curled up in a foetal position totally dependent upon others. The inevitable outcome is death but this may take very many months.

Pseudobulbar palsy is part of this clinical picture and is due to bilateral upper motor neurone lesions. There is a characteristic indistinct nasal dysarthria, but there is no wasting of the tongue and the jaw jerk is brisk. Gross emotional lability is a characteristic accompaniment. There is increasing dysphagia which is worse for liquids due to lack of speed and precision in the reflexes. This can be readily demonstrated by asking the patient to take a drink of water when she will cough and splutter due to the water 'going down the wrong way'. Aspiration pneumonia is a common terminal event.

Disturbance of postural stability

Disturbance of postural stability is the *sine qua non* of the neurology of old age (see Chapter 10). This is hardly surprising when some of the mechanisms responsible for normal postural fixation are listed viz.—visual, labyrinthine and proprioceptive afferent impulses, integrative functions and appropriate cortical and cerebellar responses. Multiple disorders of the whole network are common in the elderly.

In vascular lesions involving the dominant hemisphere walking apraxia and loss of postural control may exist even with just a minimal hemiparesis and not much sensory loss. The patient tends to fall backwards and the feet seem to be glued to the floor when attempts are made to walk. With encouragement she will shuffle a few (reluctant) steps but soon comes to a halt. The whole performance may be repeated endlessly. This is referred to as a stammering or Petren gait. These patients require long-term physiotherapy if they are to retain any degree of mobility.

Leaning backwards is also a failing of some patients with ischaemia in the vertebrobasilar territory. They cannot stand upright. Any attempt at standing or walking is ruined by leaning and falling backwards! The leaning backwards phenomenon has not yet been adequately explained. These patients and those with walking apraxia were formerly classified by neurologists as suffering from astasia abasia—i.e. an inability to walk or stand because of loss or deficiency of will power! The more closely these disorders are studied the less adequate this simplism becomes.

Treatment of diffuse cerebrovascular disease

This is unsatisfactory because although certain cerebral vasodilator drugs have shown a little promise in improving brain function in clinical trials the benefit seen in ordinary clinical practice is minimal or non-existent. Another type of drug used is that which might improve cerebral metabolism—the cerebral activators. None can be clearly recommended. On the other hand the general restlessness and querulousness of the patient can be damped down by using one of the phenothiazine tranquillizers, starting with a small dose and gradually increasing, e.g. promazine 25 mg thrice daily to start. If noctural restlessness is a problem, bigger doses (50 or even 75 mg) should be given in the afternoon and evening. Barbiturates are best avoided altogether since they are liable to increase the restlessness and mental confusion. Chlormethiazole 500 mg may be given as a night sedative if the promazine alone proves to be insufficient. For the reduction of morbidity due to cerebrovascular disease long-term prevention of atherosclerosis and control of raised blood pressure offer the most hope. The latter is already a practical possibility.

Epilepsy

Epilepsy appearing for the first time in old age is very likely to be due to cerebrovascular disease. Occasionally focal attacks occur but they often spread to become generalized (grand mal) seizures. An epileptic attack may herald a stroke, especially cerebral haemorrhage. Epileptic attacks may result from heart disease causing a sudden fall in cerebral perfusion pressure, which in other circumstances might simply produce a syncopal attack rather than a convulsion. Paroxysmal pain down the paretic side of an hemiplegic patient is sometimes an epileptic phenomenon and may respond to anticonvulsant treatment. Bouts of mental confusion and sudden akinetic attacks may have the same aetiology. In the latter the patient quite suddenly crumples to the ground but there is no loss of consciousness.

Recent onset epilepsy demands a thorough medical assessment especially of the cardiovascular and nervous systems. Cardiac dysrhythmias and cerebral tumour must be looked for and the appropriate treatment given. It is necessary to exclude hypoglycaemia or drugs (tricyclic antidepressants, phenothiazines, corticosteroids) as precipitants of the seizures. The epileptic attacks may be suppressed by the use of an appropriate anticonvulsant drug. Phenytoin (Epanutin) is a good first choice starting with 200 mg daily. It is metabolised slowly and needs be given just once in the day. A serum level of 10–20 ng/ml is effective. The level should be checked after three or four weeks and the dose adjusted accordingly. Overdose will produce ataxia, nystagmus and mental confusion. Longterm use leads to collagen overgrowth—gums, face and lymph nodes—and hepatic enzyme induction. Sodium valproate (Epilim) may replace Epanutin as the drug of first choice and indeed for younger patients many doctors already accept it as such.

The starting dose is 200 mg twice daily. Carbamazepine (Tegretol) is also popular and effective in elderly patients especially if the seizures are focal rather than general. The starting dose is 200 mg once or twice daily and the effective serum level 4–10 ng/ml. It is less sedative and less liable to cause confusion than phenytoin.

At any age the occurrence of a continuous succession of fits (status epilepticus) must be treated as a medical emergency. It may be fatal if not rapidly controlled. Energetic drug treatment to control the seizures should be accompanied by attention to the airway and the maintenance of adquate ventilation. Immediate IV diazepam (Valium) 5–10 mg given slowly over two or three minutes, repeated if necessary, or chlormethiazole (Heminevrin) by IV infusion as described in the manufacturer's literature will control the attacks in most cases. Thereafter maintenance doses of anticonvulsants will be required. There are dangers associated with the prolonged use of these drugs. Various neurological syndromes, megaloblastic erythropoiesis, disturbance of water and electrolyte balance and inactivation of vitamin D resulting in osteomalacia have all been described.

Many epileptics are satisfactorily controlled on phenobarbitone but it is better to avoid it especially in frail old people because they are very liable to develop muddle-headedness, unsteadiness of gait and falls. The long-term effects may mimic arteriosclerotic dementia. Nocturnal restlesness is often precipitated or made worse by barbiturates and abnormal sleep patterns may persist for weeks after stopping the drug. Stimulation of the liver microsomal enzymes by barbiturates is referred to in Chapter 19. Primidone (Mysoline) is chemically related to the barbiturates and has similar adverse effects.

Anticonvulsants may interact among themselves and with other commonly used drugs (e.g. phenylbutazone, phenothiazines and dextropropoxyphene) causing variously, enhanced clinical benefit, toxic effects or even inadequate treatment depending on the resultant plasma level. Phenytoin has been most often implicated in adverse drug reactions with anticonvulsants. Increased frequency of epileptic attacks may actually be due to phenytoin toxicity. Knowledge of these possibilities together with estimation of plasma drug concentration will greatly help in the management of the more complex cases. The evident dangers of treatment with these drugs must be balanced by the paramount need to control the epileptic seizures. For the majority of patients with epilepsy the risk run by accepting drug treatment is clearly the lesser evil.

CHAPTER 13 · OTHER DISEASES OF THE
NERVOUS SYSTEM

He had not suffered much from Rheumatism, or been subject to pains of the head, or had ever experienced any sudden seizure which could be referred to apoplexy or hemiplegia.

From the description of Case 1 in

An Essay on the Shaking Palsy by JAMES PARKINSON, 1817

Neurological norms in the elderly

In making a neurological examination of the aged patient there may be considerable difficulties in communication on account of intellectual failure, speech disturbance, poor vision and deafness. Furthermore, many of the accepted norms in younger people are modified or lost in old age without necessarily attracting much clinical significance. Allowance must be made for these changes in the clinical examination. Thus small pupils reacting slowly and incompletely to light and accommodation are often seen, and we have found that the corneal reflex is often absent on one or both sides without any clear explanation. Loss to greater or lesser degree of the special senses of vision, hearing, smell and taste is universal. Wasting of the small muscles of the hands, absence of the ankle jerks, abdominal reflexes and vibration sense in the feet are all common even without any obvious disease to account for the loss. **Increased angle of sway** is a function of age and so Romberg's sign is often observed. That is to say the old person sways markedly (and might even fall) if she tries to stand upright with her eyes closed and feet together.

A CNS examination in an elderly patient must be carried out at a leisurely pace. Very great patience is required by the doctor to make sure that the patient understands what she is supposed to do. Aged patients tire easily and so it may be necessary to stage the clinical examination over a series of short sessions spread even over two or three days. The young doctor must not be daunted by this nor must he make do with an inadequate assessment of his patient. In all cases it is essential to make some formal assessment of the patient's intellect. Failure to do this at the outset almost always leads to difficulties later.

Parkinson's disease

Parkinson's disease or paralysis agitans is the commonest disease of the nervous system after cerebrovascular disease. It is a disease of later life usually starting during the sixth or seventh decades and having a long course. The age of onset has been increasing steadily over the past 35 years and two main hypotheses may be considered to explain this.

1   **Cohort hypothesis.** This supposes that most Parkinson's disease is the sequel of pandemic encephalitis lethargica in the period 1918–1926. In other words idiopathic parkinsonism is actually post-infective but has a longer latent interval than the so-called post-encephalitic parkinsonism. From this hypothesis we may predict a rapid fall in the incidence of the disease in the next ten to fifteen years.

2   **Two-disease hypothesis.** This postulates that there are two main types of Parkinson's disease—the post-encephalitic type with a younger age of onset and which is dying out rapidly and another which is a disease of old age and therefore increasing along with the increased numbers of elderly. From this hypothesis we may expect an overall increase in prevalence of the disease in the next 10–15 years.

The disease starts insidiously and runs a slow, inexorable course towards disability. As Parkinson himself observed—'so slight and nearly imperceptible are the first inroads of this malady, and so extremely slow is its progress that it rarely happens that the patient can form any recollection of the precise period of its commencement'.

The Parkinson syndrome

The Parkinson syndrome (or more simply parkinsonism) is used to describe a clinical picture akin to paralysis agitans but thought to differ from it in some particulars. Practically all of the cases seen at the present time in elderly people do differ from the typical shaking palsy but there is still justification for retaining the eponym. Thus the Parkinson syndrome embraces a group of different pathological entities with marked clinical similarities (Table 13.1). Dopamine deficiency in the corpus striatum is common to all cases.

Table 13.1. Aetiology of parkinsonism

Idiopathic
Viral encephalitis
Drugs—phenothiazines, butyrophenones, reserpine, methyldopa
Heredity
Cerebrovascular disease
Trauma—the retired 'punch drunk' boxer

Parkinsonism in the elderly

Parkinsonism in the elderly differs from paralysis agitans of middle life as described by Parkinson in a notable lack of tremor and a definite tendency to dementia. The most constant manifestation is akinesia. Cerebral arteriosclerosis has long been regarded as the commonest cause of the syndrome in this age group—'arteriosclerotic parkinsonism.'

The evidence for such a nosological entity is weak and is probably no more than a chance association of the two commonest diseases of the nervous system each having its maximum incidence in old age—cerebrovascular disease and idiopathic parkinsonism. Despite the late age of onset there is evidence for an hereditary basis for some cases of the Parkinson syndrome as indeed there is for some other late onset degenerations of the brain (e.g. Huntington's chorea, senile dementia and essential tremor).

Clinical features of idiopathic parkinsonism

The syndrome of hypokinesia, rigidity and tremor is so well known that many cases are diagnosed by the patient or her relative even before the doctor is consulted! Tremor of the hand ('pill rolling') is perhaps the most obvious and the most socially embarrassing feature. However, in all but the most gross cases, it causes very little disability because it lessens on purposive movement. The tremor is usually less marked than in younger patients. It often starts in one hand and may affect no other limb for many months. It is present at rest, worsens with excitement but stops in sleep.

Table 13.2. Clinical features of parkinsonism

Hypokinesia	Mask-like face
Muscular rigidity	Chin on chest
Tremor	Dysarthria
Loss of posture control	Micrographia
Mental disturbance	Drooling saliva
Alimentary disorders	Postural hypotension

Hypokinesia or poverty of movement is often a striking feature and may be attributable in some cases to muscular rigidity, but in others it is the dominant feature even when rigidity is slight. The hypokinesia is probably the most important cause of disability yet it may not present as an obvious sign to the doctor. There is particular difficulty in the initiation of movement and while movement is in progress the patient may suddenly 'freeze' and be unable to continue. Feelings of great weakness, loss of motivation and gradual loss of phonation develop. The speech becomes low and muttering and many patients end up virtually mute. Lack of fidgeting and other spontaneous movement such as changing position in bed, crossing and uncrossing the legs while seated, smiling or even blinking are useful diagnostic clues. Paradoxically the glabella tap sign is positive—the previously unblinking eyes are unable to stop blinking in response to repeated tapping by the examiner's finger low on the forehead just above the nose. However false positives are common in patients with cerebrovascular disease. Another characteristic feature in this illness is that the patient tends to move 'all of a piece', arm swing being reduced or absent and instead of turning just the head in response to a need to look to one side the whole body turns to put the desired object in view.

Muscular rigidity appears early in the neck and may be recognizable there by the head drop test. With the patient lying supine and with no pillow on the bed, the head rests on the examiner's hand. Relaxation is encouraged and then the head is suddenly thrown up and allowed to drop back. With rigidity the normal rapid descent is slowed and in severe cases the head stays up above the waiting hand—the 'psychic pillow' sign. In the limbs, muscular rigidity may be unilateral in the earlier stages but it always becomes bilateral. Agonists and antagonists are affected equally. In the presence of tremor the rigidity is of 'cogwheel' type in the absence of tremor 'lead pipe or plastic rigidity' is observed. As the rigidity progresses the patient develops a characteristic posture with adducted flexed limbs. **Micrographia** is common; the writing becomes so small as to be illegible. The mask-like facies results from the combination of hypokinesia and rigidity. The palpebral fissures are widened and this together with the lack of spontaneous eye movements and blinking gives rise to a staring appearance.

Impairment of posture control and righting reflexes occurs. The patient given a slight push forwards or backwards may be unable to bring the centre of gravity back above her feet and so has to try to catch up with it. This **festinant (hurrying) gait** also occurs spontaneously when the patient tries to walk forward of her own volition. Getting in or out of bed or chair and even turning over in bed becomes increasingly difficult. Falls are frequent because any temporary loss of balance cannot be corrected quickly as in normal people. A stooping posture develops with dorsal kyphosis and marked neck flexion.

Mental disturbance of some sort occurs in the majority of elderly Parkinson patients. Mental depression and irritability are particularly common which is not surprising with such a tiresome disease. Dementia was specifically excluded from Parkinson's original description, but nowadays it must be regarded as part of the natural history of the disease. In one large-scale survey of parkinsonism of varied aetiology 25 per cent of patients were a burden to their families on account of dementia rather than physical disability. Even without obvious dementia, intellectual inertia is remarkably common. With these patients, despite exhortations to keep active and to keep an interest going (exhortations they appear to understand and accept) the response is entirely negative. If external drive is provided they can and they will do things. Left to their own devices they do nothing. This is a tragedy because immobility simply accelerates the decline towards dependence upon others.

Gastrointestinal complaints are also part and parcel of the disease. Dysphagia, heartburn and constipation are common. A quarter of cases have an hiatus hernia and reflux oesophagitis. Carcinoma of the stomach or colon may be suspected because of these alimentary symptoms coupled with weight loss and constipation. Loss of weight is particularly liable to occur because of the high metabolic demands consequent upon the tremor and rigidity. The patient may complain of heat intolerance and often sweats excessively. The high fluid loss from sweating and drooling of saliva (due to lack of swallowing) together with use of anticholinergic drugs worsen the tendency to constipation.

Natural history of parkinsonism

Idiopathic parkinsonism is a chronic progressive incurable disease. Twenty-five per cent of cases will be severely disabled or dead within five years of first consulting the doctor and over 60 per cent within ten years. Mortality rates are treble those of a general population of the same age, sex and race. The causes of death are bronchopneumonia, urinary tract infections and pressure sores due to the chronic wasting and the eventual bedfast state. Fractured femur and its complications is another likely cause of death.

Management of patients with parkinsonism

It is clear that the patient is fighting a losing battle but this is true of all chronic incurable diseases. There is no cure and all patients get worse. Supportive action for the whole family is required. The patient and her relatives need to know something of the nature of the disease and to know what can be done to help—by the patient, by her relatives and by the doctor. A little booklet published by the Parkinson's Disease Society is designed for this essential educative dialogue.

Nutrition needs to provide sufficient fluid, calories and roughage to counter some of the specific complications of the disease. Laxatives may be required but liquid paraffin is contraindicated especially in

Parkinson's disease because the dysphagia increases the risk of aspiration pneumonitis. Retention of urine may be precipitated by some of the anti-Parkinson drugs due to their anticholinergic action.

Physical therapy is required for the rest of the patient's life. The physiotherapist trains the patient in a specially devised physical exercise programme. The relatives are encouraged to co-operate in the training programme so that the exercises may continue to be practised at home with 'refresher' visits to the physiotherapy department. Heat and massage are soothing to the stiff painful muscles and make a good preliminary for the more active exercise including posture and gait control. When home circumstances are inadequate (e.g. lack of social support and too little space for exercises) day-hospital attendance is especially valuable.

The occupational therapist must be involved at an early stage because inevitably disabilities affecting the patient's capacity for self-care will develop. When these problems are identified they can usually be resolved by simple means. For example zip fasteners may replace buttons, Velcro fastenings replace hooks and eyes and a spring-loaded seat enable the patient to sit down and get up from a chair more easily (see Chapter 6). A home visit may be necessary to allow the occupational therapist to assess the patient in her normal environment. A few simple adaptations to the furnishing and fittings in the home could make a big improvement in the patient's ability to cope. For example, a firm mattress laid on a solid base makes it easier for her to turn over in bed, suitably placed hand-rails reduce the risk of falls and special kitchen gadgets simplify culinary activities.

Drug therapy in parkinsonism

Most cases will require drug treatment specifically for the parkinsonism and also possibly for some of the associated physical complaints and the mental depression. Current specific treatment is based on the concept of the acetylcholine/dopamine balance in the brain (Fig. 13.1). These substances act as mutually antagonistic neurotransmitters. Parkinsonism is associated with too little dopamine therefore treatment is directed towards increasing the dopamine or reducing the acetylcholine. This can be done by giving levodopa or anticholinergic drugs respectively. Both approaches may be used simultaneously to promote maximum response (Fig. 13.2).

Levodopa has replaced the anticholinergics as the drug of first choice and it represented a new concept in neurology. Previously when parts of the brain failed to function there was nothing to be done. With levodopa we can restore the deficient neurotransmitter even though the substantia nigra becomes defunct. The more recent use of bromocriptine as a

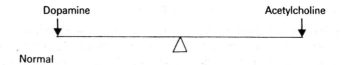

Normal

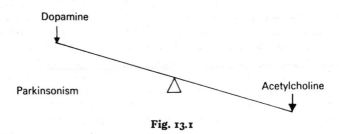

Parkinsonism

Fig. 13.1

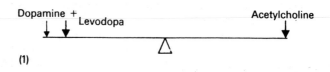

(1)

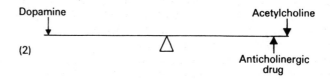

(2)

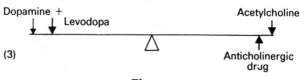

(3)

Fig. 13.2

dopaminergic stimulator is a further example of these exciting developments in neuropharmacology. Levodopa crosses the blood brain barrier and is there metabolized to release dopamine. Peripheral (extracranial) metabolism of the levodopa can be blocked by the simultaneous administration of a decarboxylase inhibitor which does not itself pass into the brain. This device minimizes the incidence of gastrointestinal intolerance and is now the treatment of choice. Proprietary preparations exist conveniently combining the two drugs in one tablet e.g. Sinemet (levodopa 250 mg and carbidopa 25 mg) and Sinemet 110 (levodopa 100 mg and carbidopa 10 mg). The alternative preparation Madopar has different nomenclature and dosages. Thus Madopar 250 (levodopa 200 mg, benserazide 50 mg) and Madopar 125 (levodopa 100 mg, benserazide 25 mg). Using the combined preparation the patient should start by taking 100 mg levodopa daily and thereafter gradually increase the daily dose (say by 50–100 mg on alternate days) until toxic effects are evident or an adequate therapeutic response is obtained. The dose is then reduced if necessary to a maintenance level which should be the lowest to allow a satisfactory response with minimal side effects. This will be in the range 100 mg–1 g daily in elderly patients but it must be kept under review because the patient's requirements may vary from time to time.

THE EFFECTS OF LEVODOPA

Levodopa is effective in all forms of parkinsonism except that induced by drugs. It may be used at any stage of the disease and be expected to improve akinesia, tremor, rigidity and even postural instability. Most patients manage initially with one or two doses of levodopa daily using a preparation containing a decarboxylase inhibitor. The benefits are usually sustained for two to three years but then further progression of the disease leads to the reappearance of early-morning akinesia, 'freezing' episodes (when the patient just seizes up in the course of some activity) and end-of-dose deterioration when the effects of the drug wear off. Ideally a sustained action levodopa preparation would be used in these cases but none is available. Reducing the size of the individual doses but progressively increasing the frequency of administration even to every hour may help. Excessive total daily dosage makes for extreme variability of symptoms and signs—the so-called 'yo-yo' effect. Some patients exhibit marked 'yo-yoing' or 'on-off' effects apparently unrelated to levodopa dosage and timing. Typically the patient swings from mobility ith wovert dyskinesia to immobility all within a period of minutes. The 'off' period persists for up to an hour or two and then just as rapidly swings to another 'on' period of similar duration. These extreme 'on-off' effects were not seen prior to levodopa treatment and probably represent a more advanced form of the disease but modified by treatment.

ADVERSE EFFECTS OF LEVODOPA

Adverse effects are common especially those due to the central action of dopamine. In the individual patient these effects are dose-related and therefore treatable by a dose reduction. Transient mental confusion, visual hallucination agitation and depression all occur. Senile dementia is one of the main limiting factors for levodopa treatment in the elderly and if moderately severe will probably preclude satisfactory use of the drug. Appropriate simple psychometric testing should always be done in the initial work-up of the case. Abnormal movements, especially facial dyskinesia, postural hypotension and tachydysrhythmias may also limit treatment. In these cases a lower dose of levodopa might still give a worthwhile improvement but without the troublesome side effects.

CONTRAINDICATIONS TO LEVODOPA THERAPY

The presence of dementia, pyschoneurosis, ischaemic heart disease, glaucoma, prostatism, peptic ulcer and severe renal or hepatic disease are all relative contraindications. Levodopa must not be used concurrently with monoamine oxidase inhibitors (the authors see virtually no role for MAOIs in geriatric practice!). Pyridoxine (vitamin B_6) facilitates decarboxylation of levodopa and is contraindicated when using levodopa alone, but not when using levodopa in combination with a decarboxylase inhibitor. Many proprietary antiemetic/antinauseant preparations, as well as compound vitamin tablets, contain pyridoxine. Levodopa is not indicated in drug-induced parkinsonism.

Amantadine (Symmetrel) given in 100 mg capsules once or twice daily is worth a try when the patient cannot tolerate levodopa. Bromocriptine may also provide an alternative to levodopa. It is an ergot alkaloid which activates dopaminergic receptors and has other uses in the suppression of lactation and the treatment of acromegaly. It is expensive and commonly causes adverse reactions similar to those of levodopa and which are dose dependent. Some additional bizarre reactions affecting eyes (smarting and diplopia) and ankles (erythema, oedema and tenderness) have also been reported.

ANTICHOLINERGIC AND ANTIHISTAMINE DRUGS

These were the main drugs used prior to the introduction of levodopa. They still have a role as an alternative when levodopa is ill tolerated and also as an adjunct to levodopa. They are the drugs of choice for drug-induced parkinsonism. However, anticholinergic drugs are poorly tolerated by frail old people more especially in the presence of dementia. Any drastic increase or reduction in dosage is dangerous. Common adverse effects are blurred vision, increased constipation, retention of urine and toxic psychosis with delirium. The risk of precipitating glaucoma seems to be more theoretical than real. Commonly used synthetic anticholinergics are benzhexol (Artane or Pipanol) and benztropine mesylate (Cogentin). Benztropine mesylate is a potent analogue of atropine and can be used in conjunction with levodopa or benzhexol. It has a long duration of action and is cumulative so that a bedtime dose can be given to relieve morning rigidity. A suitable starting dose is 0·5 mg. The daily dose may be increased by 0·5 mg at weekly intervals to a maintenance dose of 2–4 mg daily. This drug is also available as a parenteral injection (2 mg per 2 ml ampoule) for the rapid relief of drug-induced parkinsonism.

Surgical treatment

Observations on brain-damaged patients have suggested that tremor and rigidity might respond to appropriately placed destructive lesions in the basal ganglia. Stereotactic techniques are employed to ensure correct placement of the lesion but autopsy follow-up has shown that some inaccuracy is not rare. The 'ideal' case for brain surgery would be a (biologically) young patient with slowly progressive disability due to unilateral tremor and rigidity and not responding satisfactorily to appropriate levodopa treatment. These cases are rarely seen in geriatric practice.

Other disorders with involuntary movements

Essential tremor

Essential tremor is an involuntary fine or coarse rhythmical movement appearing late in adult life. It is transmitted by dominant inheritance and affects the head (always), face, tongue, arms and legs. As with the tremor in Parkinson's disease the movements are present at rest and are exaggerated by stress. It is made less obvious by voluntary movement and ceases in sleep. There are no other symptoms and signs of parkinsonism and in particular no rigidity and no disablement. Essential tremor is a benign condition usually unresponsive to treatment, but it occasionally responds to beta-blockers or tetrabenazine.

Intention tremor

Intention tremor is not present at rest but comes on with movement such as buttoning clothes, using cutlery or writing. There is a lack of the other CNS signs seen in multiple sclerosis and degenerative cerebellar disorders. No medical treatment is indicated.

Hemiballismus

This is characterized by unilateral involuntary movements of face and limbs due to a lesion (usually vascular) of the subthalamic nucleus on the opposite side. The movements affect especially the proximal segments of the limbs and may be so severe that the patient even throws herself out of bed. They stop in sleep, can be abolished by stereotactic surgery and usually resolve spontaneously in four to six weeks. Thiopropazate (Dartalan) may be effective in doses of 30–60 mg daily. Another effective drug is tetrabenazine (Nitoman) starting with 25 mg thrice daily.

Progressive cerebellar degeneration

Cerebellar degeneration may occur as an hereditary disorder but it also occurs sporadically later in life, even in the seventh decade. The clinical picture depends on which parts of the cerebellum and adjacent structures are affected. There is a gradual onset of dysarthria, intention tremor and ataxia. Nystagmus is usually absent. The limbs become hypotonic and the tendon reflexes are usually depressed or lost. Voluntary power is well preserved. Mental deterioration and loss of sphincter control are late features. Physiotherapy should be instituted to delay the inevitable loss of mobility and eventual confinement to bed or chair. Subacute combined degeneration of the cord, cerebellar degeneration secondary to carcinoma of the lung and cerebellar tumour (usually a metastasis) should be excluded by the appropriate tests.

Progressive supranuclear palsy

This uncommon disorder, of unknown aetiology, occurs in the sixth or seventh decade. It is characterised by progressive loss of conjugate (especially upward) gaze associated with unsteadiness of gait and intellectual failure. Pseudobulbar palsy and dystonic rigidity develops and death occurs in a few years. Widespread degeneration is found in the brain. No specific therapy is available.

Drug-induced extra-pyramidal disorders

Drugs which interfere with normal catecholamine metabolism in the brain may cause extra-pyramidal disorders. A picture very like Parkinson's disease may develop with hypokinesia, weakness, immobility and drooling but usually with no tremor. The old lady just 'goes off her feet' or becomes 'unwilling to help herself'. This adverse reaction is especially liable to occur with the butyrophenones (e.g. Haloperidol) and phenothiazines (e.g. chlorpromazine and thioridazine). **Akathisia**—'the jitters'—a compulsive motor restlessness with an associated anxiety can also be due to phenothiazines especially those with a piperazine side chain (e.g. prochlorperazine or Stemetil and perphenazine or Fentazin). Even a single dose can produce restlessness. With

Table 13.3. Drug-induced extra-pyramidal disorders

Akathisia	— 'the jitters'
Dystonia	
Parkinsonism	
Tardive dyskinesia	

bigger doses dystonic movements especially of face, head and neck occur. The phenothiazines with a trifluoromethyl group (e.g. trifluoperazine or Stelazine and fluphenazine or Moditen) seem more likely to produce acute dystonic reactions. Akathisia may come on in a matter of days after starting the offending drug whereas the parkinsonian picture usually takes weeks to develop. A most bizarre development may be seen after months of treatment—persistent **'tardive dyskinesia'** —affecting the mouth and face. There is smacking of the lips, grimacing, abnormal tongue movement and grunting—causing more distress to the observer than to the patient. Acute dystonic reactions including oculogyric crises have been observed mainly in younger patients. Drug-induced parkinsonism, akinesia and facial dyskinesia occur commonly in elderly patients but are easily overlooked even in their more gross forms if the doctor is not familiar with the problem. This is so especially with akathisia where the motor restlessness and anxiety, induced by a phenothiazine, is met by the prescription of increasing doses of the offending drug. If any one of these adverse reactions is suspected the noxious drug should be withdrawn. Recovery then usually occurs but more rapid reversal results from the use of certain anti-Parkinson drugs especially the anticholinergic drug benztropine (Cogentin). Levodopa is not effective in drug-induced parkinsonism. A reduction of dose possibly combined with low doses of benztropine may be required for example in certain psychiatric disorders where long-term medication with a phenothiazine or butyrophenone is indicated despite the adverse extra-pyramidal effects.

Subdural haematoma

The veins traversing the subdural space are especially liable to tear in old people because of the mobility of the shrunken brain within the skull.

Subdural haematoma is an encysted collection of blood between the dura mater and the arachnoid; it may be traumatic or spontaneous. Head injury is very common in the elderly because of the frequency of falls; thus subdural haemorrhage reaches its second and major peak of incidence in old age. Infancy represents the first peak. In the elderly quite trivial trauma (without any clinical evidence of bruising or laceration of the scalp) may be sufficient to cause the bleed and occasionally no history of injury is obtained. The haematoma is often bilateral and this heightens the difficulty in diagnosis. Chronic alcoholism, treatment with anticoagulants, thrombocytopenic purpura and scurvy are all causes to be considered. Shrinkage in the volume of the brain associated with ageing gives extra space for the development of the haematoma which may develop to a considerable size before the onset of symptoms and signs. This may take days or weeks. A rapidly progressive illness will suggest the more usual cerebral infarction whereas slow progress may suggest a brain tumour. Subdural haematoma may present with intellectual deterioration and personality change but the duration of the illness is rarely greater than three months. Fluctuating neurological signs and symptoms, previously regarded as characteristic, occur in less than a third of cases. Hemiparesis is the presentation in about a quarter of all cases. Inequality of the pupils is often present; the larger pupil on the side of the lesion often associated with slight ptosis. A high index of suspicion is necessary to make the diagnosis and many cases are missed clinically. A careful examination of plain X-ray films of the skull may show displacement of the choroid plexus or the pineal confirming the presence of a space occupying lesion. Isotope brain scan and CAT scan both play a useful part in the diagnosis of subdural haematoma. LP is not of much value because the CSF is usually normal.

Referral to the neurosurgeon is mandatory if there is any thought of positive treatment but not all cases will respond satisfactorily to his ministrations. Nevertheless some dramatic improvements have followed evacuation of the blood even in very elderly patients. A shallow haematoma not progressing is not benefited by surgery.

Cerebral tumour

Cerebral tumours, primary and secondary, are not common in the elderly but the true incidence is difficult to assess because reported autopsy and neurosurgical series relate to highly selected material. Many elderly patients with cerebral neoplasm must die with a diagnosis of cerebrovascular disease or senile degeneration of the brain. The clinical presentation is often atypical with the tumour attaining a large size before the onset of signs and symptoms. Later there may be a relatively sudden deterioration in cerebral function with the onset of coma and the likely misdiagnosis of cerebrovascular accident. This occurs when the normal CSF circulation and venous drainage are impaired to a critical degree. Papilloedema is rarely seen. In chronic or subacute presentations cerebral tumour may mimic senile dementia.

In Cambridge, elderly patients referred with a diagnosis of cerebral tumour for specialist investigation most often have metastases—cerebral or cerebellar. Of the primary brain tumours the gliomas and meningiomas account for the majority. Acoustic neuromas are not often seen.

Meningioma

Meningioma is the commonest primary cerebral tumour in the elderly but it is often asymptomatic and discovered merely as an accidental finding at autopsy. By contrast symptomatic meningioma is commonest in the fifth decade. Meningioma is a slowly growing neoplasm developing over months and years and will only be suspected if it is in a location likely to produce focal neurological signs or if epileptic convulsions occur. X-ray of skull may show displacement of pineal or choroid plexus, erosion of the dorsum sellae, bone destruction or calcification. An isotope or CAT scan will delineate the tumour. The next step will be neurosurgical referral.

Gliomas

The gliomas are infiltrative growths of varying grades of malignancy arising from the supporting tissues of the brain. The astrocytoma is relatively benign the course extending over years rather than months. It tends to occur in younger patients. Much more commonly seen in the elderly is the highly malignant glioblastoma multiforme. This is characterized by rapid growth with diffuse cerebral signs and raised intracranial tension developing over weeks rather than months. Epileptic convulsions are common. Brain scanning will demonstrate the tumour.

Surgical excision is not feasible and radiotherapy is simply palliative in this highly malignant neoplasm. Dexamethasone therapy is worth giving to try to secure temporary respite from symptoms.

Cerebral metastases

The majority of cerebral metastases come from the lungs (35–40 per cent), some from the breast and a few from the colon, rectum and kidney. The cerebral hemispheres are usually affected. The clinical picture resembles that of glioblastoma multiforme and the prognosis is poor. The CAT scan may show multiple defects.

Acoustic neuromas

The acoustic neuroma is a benign, very slowly growing tumour occurring in isolation or as part of a generalized neurofibromatosis. The auditory nerve alone may be involved giving rise to increasing deafness, tinnitus and giddy spells. The CSF protein is markedly raised. Surgical resection is the treatment whenever feasible.

Non-metastatic neurological complications of carcinoma

In certain malignant diseases in the absence of metastases symptoms and signs may develop in the CNS even before there is any local evidence of the tumour itself. The cause is obscure but a conditioned deficiency of some important metabolite such as folic acid or neurological damage due to tissue sensitization has been postulated. The

Table 13.4. Neurological complications
of carcinoma (non-metastatic)

Symmetrical peripheral neuropathy
Subacute cerebellar degeneration
Myopathy
Cerebral degeneration

oat-celled type of bronchial carcinoma is the commonest cancer to present in this way but neurological complications may also occur with cancer of stomach, large bowel, uterus and ovary. The neurological disorder usually precedes the discovery of the neoplasm but the reverse may obtain. The clinical presentations include symmetrical sensory **neuropathy** or mixed sensory and motor neuropathy, subacute cerebellar degeneration and cerebral atrophy. The latter produces a fairly rapid onset of dementia; with obvious deterioration over weeks or months to distinguish it from senile dementia. In the cerebellar degeneration also the fairly rapid progress serves to differentiate it from the very slowly progressive late cerebellar atrophy of old age.

Myopathy also occurs in association with these malignant diseases and may mimic myasthenia gravis but with only a partial response to anticholinesterase drugs such as neostigmine and pyridostigmine. The electromyographic picture differs from that of myasthenia gravis. The weakness and ready fatiguability of the proximal limb muscles may be a striking feature even before there is clinical evidence of muscle wasting.

Autonomic dysfunction

Autonomic dysfunction is common in the elderly. Control over body temperature, blood pressure, gut motility, functions of bladder, pupil and exocrine glands is mediated by the autonomic nervous system. The control is largely reflex in nature. The autonomic nervous system (ANS) has two subdivisions which to a large extent are mutually antagonistic in function and which have anatomically separate pathways. The parasympathetic system is cholinergic via cranial nerves 3, 7, 9, and 10 and the sacral nerves 2, 3 and 4. The sympathetic system is mostly adrenergic via the thoracic and lumbar nerves but the sudomotor fibres are cholinergic.

Table 13.5. Autonomic nervous system dysfunction

Orthostatic hypotension
Impaired thermoregulation
Disordered gut motility
Impaired bladder control
Impotence

Autonomic dysfunction is commonly seen in association with diabetes mellitus and may be manifest clinically by diarrhoea, depressed oesophageal and gastric motility, retention of urine and postural hypotension. Impotence commonly occurs. ANS disorders are seen frequently in parkinsonism; furthermore primary degeneration of the ANS occurs as a separate disease entity with severe persistent orthostatic hypotension followed after months or years by parkinsonism (Shy-Drager syndrome). It also seems likely that ANS degeneration occurs as an ageing phenomenon in the absence of other identifiable disease.

Postural hypotension

This is a very common problem affecting many elderly patients. It occurs when the baroreceptor reflex arc mediated by the ANS is not

working satisfactorily. Drugs are often implicated in postural hypotension (Table 13.6) and another aetiological factor is hypovolaemia.
Normally the baroreflexes maintain blood pressure on standing up but
with ANS dysfunction the systolic pressure will drop 20 mmHg or
more and the patient may feel faint or even lose consciousness if the
mean systolic pressure falls below the critical level of 80–90 mmHg,
see also Chapter 12. The symptoms are often worst first thing in the
morning and may be described as weakness, 'feeling muzzy in the head',
or just unable to manage. Orthostatic hypotension or hypotension
induced by exercise is probably the commonest cause of syncope and
of the legs giving way in elderly patients. Often the relatives or nurses
say that the patient just does not try to help herself!

Management of postural hypotension

Drugs likely to lower the blood pressure should be stopped where
possible, e.g. sedatives, tranquillizers, diuretics and hypotensive agents.
Frequent changes of posture are indicated to retrain the baroreceptor
reflexes which become less effective if they are not used as for example in
prolonged recumbency. Progressive elevation of the head of the bed

Table 13.6. Drugs implicated
in postural hypotension

Hypotensive agents
Diuretics
Tranquillizers
Antidepressants
Hypnotics
Vasodilators
Levodopa
Beta-blockers

and the use of a tilting chair allows semi-recumbent positions in order to
induce reactive vasoconstriction in the peripheral vessels as well as
sodium retention (excess sodium loss is also associated with recumbency). Firm elastic stockings should be worn by day and also at night.
Getting out of bed at night must be regarded as a normal human
activity. The mineralocorticoid 9-alpha-fluoro-hydrocortisone or
fludrocortisone increases sodium retention and hence plasma volume
and it also has vasoconstrictor effects. It should be started in a dose of
0·1 mg daily and if necessary be increased to 0·2 or even 0·3 mg daily
while keeping a watch for signs of fluid retention.

Thermoregulation

Control of body temperature is dependent on the intact ANS. Exposure to cold results in conservation of heat by cutaneous vasoconstriction and an increase in heat production by shivering in addition to conscious activity to achieve the same ends. Exposure to heat has converse effects. Accidental hypothermia is described in Chapter 16. As with postural hypotension multiple factors are involved including ANS dysfunction, cold environment, drugs, decreased basal metabolism and immobility. It has been demonstrated that elderly survivors of accidental hypothermia commonly have ANS dysfunction as judged by lack of shivering and defective skin vasoconstriction in the face of moderate cooling.

Disorders of gut and bladder motility

Some degree of oesophageal dysfunction is not uncommon in elderly patients with disorganization of the normal swallowing mechanism. Non-propulsive repetitive contractions occur giving rise to the 'corkscrew oesophagus' appearance on barium swallow examination.

Intractable constipation often with gross dilatation of the colon may be seen but whether this represents autonomic dysfunction or is the result of long-term constipation with or without abuse of purgatives (cathartic colon) is not clear.

The usual disorder in bladder motility is the pattern of the uninhibited neurogenic bladder secondary to gross brain damage. Only in a minority of elderly patients is ANS dysfunction the main determinant in the bladder disorder.

Herpes zoster

Herpes zoster is an acute virus infection affecting the peripheral sensory neurone and the area of skin it supplies. Occasionally the motor neurone is also involved, e.g. facial nerve. One or more adjacent segments may be affected but it is rarely bilateral. It often occurs in small outbreaks and mostly the elderly are affected. However the majority of cases are probably due to the reactivation of the varicella virus which, following an attack of childhood chicken pox, has lain dormant in the posterior root ganglia or their cranial nerve equivalents for sixty or seventy years. This reactivation may occur spontaneously possibly as a result of the waning of childhood immunity (idiopathic zoster). Alternatively it may be precipitated by trauma or by the disturbance of immune mechanisms by disease (lymphatic leukaemia, myeloma) or the use of immuno suppressive drugs; this is referred to as 'symptomatic zoster'. Zoster may occasionally follow exposure to varicella but the reverse is much more frequently seen. Although the general symptoms of the disease are usually mild they may be quite severe in the aged and also in them the risk of severe intractable post-herpetic neuralgia is higher.

Herpes zoster usually begins with burning pain in the segment or segments involved. Three or four days later a papular rash develops which then becomes vesicular. The eruption fades in a matter of days leaving the skin permanently scarred at the site of the vesicles and to a variable degree anaesthetic. The affected area may be the site of chronic pain lasting for months or indefinitely; this is 'post-herpetic neuralgia'. The sensory divisions of the trigeminal nerve are not uncommonly affected. This is particularly distressing in the case of the ophthalmic division because the eye may be involved.

There is no specific treatment of proven value which can be given in the acute stage to prevent the occurrence of persistent neuralgia. Injections of large doses of vitamin B_{12}, full doses of corticosteroids and radiotherapy have all been tried and found wanting. Currently idoxuridine (IDU) is recommended if the patient is seen early and certainly before crusting of the lesions has occurred. The IDU is made up in a 5 per cent solution with dimethylsulphoxide. It is applied to the whole dermatome 4 hourly for 2–4 days and is said to hasten recovery, reduce pain and lessen the severity of post-herpetic neuralgia.

IDU in dimethylsulphoxide as used on the skin must not be used in the eye. If the eye appears to be involved by the virus the pupil should be kept dilated by using atropine eye drops thrice daily. The use of prednisolone eye drops and idoxuridine eye drops (0·1 per cent aqueous solution) is also advocated. Corneal ulceration, uveitis and secondary glaucoma may result from zoster affecting the eye and so urgent referral to the ophthalmologist is indicated.

In the chronic stage although the affected area of skin has reduced sensitivity to both pain and temperature, persistent neuralgic pain may make the patient's life a misery. Notwithstanding the evil reputation of this disease it must be remembered that the majority of patients recover without any residual symptoms although the scarring and hypoaesthesia are permanent. Yet other cases have pain but manage quite well with regular simple analgesics, e.g. paracetamol (Panadol) tablets 1 g four times a day or dihydrocodeine tartrate (DF 118) tablets 30 mg three or four times daily. The latter may exacerbate constipation and drug dependence has been reported. Even if these drugs do not adequately relieve the pain the stronger analgesics related to morphine (e.g. pethidine, methadone and pentazocine) and morphine itself must be avoided because of the long-term need for treatment and the consequent risk of addiction. Chlorpromazine 25–50 mg twice or thrice daily will potentiate the mild analgesics but it may cause the patient to be unacceptably drowsy or to have other adverse effects. Phenytoin or carbamazepine may be tried. With severe intractable pain deep X-ray irradiation of the spinal cord and nerve roots has been employed but the effect is short lived. Division of the sensory roots or their destruction by phenol injections is not better. The use of a cooling spray or the application of an electrical vibrator to the painful area for 15–20 minutes three or four times in the day for weeks or months appears to help some patients. The mental depression which accompanies the chronic pain also requires treatment by means of attendance at a day centre, diversional occupational therapy and the use of antidepressant drugs (see Chapter 7).

Motor neurone disease

The usual age of onset of motor neurone disease (MND) lies between 50 and 70 years and the usual duration of the illness is between two and three years. Some longer survivals have been reported but the disease appears to be invariably fatal and there is no effective treatment to delay the characteristic remorseless wasting and weakness. No satisfactory explanation has been found for the disintegration of the motor neurones but the possibility of a slow virus infection has been mooted.

The physical patterns of the disease depend upon variable combinations of upper and lower motor neurone (UMN and LMN) signs in the bulbar, arm and leg muscles. The commonest pattern is of predominantly LMN signs in the arms, predominantly UMN signs in the legs and a mixture of the two in the bulbar muscles (e.g. tongue). Fasiculation of the affected muscles is common but not pathognomonic. The hallmark of MND is the simultaneous presence of LMN and UMN signs in any one limb in the absence of sensory loss. Muscular pains are a frequent complaint in MND but there is no evidence of peripheral neuropathy and there is never any sensory impairment. Respiratory distress is invariable in the terminal stage.

Treatment is essentially supportive in psychological, social and physical terms. The patient's intellect is well preserved and the gradual impairment of mobility, personal independence and (eventually) swallowing, and breathing cause great emotional disturbance with fear, resentment and depression. Those caring for the victim suffer also as indeed they do with so many incurable diseases. They face the difficulty of problems and questions to which there is no answer and eventually they may have to cope with a patient whose intellect is preserved but who cannot talk, write or make signs but can only listen. The patient wants to hear words of understanding, encouragement and hope, but who can speak them?

As deglutition and respiration fail there will be ethical problems to consider. Should the patient be tube fed or a gastrostomy performed? Should the epiglottis be closed and a tracheostomy provided to prevent inhalation of food? Should the patient be put on a respirator to relieve the breathlessness? With the growing use of sophisticated intensive care facilities in our hospitals a nice sense of balance is required to ensure that the medical approach is also the most humane approach to this and other very distressing illnesses.

Peripheral neuropathy

Peripheral neuropathy is very common in the elderly. Indeed there is a steady rise in frequency with advancing age. Many cases cannot be ascribed to any particular cause but high on the list of recognized causes are diabetes and malignant disease—especially bronchial carcinoma.

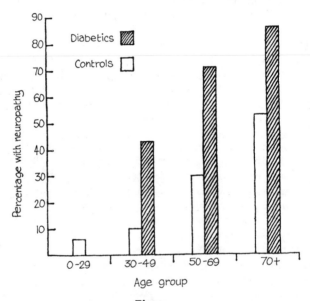

Fig. 13.3

Neuropathy due to ischaemia, rheumatoid disease and drug toxicity are other important possibilities. At any age in the presence of diabetes the signs of neuropathy appear earlier and the incidence is higher than in non-diabetics (Fig. 13.3). Thus in elderly diabetics the incidence of peripheral neuropathy approaches 90 per cent. As was mentioned earlier

ANS degeneration is also much more common in diabetics. The cause of the neuropathy is unknown. Many cases (about 50 per cent) have a raised CSF protein level.

A sensory or mixed sensorimotor peripheral neuropathy of glove and stocking distribution is the common neuropathy of diabetes. The ankle and knee jerks are lost and the lack of sensation in the foot in association with ischaemia, trauma and sepsis sets the scene for diabetic gangrene. Pains in the lower limb and pelvic girdle are common and ANS involvement may lead to loss of bladder control. Amyotrophy, especially weakness and wasting of the thigh muscles, and isolated nerve palsies are usually associated with poor diabetic control.

Careful correction of the diabetes mellitus is the recommended treatment. Many cases improve after a period of good diabetic control. For other aspects of diabetes and the management of the diabetic foot see Chapters 14 and 16.

Trigeminal Neuralgia

This is characterized by severe recurrent paroxysms of pain confined to one or more divisions of the fifth cranial nerve. The ophthalmic division is not usually affected, there are no objective signs and the aetiology is unknown. Elderly people are the usual victims and similar symptoms in younger folk should suggest some underlying disease, e.g. multiple sclerosis.

The drug of choice is carbamazepine (Tegretol) starting with a dose of 200 mg once or twice daily. Phenytoin is also used (see Chapter 12, use in epilepsy). Some cases fail to respond to drug treatment and require surgical intervention by injections or section of the pain fibres. The surgeon aims to produce anaesthesia in the affected area but to spare the nerve supply to the cornea if at all possible.

'Restless legs' syndrome

A number of elderly patients, in the absence of obvious vascular disease, complain of aches and even cramps in the leg muscles coming on with rest in bed or chair. They have to get up and walk about to secure relief. The aetiology is unknown and there are no abnormal physical signs. The symptoms may be relieved by simple analgesics or by chlorpromazine 25–75 mg at night. Alternatively diazepam 5–10 mg may be tried. There is no underlying disease of muscle or peripheral nerves.

Entrapment Neuropathy

Where peripheral nerves run in confined spaces they may be subjected to damage from pressure. Initially pain, but later loss of sensation and motor function occurs. Early recognition and release of the entrapment gives complete relief unless the axons are interrupted. These entrapment lesions are quite common and are predisposed to by a variety of factors especially rheumatoid arthritis, which not uncommonly causes pressure on the median nerve in the carpal tunnel and malalignment following fractures, e.g. at wrist, elbow or humerus. The diagnosis is made on the history and examination but motor nerve conduction studies will pinpoint the site of the lesion with great accuracy. Mild cases respond to hydrocortisone injections with rest to the affected part. More severe cases require surgical decompression.

Peripheral nerves affected by vasculitis or diabetes are particularly vulnerable to the effects of pressure. Entrapment of the lateral cutaneous nerve of the thigh in the inguinal ligament gives pain and paraesthesia over the lateral aspect of the thigh (meralgia paraesthetica).

Cervical Spondylosis

This results from chronic intervertebral disc degeneration and affects especially those in their sixties and seventies. Lateral herniation of discs with osteophyte encroachment on the intervertebral foramina produces pressure on one or more nerve roots causing initially pain and paraesthesia and later mixed motor and sensory loss of the appropriate segmental distribution. Acute attacks tend more to affect the middle aged but acute, subacute and chronic features may all occur at different times in the same patient. Chronic dorsomedial disc lesions calcify to produce solid transverse bars and by pressure on the anterior spinal artery impair the blood supply to the anterior two thirds of the cord. Additionally there may be direct pressure on the anterior surface of the cord and cervical myelopathy develops. This may mimic tumour of the cord, motor neurone disease or subacute combined degeneration of the cord. Radiological examination will confirm the presence of narrowed disc spaces, encroachment on the intervertebral foramina and narrowing of the anteroposterior diameter of the spinal canal. The clinical picture varies with the precise level and severity of the lesions but often includes insidious weakness of the legs with brisk jerks and dermatome sensory loss in the upper limbs. Involvement of the spinothalamic tracts will cause disturbance of pain and temperature sense in the legs.

Treatment is based on immobilization of the neck in a light metal or plastic collar. Decompressive surgery is rarely required.

Cervical Spondylitis

Inflammatory disease of the cervical spine (excluding infections) is most commonly due to rheumatoid arthritis. Synovitis may damage the occipito-atlanto-axial articulation with the danger of atlanto-axial subluxation which is said to occur in some 25 per cent of rheumatoid patients attending hospital. Surprisingly little pain may result from this and only a minority develop a neurological lesion. Ischaemic myelopathy may develop from mid and lower cervical lesions as in cervical spondylosis.

Management is as for cervical spondylosis in addition to the usual treatment of the rheumatoid disease. Progressive neurological impairment may demand surgical fusion to stabilize the neck. All who are involved in handling the patient (anaesthetists, nurses, physiotherapists, porters etc.) should be warned of the potential danger of mishandling the head and neck, especially with rheumatoid patients who are to undergo surgery.

CHAPTER 14 · DISEASES OF THE HEART, BLOOD VESSELS, AND LUNGS

> You must eat less, or use more Exercise, or take Physick, or be sick.
>
> Advice from Sir Charles Scarbouragh to the Duchess of Portsmouth; in *Essay of Health and Long Life*, by
>
> GEORGE CHEYNE, 1725

Atherosclerosis

Atherosclerosis is a process which has started in all men and nearly all women in the developed countries by the age of twenty, and whose progress throughout life accounts for more male deaths than any other factor from their mid-thirties onwards. It is also responsible for an enormous amount of morbidity and mortality in both sexes in old age. It is associated with subintimal thickening by crystalline cholesterol and fibrous tissue and often small haemorrhages to form atheromatous plaques. It affects initially the aorta but subsequently all medium-sized arteries. Its effects lead to ischaemic heart disease (IHD), the majority of strokes, a large proportion of peripheral vascular disease, and more rarely, mesenteric and renal vascular disease. In advanced age, the majority of people die of the effects of atherosclerosis.

Aetiology

Among the numerous aetiological theories propounded, three major risk factors have been identified—hypertension, cigarette smoking, and plasma lipids.

HYPERTENSION

Hypertension carries an increased risk of left ventricular hypertrophy and ischaemia, and cerebrovascular disease. Contrary to previous belief, the Framingham (USA) study has demonstrated that elevation of the systolic pressure, in particular, is closely correlated with clinical evidence of atherosclerotic disease. It has also been shown that a reduction in the blood pressure of hypertensive subjects is followed by a decrease in morbidity from atherosclerotic events.

CIGARETTE SMOKING

A cigarette consumption of over twenty per day carries a considerable increase in cardiovascular risk. Cessation of smoking is followed by a reduction of this risk.

PLASMA LIPIDS

When communities are compared, the mean serum cholesterol correlates with coronary disease incidence better than any other factor. Within communities, the serum cholesterol is a major determinant of coronary and atheromatous risk. Unfortunately, the individual cholesterol level correlates poorly with the individual diet, but it may be linked with the intake of animal fat. There is some evidence that an increase in the proportion of polyunsaturated fats, mainly of plant origin, can retard the progress of atherosclerosis. It has recently been shown that the small fraction of cholesterol which is transported attached to high density lipoprotein (HDL cholesterol) exerts a **protective** influence against coronary heart disease: a high concentration of low density lipoprotein cholesterol (LDL cholesterol) predisposes to it.

MINOR FACTORS

Among these may be mentioned:

Diet

Besides the quantity and type of fat consumed, other constituents have been implicated. A high intake of sucrose may be harmful. An overall excess intake of calories, leading to obesity, appears to be associated with a tendency to atherosclerosis. A low dietary fibre intake may be associated with ischaemic heart disease.

Life-Style

Lack of exercise may contribute to the pathogenesis of arterial disease, and physical exercise (preferably dynamic rather than isometric) certainly seems to raise the HDL cholesterol. Stress is a popular culprit, and there is some evidence linking Type A (striving) behaviour with coronary artery disease. A soft water supply is associated with increased risk.

Underlying Disease

The hyperlipidaemias are a potent, though comparatively uncommon, cause of premature vascular disease. Diabetes mellitus is associated with widespread arterial disease. The arterial complications of diabetes have in fact been described as an acceleration of the normal ageing process: they are perhaps better regarded as an acceleration of the abnormal ageing process.

Heredity

In some instances a striking familial tendency to vascular disease is found in the absence of other recognizable factors. The influence of heredity remains more a clinical impression than an established mechanism, and may be related to other features such as hyperuricaemia, the possession of blood group A, or geographical location. It may exert its influence in indirect ways, for example through the dietary habits of the family or of the ethnic group. Heredity is more clearly implicated in some of the hyperlipidaemias, whether primary or secondary to disorders such as diabetes mellitus.

PROPHYLAXIS

However great the increase in the workload of the geriatrician, the objective must be to delay the process of atherogenesis so that its effects do not make themselves felt until old age. The measures which offer the best chance of achieving this aim are the avoidance of cigarettes, the treatment of moderate and severe hypertension, cutting down on saturated animal fats, and taking regular exercise.

The effects of arterial disease

The precise pathological events leading to clinical manifestations seem to be various. They include gradual occlusion by atheroma, sudden occlusion by subintimal haemorrhage, embolization by platelet thrombi which form on atheromatous plaques, and insufficiency to cope with demands for an increased oxygen supply.

Clinically, the effects make themselves felt in the organs supplied and these effects may result from infarction or ischaemia, depending on the severity and suddenness of the impairment of the blood supply.

THE CORONARY ARTERIES

If the coronary vessels provide an adequate blood supply to the myocardium at rest, but are incapable of augmenting it to meet the increased oxygen demands of exercise, the myocardium protests by producing the symptom of angina of effort. Complete occlusion results in the varied clinical picture of myocardial infarction. Between these extremes lie the intermediate syndromes of coronary insufficiency and Prinzmetal's variant angina, thought to be due to spasm rather than disease of the coronary vessels, in which the pain occurs at rest and the subject can often exercise freely: however, there is a liability to ventricular arrhythmia and infarction. In older subjects the collateral circulation has been allowed time to expand, and this may explain the comparatively favourable prognosis of infarction in this age group, and possibly also its relative painlessness.

THE PERIPHERAL ARTERIES

Sudden occlusion of the popliteal artery is likely to lead to gangrene of the extremity. Narrowing of the iliofemoral vessels may be compatible with adequate vascularization of the calf muscles at rest but may produce intermittent claudication when walking, and this symptom often improves with time as collateral channels open up. Rest pain, however, is rightly regarded as a danger signal.

THE CEREBRAL VESSELS

The distinction here is less clear, because cerebral exertion does not appear to lead to symptoms or signs of ischaemia. Infarction is a better understood phenomenon than the transient ischaemic attacks which may herald it.

THE MESENTERIC VESSELS

1 Small intestine

Thrombotic or embolic arterial occlusion leads to the dramatic, and often fatal, picture of infarction of the small bowel. The onset is rapid with severe pain, vomiting, absent bowel sounds, and shock. The less common syndrome produced by progressive arterial narrowing is mesenteric angina, characterized by the triad of post-prandial abdominal pain, weight loss and diarrhoea, which may be due to frank steatorrhoea. Stricture formation or infarction often ensue.

2 Large intestine

Large bowel ischaemia may give rise to local mucosal infarction, often at the splenic flexure, with a clinical picture of haemorrhagic colitis (chapter 15). This may resolve, or stricture formation may follow.

Sudden complete occlusion of a major vessel may lead to massive infarction.

Ischaemic heart disease

Coronary artery disease may present in the two classical ways which occur in younger patients—angina of effort, and myocardial infarction. In the middle-aged, the clinical picture of infarction varies from sudden death, to cardiogenic shock and severe central chest pain, to mild twinges of discomfort ascribed to indigestion. It is the concern of this book to enlarge upon the form that disease processes tend to adopt in older subjects, and the classical picture of acute myocardial infarction is not the rule in geriatric medicine.

Angina pectoris

Central chest pain may be due to cardiac ischaemia, but left ventricular hypertrophy and T wave inversion in the electrocardiogram do not prove that it is. Nor does radiographic demonstration of an hiatus hernia prove that it is not! Multiple pathology highlights the importance of taking a full history, but even the history is all too often either misleading or grossly defective. Episodes of breathlessness on minor exertion, probably due to mild left ventricular failure, are sometimes encountered instead of angina. A vague sensation of discomfort in the chest may be experienced simultaneously, but is overshadowed by the dyspnoea.

Myocardial infarction

Like any other sudden illness in old people, a myocardial infarct often presents as a toxic confusional state. On the other hand the fall in blood pressure and cerebral perfusion can result in a fall, or a syncopal episode, TIA or stroke. Often there is no chest pain and sometimes it is such a minor feature that it is only mentioned on specific questioning.

Management of Myocardial Infarction and Angina

In general, the uncomplicated myocardial infarct in an elderly subject can probably be better managed at home than in hospital, provided that the home circumstances permit. An initial short period of bed rest may be dictated by the patient's general condition but need not otherwise be advised. Adverse factors include cardiogenic shock, which carries a very grave prognosis. Defects of rhythm and conduction are managed similarly to such events in younger patients. Intensive coronary care, with monitoring and resuscitation, may well be appropriate in previously fit subjects in their late sixties and seventies. Indeed, it has been reported that the results following successful resuscitation from cardiac arrest may be better among the elderly, perhaps because of better collateral channels. The possibility has recently emerged of improving survival following acute myocardial infarction in younger

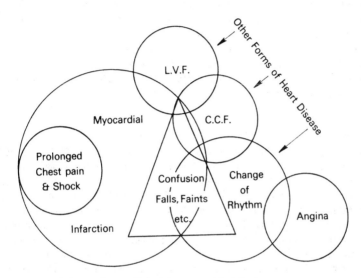

Fig. 14.1. Some clinical features of I.H.D. in the elderly

subjects by prolonged drug therapy. The intention is to reduce the incidence of reinfarction, sudden death, and dysrhythmia, and the agents reported to be effective include beta blockers, sulphinpyrazone, and aspirin. These measures would be very seldom justified in persons over the age of seventy.

Patients whose activity is curtailed and whose life is plagued by severe, frequent, or prolonged attacks of angina often respond well to beta blockade. If this is contra-indicated by heart failure or chronic lung disease, alternatives include nifedipine, verapamil and perhexilene. Sometimes an episode of infarction can produce one of the clinical pictures described below which can equally be caused by IHD without actual infarction, or indeed by totally different pathologies, so non-specific are the effects of cardiac disease (Fig. 14.1).

ABNORMALITIES OF RHYTHM AND CONDUCTION

Even at an advanced age, the heart usually remains in sinus rhythm.

However it is common to find ectopic beats. Coronary artery disease, with or without infarction, and many other disorders of the heart, can lead to a wide variety of disturbances of rhythm and conduction.

Atrial fibrillation

Atrial fibrillation may occur paroxysmally but generally becomes established sooner or later during the course of most serious cardiac conditions. In the elderly it is most often the result of IHD but occasionally previous hypertension has played a part. The other important possible cause is thyrotoxicosis, and this should always be considered. The factor precipitating the onset of this rhythm may be a chest infection, and the patient is often initially seriously ill because the uncontrolled ventricular rate is often well in excess of 120 per minute, which is incompatible with an adequate cardiac output. Digitalization is required to reduce the ventricular rate to 80 or 90 per minute, and can be achieved by giving oral digoxin in a dose of 0·25 mg twice daily for the first 48 hours. The initial dose can be given intramuscularly if the patient is vomiting or has difficulty with swallowing. Thereafter maintenance therapy is required for as long as the fibrillation persists, but a very small dose is usually sufficient, such as 125 micrograms daily. Atrial fibrillation is occasionally refractory to control by digoxin, particularly if it is due to hyperthyroidism, but may respond satisfactorily to one of the beta-adrenoreceptor blocking drugs.

The onset of atrial fibrillation is frequently the event which tips the patient into cardiac failure. Once controlled, it is compatible with a symptom-free life for many years, and in the elderly there must be very few indications for attempting to convert to sinus rhythm as the underlying heart disease is likely to be permanent. Many elderly patients have an acceptable ventricular rate without any medication at all.

Other supraventricular rhythms

Atrial tachycardia and flutter should be attributed to digoxin if the patient is taking this drug: and if not, thyrotoxicosis should again be suspected. Digitalis is a dangerous drug in all ages, because the therapeutic level is so close to the toxic level. In old age and in the small in stature and the frail, especially in the presence of impaired renal function, it is particularly likely to cause vomiting, mental confusion, and dangerous arrhythmia. If in doubt, the drug should be withdrawn pending the results of blood level estimation.

Supraventricular tachydysrhythmia resistant to digoxin, or possibly attributable to it, may respond to a beta blocker or verapamil. Either of these drugs may precipitate severe hypotension.

Ventricular tachycardia

This very serious ectopic rhythm is generally due to myocardial infarction but may also be the result of digitalis toxicity. It may be heralded by frequent ventricular extrasystoles (six or more per minute), particularly when the R wave of the extrasystole occurs during the T wave of the preceding normal beat. The usual treatment is the intravenous injection of a 'bolus' of 50 to 100 mg of lignocaine, followed by an infusion of the same drug at a rate of 1–4 mg per minute. If there is a poor response to lignocaine, mexiletine, disopyramide, or a beta blocker should be tried, but they are liable to produce hypotension, heart failure, and bradycardia.

Conduction defects

The conducting tissues of the heart can be affected by IHD with or without infarction. They commonly undergo fibrosis in advanced age in the absence of significant coronary disease. Digitalis should also always be borne in mind as a possible cause of heart block of any degree.

The sino-atrial node and atria. Sinus arrest or sino-atrial block may lead to dropped beats. If the sinus is not functioning properly, beats may be initiated from various ectopic foci throughout the atria and the P waves will be of varying shape and size and the PR interval also will be variable. This wandering pacemaker leads to a multifocal atrial rhythm which may be punctuated by paroxysms of multifocal atrial tachycardia.

The sick sinus syndrome (Fig. 14.2) is also characterized by defective elaboration of sinus impulses with chaotic atrial activity and

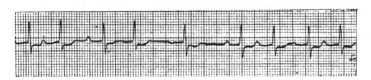

Fig. 14.2

changing P waves but with intermittent or persistent bradycardia. Episodes of rapid supraventricular arrhythmia may supervene.

These conditions lead to such non-specific complaints as dizziness, falls, and faints, as well as palpitations. The diagnosis is sometimes only established by a 24 hour rhythm tape obtained by continuous ambulatory monitoring. Drug treatment is often unsatisfactory but pacing may relieve the symptoms.

Atrioventricular block—heart block. Complete heart block with a slow regular idioventricular rhythm is characterized by the additional physical sign of a collapsing pulse due to increased diastolic filling and a high stroke output. There is also a variable first heart sound in the presence of normal atrial activity because if the ventricle contracts very soon after the atrium, the valve cusps will still be wide open instead of floating together, and the sudden increase in ventricular pressure will shut them with a much louder bang. Similarly, if the atrium happens to contract at a time when the AV valve is closed, there will be a steep rise in intra-atrial pressure, seen in the neck as a cannon wave.

If the increased stroke volume fails to compensate for the slow rate, the cardiac output will fall, thereby limiting the exercise tolerance, resulting in severe failure. The other major complication is the Stokes-Adams attack, which may occur in any degree of AV block or even bundle branch block: the underlying defect of conduction may be paroxysmal in nature, causing diagnostic difficulties. Stokes-Adams attacks are most common in established complete heart block, and any one of these attacks may prove fatal. A poor output and Stokes-Adams attacks are the two main indications for advising a pacemaker, which may be of enormous benefit in patients well into their eighties or even nineties. It is usual to try the effect of long-acting isoprenaline (Saventrine) in the first instance, starting with 30 mg twice a day and increasing the dose to 30 mg four times a day. Although this may increase the ventricular rate, it is very doubtful if it improves the life expectancy.

Stokes-Adams attacks. These attacks are caused by the sudden onset of ventricular asystole or rapid ventricular tachycardia leading to the cessation of effective cardiac activity and a fall in cardiac output to virtually zero. They are thus characterized by loss of consciousness sometimes associated with convulsions. The typical sequence of colour changes is from pallor to cyanosis with subsequent flushing due to reactive hyperaemia. Spontaneous recovery normally occurs within half a minute or so. However, in the individual attack there is no guarantee of the resumption of an effective circulation, so measures should be taken appropriate to cardiac arrest. If elevation of the legs and a blow to the praecordium are not effective, external massage is instituted, followed by DC shock treatment with the arrival of the resuscitation team.

CONGESTIVE CARDIAC FAILURE

Heart failure is a very common manifestation of IHD in old people. Indeed, severe occlusive disease of the coronary vessels may present as a congestive cardiomyopathy with painless severe biventricular heart failure, a low output, and a very large heart. It should be noted that massive dependent oedema often occurs without cardiac failure due, for example, to such simple causes as sitting motionless for long periods (Table 14.1).

Table 14.1. A general classification of oedema

Generalized fluid retention
  Oliguric renal failure   Drugs—steroids   carbenoxolone
  Congestive cardiac failure   oestrogens   phenylbutazone
                                                 methyldopa
Increased venous pressure
  General—congestive cardiac failure
  Local—venous insufficiency or thrombosis or external compression by
        tight clothing
  Lack of muscle pump action—stroke & immobility

Hypoalbuminaemia
  Deficient intake—malnutrition
  Defective synthesis—liver disease
  Excessive loss—e.g. via kidney (nephrotic syndrome) or bowel

Lymphatic obstruction
  Malignant disease and lymphoma
  Parasitic
  Hereditary

Local defect in capillary wall
  Inflammation, angioneurotic oedema

Non-oedema (included in differential diagnosis of 'billiard table legs')
  Fat (simple obesity, lipodystrophy, Dercum's disease, lipomatosis etc.)
  Mucinous oedema (myxoedema)

Heart failure is the final common path of virtually every form of cardiac pathology, and the precipitating factor may be a respiratory infection, an episode of infarction, or a change of rhythm. It may present in the classical way with breathlessness on exertion and on lying flat, but in the old it often leads to the onset of mental confusion.

The management of heart failure has traditionally included the use of digitalis for its inotropic effect of increasing contractile power and thus the stroke volume and cardiac output. Digoxin is now mainly indicated for its chronotropic action in controlling the ventricular rate in atrial fibrillation, and diuretics are the mainstay of treatment of the failing but regular heart. The potent loop diuretics (frusemide 40 mg or more: bumetanide 1 mg or more) are popular and effective, but may cause incontinence, retention of urine, dehydration and electrolyte imbalance. In milder cases, the benzothiadiazines (e.g. bendrofluazide 10 mg) may be sufficient.

Elderly patients on diuretics are especially vulnerable to potassium depletion because their intake is often poor. These drugs tend to produce a hypochloraemic alkalosis, so effervescent chloride-containing potassium supplements such as Kloref or Sando-K are usually given. An alternative, in cases of resistant oedema, is to potentiate the action of the diuretic by the use of a potassium-conserving agent such as the aldosterone antagonist spironolactone (25 mg thrice daily), or triamterene (50 mg thrice daily), or amiloride (5 mg twice daily).

Pulmonary oedema

Acute pulmonary oedema is one of the common medical emergencies in the elderly. It is most frequently attributable to IHD. Although it is traditionally taught that this condition is easily distinguished from severe breathlessness due to bronchopneumonia or airway obstruction, in practice the three quite commonly coexist in older subjects and the chest is a veritable orchestra of bubbles and squeaks. Intravenous frusemide 20–40 mg and perhaps intravenous aminophylline (250 mgs) is the treatment of choice, together with antibiotics and oxygen.

Milder degrees of pulmonary oedema occurring at night give rise to paroxysmal nocturnal dyspnoea, and this can cause nocturnal restlessness or confusion. It is worth trying an early evening dose of a diuretic, preferably a short-acting one such as bumetanide 0·5 mg, in such cases.

Other forms of heart disease

Degenerative (calcific) valve disease

Aortic valve disease of rheumatic, syphilitic, and other inflammatory origin is less often seen nowadays, although calcification in a congenitally bicuspid valve may be found at autopsy. Aortic sclerosis is usually benign and may be recognized by the presence of an ejection midsystolic murmur, sometimes accompanied by a thrill, classically basal but sometimes mainly apical, radiating up into the neck. An early diastolic murmur may also be audible. Although there is usually clinical evidence of left ventricular hypertrophy, the pulse pressure is wide due to the presence of atherosclerosis (a locomotor brachial artery can often be seen), and this distinguishes the condition from haemodynamically significant aortic stenosis.

Calcific **mitral** valve disease, on the other hand, does cause significant mitral regurgitation. It is commoner in women, unlike other forms of degenerative heart disease, and its incidence rises with age. Both these disorders may predispose to infective endocarditis, and both may produce radiographically visible calcification in the valve rings.

Hypertensive heart disease

There is a considerable overlap between hypertensive heart disease (HHD) and IHD, and indeed the former is often a precursor of the latter. The effects of longstanding hypertension are therefore often observed at post mortem.

In geriatric practice, the ravages of hypertension most often make themselves apparent in the central nervous system. Cerebral haemorrhage is a direct result of the disease. Men with diffuse cerebrovascular disease are also commonly encountered, showing the clinical picture of intellectual impairment, pseudobulbar palsy, and bilateral pyramidal signs.

It is to be hoped that as a result of widespread screening and modern drugs, an increasing number of males will reach the geriatric age range on long term antihypertensive therapy. The treatment should be continued, under regular surveillance so that it can be cut down or stopped if the blood pressure falls too low due to increased sensitivity to the drug or due to intercurrent myocardial infarction.

It is probably seldom desirable to start anybody over the age of seventy-five on antihypertensive therapy, because the side-effects are likely to outweigh any potential benefit. The sphygmomanometer reading is, in any case, prone to error in this age group because the stiffness of the arterial wall may cause the diastolic pressure as measured by the cuff to be up to 30 mm higher than the true intraluminal pressure measured directly. The correct management of the newly discovered hypertensive in the 65 to 74 age range is controversial. The Framingham study has shown that the considerably higher mortality suffered by men with a systolic pressure over 160 mm compared with their contemporaries with a systolic pressure below 130 mm, persists into this decade. The reversibility of this trend with treatment remains unproven. Until the debate is resolved, a course must be steered between the Scylla of therapeutic nihilism and the Charybdis of meddlesome interference.

Postural hypotension

Postural hypotension is a serious finding, because it can easily lead to light-headedness on standing, and thus to falls. Here it is the systolic level which is of greater importance, and symptoms are unlikely to result unless the drop is greater than 40 mmHg and the standing level 120 mmHg or less.

The causes of this condition include the following:

Hypovolaemia due to blood loss or salt and water depletion.

Loss of normal baroceptor reflexes due to recumbency.

Loss of normal baroceptor reflexes due to autonomic neuropathy—e.g. diabetes mellitus: extra-pyramidal disease (Shy-Drager syndrome).

Reduced cardiac output.

Drugs—antihypertensive agents including diuretics
        phenothiazines.
        levodopa.
        tricyclic antidepressants.

The first step in the treatment is the identification and correction of the cause. If this is impossible, elastic stockings are worth trying, or it may be necessary to have recourse to 9-alpha fluorohydrocortisone (0·1 mg once, twice or thrice daily). In mild cases, all that may be necessary is a simple warning of the danger of suddenly getting out of a bed or a warm bath. Some cases are very recalcitrant, but a recent report indicates that indomethacin may prove to be effective, possibly by inhibiting the synthesis of vasodepressor prostaglandins.

Mucoid degeneration of the mitral valve: the floppy mitral valve

In this degenerative condition of old age, the posterior cusp of the valve enlarges in area due to infiltration of its dense fibrous tissue with mucopolysaccharide. Ballooning of the cusp leads to prolapse and mitral regurgitation, the apical murmur often being late rather than pansystolic. The mitral incompetence is often well tolerated unless complicated by rupture of the chordae tendinae, when it may become torrential and culminate in severe heart failure and pulmonary oedema. The diagnosis can often be confirmed by echocardiography.

Cardiac amyloidosis and brown atrophy

Senile cardiac amyloidosis is a type of primary amyloidosis commonly seen at autopsy among the old, and in fact it has been recorded as having an incidence of over 50 per cent in subjects aged over 90. It is virtually impossible to diagnose during life, and indeed its clinical significance remains uncertain.

'Brown atrophy' due to deposition of pigment in the myocardial fibres, is another prevalent post-mortem finding in old age. It probably represents an age change of no clinical importance.

Thyrogenic heart disease (see Chapter 16)

Cardiac failure of obscure origin in the elderly, especially if precipitated by a supraventricular tachy-arrhythmia, should arouse suspicion of thyrotoxic heart disease. In atrial fibrillation, the ventricular rate may be very resistant to control by digoxin and beta-adrenergic blocking drugs will then act more quickly than antithyroid agents, although many of them carry the risk of aggravating fluid retention.

Hypothyroidism may cause bradycardia, pericardial, pleural or peritoneal effusions, and angina. Replacement therapy with thyroxine has to be instituted extremely slowly because of the danger of cardiac arrest. Although angina is an indication to proceed with even more circumspection than usual, preferably with the patient in hospital, treatment should not be withheld on this account because an improvement in exercise tolerance and in the electrocardiogram may be hoped for.

Endocarditis

With the diminishing incidence of rheumatic heart disease in the young, infective endocarditis has shifted its emphasis towards older age groups, affecting sclerotic or even previously normal valves. Urinary tract and other infections, and procedures such as catheterization are likely sources of bacteraemia in elderly people. The clinical picture is often atypical, and in particular, fever may be absent and the murmurs may be non-specific, so that it is essential to maintain a high index of suspicion. An aphorism which applies to so many diseases in geriatric medicine!

Non-bacterial thrombotic endocarditis is a condition which is occasionally seen in association with mucous-secreting adenocarcinomata of the bronchus, stomach or colon, and is more inclined to afflict the elderly. Vegetations occur on the aortic or mitral valve and may lead to systemic or coronary embolization. It is sometimes associated with evidence of disseminated intravascular coagulation.

Peripheral vascular disease (Fig. 14.3)

The clinical consequences of degenerative disease of the femoral, popliteal, and tibial vessels, are distressing and recurrent sources of admissions to the geriatric wards. The vital importance of foot hygiene in the elderly cannot be stressed enough. Three or four-monthly visits to (or from) a chiropodist are necessary, particularly in diabetics and those with vascular disease. Old people often find it very difficult to look after their own feet because of failing vision, because of poor co-ordination of the hands, or because they cannot bend spine, hips or knees sufficiently to bring their feet within range.

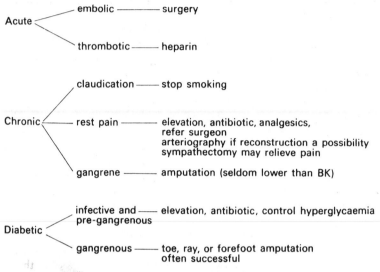

Fig. 14.3. Scheme of management of the ischaemic limb

Acute ischaemia causes a cold, painful, blotchy, blue and white leg which becomes anaesthetic and then paralysed. If the onset is very sudden, particularly in the presence of atrial fibrillation or recent myocardial infarction, **embolism** should be suspected, in which case surgery within eight hours offers a good prospect of salvaging the limb. The differential diagnosis is **thrombosis** in a narrowed atherosclerotic vessel, more probable if there is a previous history of claudication. The most helpful treatment is conservative and the limb is cooled and the patient heparinized.

Arterial insufficiency is usually a more gradual process, and may take several forms. **Intermittent claudication** carries a compara-tively favourable prognosis, some 70 per cent of younger patients being unchanged or improved after five years: of the 30 per cent whose symptoms grow worse, only a third come to amputation. Management is by reassurance, stopping smoking, and providing a walking stick. Weight reduction may be helpful. Walking and cycling are encouraged, and the symptoms will clear up over a period of months or years in 25 per cent of cases.

A syndrome which should be mentioned here is **neurogenic claudication**, in which similar symptoms are caused by disease of the spinal arteries, sometimes in association with a local compressing lesion. The pain is sometimes accompanied by neurological signs occurring on exercise (foot drop, loss of reflexes), and laminectomy is often beneficial. When concurrent disease of the foot vessels has obliterated the pulses, the differential diagnosis is very difficult, and arteriography and myelography may be required to establish the cause.

Rest pain is generally felt in the foot rather than the leg, and is worst at night. Its onset, especially when accompanied by patches of ulceration or necrosis, indicates that gangrene will inevitably follow unless surgical treatment is practicable. The patient is rested with the foot exposed while the opinion of the vascular surgeon is sought. Adequate analgesia is essential, and powerful drugs such as heroin may well be required. Rest pain is frequently due to infection complicating an ischaemic extremity, so that appropriate antibacterial and antifungal therapy can be given. Many of these patients find that they are most comfortable when the foot is dependent, perhaps by enlisting the aid of gravity in maintaining the blood supply. Unfortunately, this is the best way to precipitate gangrene. The foot **must** be elevated to drain infection and oedema, even though elevation increases the pain.

Arteriography is usually required especially if the surgeon considers that arterial reconstructive surgery may be feasible. Disease of the aorto-iliac or femoropopliteal vessels offers better prospects than occlusions below the knee. Major reconstructive arterial surgery is a formidable undertaking in the old; not only is it associated with all the usual risks inherent in major surgery in this age group, but there is also the likelihood that the atheromatous process affects the cerebral, coronary and renal vessels as well as those of the leg—and the other leg, too.

Conservative measures often fail materially to influence the outcome, and many of these patients come to some form of amputation. Lumbar sympathectomy is effective in the relief of rest pain if there is no gangrene beyond a small patch of necrotic skin. **Gangrene** of the toes or foot is a common sequel despite all these measures, and will necessitate amputation. This should be regarded as a positive and helpful measure, not as an act of despair, for the improvement in health and morale following the removal of a painful, infected, and contracted limb is often dramatic. The operation offering the best hope for rehabilitation is below knee, but if it fails to heal a further amputation may have a disastrous effect on the patient's morale. Through knee and Gritti-Stokes amputations are relatively atraumatic and carry a low mortality. All too often, the poor viability of the limb necessitates an above knee (e.g. mid-thigh) operation in order to ensure good healing, although it carries a higher mortality (about 1/3) and a low rehabilitation success-rate (about 1/3). About half the survivors will lose the other leg within three years. Following surgery, the early fitting of a pylon or prosthesis and energetic rehabilitation can be very rewarding.

The **diabetic foot** is particularly vulnerable to arterial insufficiency, often predominantly distal, but neuropathy and infection are also likely to be contributory factors. Osteomyelitis of the metatarsal heads is a frequent feature. Conservative measures aimed at reducing oedema, correcting hyperglycaemia, and clearing up cellulitis, may at least temporarily save the limb. When gangrene does occur, local amputation of toes or forefoot is often successful in diabetics, but seldom in straight-forward atherosclerosis. This is because in diabetics, the cause of the gangrene is trophic—for instance due to pressure of corns on insensitive tissues with a reasonable blood supply. Where diabetic gangrene is associated with occlusion of major vessels, local treatment is ineffective. Ischaemia of the toes with a palpable popliteal pulse is a diabetic foot; without a popliteal pulse, it is straightforward atherosclerosis in a diabetic.

Abdominal aortic aneurysm

Routine palpation of the abdomen often reveals enlargement of the aorta, and it may be difficult to be sure when this has reached aneurysmal proportions. Calcification on the lateral X-ray may help to determine the size and extent of an aneurysm. These aneurysms are of athero-sclerotic origin, and carry a high risk of leaking, or, more catastrophi-cally, rupturing. Many vascular surgeons therefore advise a prophylactic elective operation as soon as the diagnosis is made.

Connective tissue disease

Gangrene of the digits occasionally occurs in old people as a mani-festation of polyarteritis nodosa. Evidence of the disease should be sought in other systems, notably the kidneys, joints and lungs, and if the diagnosis seems probable, treatment with large doses of cortico-steroids is instituted. A similar arteritis may complicate rheumatoid disease.

A related disorder is **giant cell arteritis** in which there are marked inflammatory changes in the media with focal necrosis, granulomata, and numerous giant cells. This disease classically affects the superficial temporal vessels causing headache and extreme tenderness; there may be visible nodules along the vessel, or it may be pulseless. Constitutional disturbances such as fever and weight loss are usual, and the sedi-mentation rate is elevated, usually to over 50 mm per hour. The disease often spreads to involve other vessels, particularly the ophthalmic artery and its branches, with consequent loss of vision, so it is mandatory to give steroids in large doses as soon as the diagnosis is made. Prednisone can be used in an initial dose of 45 mg daily, reducing to a maintenance dose over a prolonged period as dictated by the ESR.

Unlike polyarteritis nodosa, giant cell arteritis is primarily a disease of the elderly, and its onset may be heralded by polymyalgia rheumatica —a syndrome characterized by the rapid onset of severe non-articular aches and pains in association with marked morning stiffness. The response to steroid therapy is most gratifying.

Thrombo-embolic disease

Deep-vein thrombosis of the leg is a common and ominous occurrence in the elderly. Among predisposing factors may be mentioned recumbency and immobility—it has been estimated that at least 60 per cent of hemiplegics suffer a thrombosis on the affected side. The figure for fractures in the region of the hip joint is probably similar, unless prophylactic heparinization is used pre-operatively. Sometimes there is a previous history of venous insufficiency or varicose veins, or perhaps a 'white leg' during pregnancy. When a deep-vein thrombosis occurs out of the blue, an occult carcinoma of the stomach, bronchus or pancreas is strongly suspected. The physical signs of venous thrombosis are often misleading and it may be advisable to confirm the diagnosis by techniques such as ^{125}I—labelled fibrinogen, venography, Doppler ultrasound, or cuff impedance plethysmography.

Pulmonary embolism is exceedingly prevalent in old age. Just how prevalent, is only beginning to emerge now that lung scanning has become so widely available. It often occurs in the absence of any clinical evidence of venous thrombosis, and without predisposing factors such as immobility or recent surgery. A high index of suspicion is required, for it can masquerade in many guises (Table 14.2) and it is clear that many pulmonary emboli have in the past been mistaken for respiratory infections and myocardial infarcts. An early lung scan is desirable and it may be necessary to perform both perfusion and ventilation scans in the hope of demonstrating areas where there is ventilation but no perfusion. When a segment of lung has undergone infarction, it ceases to be ventilated, and the result of the scan is likely to be equivocal.

The investigation and management of venous thrombosis and pulmonary embolism does not differ materially in the old. Although the hazards of anticoagulants are greater, they should not be withheld on account of age alone, because the untreated disease is so dangerous.

Table 14.2. Presentation of pulmonary embolism

Sudden death
Shock and collapse
Pleurisy and haemoptysis
Pleural effusion
Change of cardiac rhythm
Breathlessness, heart failure, pulmonary hypertension
Episodic cough
Faints, falls, funny turns
Going off, failure to thrive, inanition
Hypotension and tachycardia

Strict control of the dosage is essential, so no changes should be made in any other drug regime in case it alters the effectiveness of the anticoagulant. The latter should in any case be withdrawn as soon as possible (see Chapter 19).

Other lung diseases

Many important lung diseases such as pneumoconiosis and bronchiectasis turn up in the geriatric department from time to time, but more as the legacies of youth than as currently active problems. In addition to pulmonary embolism, there are one or two respiratory conditions in old people which deserve special mention. Most of them are commoner in men than women, a departure from the usual pattern of geriatric practice.

The wheezy old man

The differential diagnosis may be quite difficult on clinical grounds but must be attempted because it affects management and prognosis (Table 14.3).

I   CHRONIC BRONCHITIS

Probably more than half of all old men smoke, and about half of these will have consequently developed chronic bronchitis within the Medical Research Council definition. That is to say that the irritant effect of the smoke has caused hyperplasia of mucus-secreting cells throughout the bronchial tree, with hypersecretion of mucus. This has progressed to the extent that there has been expectoration of mucoid sputum on most days

Table 14.3. The wheezy old man—N.B. a mixed picture is common

	Chronic bronchitis	Emphysema	Late onset asthma
Dyspnoea	Variable—from absent to severe	Severe on exertion	Occurs at rest. Variable, often worst at night
Sputum	Mucoid with purulent exacerbations	Scanty	May contain eosinophils
Clinical picture	Smoking, blue bloater	Pink, smoking, puffing old buffer: frequent weight loss	Wheezy old geezer Nocturnal cough
Prognosis	Years—may recover from recurrent bouts of respiratory failure	Years—but only weeks from onset of respiratory failure	Good with treatment
Treatment	Antibiotics bronchodilators	None effective	Corticosteroids + bronchodilators

for at least three months of the year during the preceding two years. From time to time, especially during winter this is likely to be complicated by acute infective exacerbations (usually caused by H. influenzae or the pneumococcus) and the sputum will then become purulent. It may also be complicated by airway obstruction, often largely by secretions. One likely outcome is death from bronchopneumonia and respiratory failure, although if resuscitated from such an episode the prognosis is often surprisingly good. Alternatively, the condition may progress to the 'blue bloater' with polycythaemia, pulmonary hypertension and right heart failure.

The acute exacerbation is treated with broad spectrum antibiotics as soon as the sputum becomes purulent—generally amoxycillin, co-trimoxazole, or doxycycline in the first instance, without waiting for the results of sputum culture. Simple bronchodilators are helpful, but the mucolytic agents do not appear to be strikingly beneficial in practice. Oxygen is often required, but may be lethal in high concentration: it should therefore be given by a method which permits low, known concentrations, such as the Venturimask (under most other circumstances oxygen seems to be best tolerated by the aged when given by nasal cannulae at a flow rate of two litres per minute, giving an inspired oxygen concentration of 30 to 35 per cent). Physiotherapy is essential in order to get rid of the secretions. It is essential to avoid all sedative or hypnotic drugs during an exacerbation of chronic bronchitis.

2   EMPHYSEMA

Although defined in pathological terms, emphysema may be suspected clinically when there is long-standing severe breathlessness on exertion with comparatively little variation and with little or no sputum. In the later stages it is often associated with considerable weight loss. The clinical picture is classically that of the 'pink puffer' who tends to breathe through pursed lips. The chest X-ray shows low flat diaphragms and a narrow mediastinal shadow. There is no really effective therapy and the outlook following an episode of respiratory failure is so poor that heroic therapeutic measures are seldom justified.

3   LATE ONSET ASTHMA

This is increasingly recognized as an entity in its own right as a cause of wheezing and dyspnoea coming on over the age of sixty. It is probably an intrinsic variety of asthma, and may or may not follow a history of bronchitis. The dyspnoea occurs at rest, and is variable: characteristically it is worse at night often with paroxysmal cough, and there are episodes indistinguishable from paroxysmal nocturnal dyspnoea associated with coughing. The wheezing is often described as a tightness of the chest, so that angina, left ventricular failure, emphysema and bronchitis all have to be considered in the differential diagnosis. There may be a past history, or a family history, of allergy, and eosinophilia in the blood film is also suggestive. Eosinophils should also be sought in the sputum.

The first line of treatment is to try simple sympathomimetic bronchodilators, preferably one with beta-2 stimulant activity in order to avoid serious cardiac effects. Salbutamol (Ventolin) can be taken in tablet form (2 mg thrice daily), rather better by metered dose aerosol delivering 100 mcg per actuation (one or two inhalations thrice daily), or, best of all, by inhalation of a dry powder preparation from a 'rotacap' (200 or 400 mcg thrice daily). Unfortunately, only a small minority of old people prove adept at acquiring the skill of using an inhaler.

Failing these measures, there is often a very gratifying response to corticosteroids, which should be tried despite their dangers whenever the diagnosis is seriously entertained. Side effects are less severe if given by inhalation rather than systemically, and while some cases respond well to this route of administration, others may be able to graduate onto it from oral therapy for subsequent maintenance. The Becotide metered dose aerosol inhaler delivers 50 mcg beclomethasone per actuation, and 600 to 800 mcg may be required daily in the acute attack, reducing to 100 mcg thrice daily thereafter. When oral steroids are necessary, prednisolone is given in a starting dose of 30 to 45 mg daily. The response is monitored by serial readings on the peak expiratory flow gauge and the dose judiciously reduced to a maintenance level, or inhalations substituted.

Respiratory failure

Respiratory failure is a not uncommon emergency in the geriatric department and is characterized by a fall in arterial oxygen saturation with or without CO_2 retention. If blood-gas analysis shows a raised CO_2 tension, oxygen must be given in low concentration (e.g. 24 per cent by Venturimask) continuously until the patient has improved.

Although the cause may be an obvious attack of bronchopneumonia, respiratory failure is sometimes precipitated by the injudicious use of sedative or hypnotic drugs. Sometimes, however, it supervenes insidiously on one of the chronic disorders mentioned above. In the absence of a satisfactory history, there may be very few pointers to the lungs as the source of the trouble. Presenting manifestations recently seen in our department have included acute confusion, stupor, fits, profound lassitude and intractable cardiac failure with massive oedema.

Tuberculosis

The decline in the incidence of tuberculosis in this country has been much less marked in the old than in the young with the result that it has become a disease of immigrants and of old people. It particularly affects those living in conditions of deprivation, especially old men, and malnutrition and poor housing are probably contributory factors. Most cases are thought to be caused by reactivation of old, healed lesions. The clinical picture may be reasonably typical, or it can be highly non-specific. The most worrying form has become known as 'Cryptic' miliary tuberculosis, which appears to be as common as the overt variety in people over sixty. The cryptic type takes the form of insidious, progressive non-specific malaise, perhaps with a mild intermittent fever and weight loss, but with a clear chest X-ray. It especially attacks those on steroid therapy. It is usual to perform laryngeal swabs and even to culture biopsy material from the bone marrow or liver, but a therapeutic trial of antituberculous chemotherapy is often the only way to proceed.

Streptomycin and PAS are both obsolete—certainly for the treatment of elderly patients in this country. Isoniazid remains a safe and effective first-line drug and is very well tolerated in conjunction with rifampicin: the administration of ethambutol as well for the first two months complies with the principle of starting off with triple chemotherapy.

It is necessary to continue treatment for a period of twelve months. The usual doses and likely side effects are given in Table 14.4.

Table 14.4. Chemotherapy of tuberculosis

Drug	Daily dose	Single or divided dose	Toxicity
Isoniazid	300 mg	divided	Peripheral neuropathy (prevented by pyridoxine)
Rifampicin	450–600 mg	single	Jaundice
Ethambutol	15 mg/kg body weight	single	Retrobular neuritis

Bronchopneumonia

Pneumonia is a very common illness of the old, in whom it generally takes the form of bronchopneumonia rather than the lobar variety. Bronchopneumonia is a disease of the extremes of life, and tends to affect the frail and the ill. The predisposing factors include immobility, when it may be termed hypostatic pneumonia, and difficulties with swallowing which lead to aspiration—this is a likely consequence of pseudobular palsy, for example. Heart failure, infections of the upper respiratory tract and generalized infections such as influenza are especially liable to culminate in bronchopneumonia. Physical signs are often lacking, and cough and fever may be slight or absent. Indeed, a confusional state with rapid respiration is a common clinical picture when the patient is in fact in the throes of her terminal illness. Although sputum is often unobtainable for culture, Haemophilus influenzae and the pneumococcus are the commonest causative organisms. The usual treatment is with oxygen (which should generally be given in high concentration to the elderly as CO_2 retention is an uncommon complication in the absence of severe chronic lung disease) and with a broad spectrum antibiotic such as ampicillin or septrin. Tetracycline is likely to cause diarrhoea and is dangerous in the presence of renal failure which it may exacerbate; doxycycline is safe.

Friedlander's pneumonia

Pneumonia due to Klebsiella pneumoniae is another disease of elderly, malnourished, and sometimes alcoholic men. It causes a pneumonia of acute onset, characteristically involving one or both lobes with confluent foci of consolidation often breaking down in the centre to form abscess cavities and sometimes progressing to local fibrosis. There may be a close radiological similarity to pulmonary tuberculosis, but in this condition streptomycin may have to be given in order to save life. It is sometimes used in combination with tetracycline.

Legionnaires' disease

The first reported outbreak of this severe pneumonic illness occurred in Philadelphia in 1976, although previous minor epidemics of a probably identical disease have been identified retrospectively. Since then, increasing numbers of cases occurring both in outbreaks and sporadically have been reported from America, Britain, Spain, and other countries. The age range is wide, but there may be a predilection for the elderly and those with chronic respiratory disease who certainly suffer a higher mortality than other victims. The causative organism is a Gram negative coccobacillus.

The initial phase of the illness is non-specific with fever, headache, confusion, drowsiness, prostration, and commonly diarrhoea. After two or three days dyspnoea and unproductive cough become the predominant features and the X-ray shows segmental or lobar consolidation. There is often a leucocytosis, and serological tests are being developed. It is conventional to prescribe a course of erythromycin, although its efficacy remains speculative.

Carcinoma of the bronchus

Bronchogenic carcinoma is a great imitator in geriatric medicine because it can mimic almost any other disease. It is very common, being the legacy of a lifetime's devotion to the cigarette habit, and usually takes either the squamous or the poorly differentiated oat-cell form. By the time it is discovered, it has often metastasized to lymph nodes, bone, brain, liver, skin or elsewhere, and may have involved the pericardium by direct spread. It is also notable for occasionally causing the various non-metastatic syndromes due to hormonal and other metabolic products of the tumour. If there is histological or cytological evidence of a squamous cell type of growth, and if there is no apparent spread, and if the patient's general condition permits, and if overall lung function is good, resection offers the only hope of a cure. Far more often, palliation is all that can be offered in elderly patients, and radiotherapy may dramatically relieve pain in the chest or bones or the effects of metastases on the nervous system. By shrinking the tumour, radiotherapy is also extremely effective in the relief of superior mediastinal obstruction. It is not uncommon for secondary deposits or metabolic effects to make their presence felt before the primary tumour is radiologically apparent, and the true diagnosis is often established at autopsy. Among the very elderly, therefore, this disease offers little prospect of therapeutic achievement, although it may sometimes adopt an extremely slowly progressive course over a period of months or occasionally years.

Cheyne-Stokes respiration

Cheyne-Stokes respiration or periodic breathing seems to be due to over-reaction by the respiratory centre to changes in pCO_2: the effect is like a novice helmsman who grossly over-adjusts the tiller in response to every fluctuation in the breeze and then has to correct his corrections and so, steers a zig-zag course. It is a common finding among the sick elderly and may be due to a number of causes including strokes, heart failure, and severe respiratory disease. Although it is usually regarded as of sinister import, the occasional chronic Cheyne-Stoker is followed up over a period of years in geriatric out-patient clinics.

CHAPTER 15 · GASTROINTESTINAL DISEASE

Always remember that aged men should eat often, but
little at a time for it fareth by them, as it doth by a lamp
the light whereof is almost extinct, which by pouring in
of oil little and little, is long kept burning: and with
much oil poured in at once, it is clean put out.

THOMAS ELYOT, *The Castel of Health*, 1534

Introduction

Pathology in the gastrointestinal system is common in old age. A
review of new patients attending a geriatric out-patient clinic, has
shown that 18 per cent of the significant problems detected were due to
changes in the alimentary tract. As the diseases of adolescence and
middle age can all occur in the elderly, a fully comprehensive account
of gut disease afflicting the aged, cannot be given in a book such as this.
The aim here will be to give a brief outline of conditions which are
common in old age, or present in an unusual fashion, or require special
skill and consideration in their treatment when the patients are elderly.
It should be remembered that the common emergencies which affect
the young, such as appendicitis and strangulated herniae, remain as
serious hazards, even to the old.

Dysphagia

Dysphagia is a symptom which must always be taken seriously, and
its investigation is usually simple. Direct examination of the mouth will
reveal areas of soreness or carcinoma. Indirect examination of the
larynx and pharynx in search of malignant lesions, postcricoid webs and
infections is best carried out by experts.

Oesophageal lesions (carcinoma, strictures, diverticula or spasm)
can all be demonstrated on barium swallow. Monilial infection in the
frail elderly patient is a possible cause for dysphagia, especially after
antibiotic treatment, and may be diagnosed during a barium swallow.
Extrinsic lesions such as enlarged hilar glands, a retrosternal goitre or
an unfolded aorta may all be visible on a straight X-ray of the chest.

Holdup at the oesophageal/gastric junction may be due to a hiatus
hernia (see below) or a carcinoma of the cardia extending upwards.

Many elderly patients on investigation for dysphagia will be found to have no evidence of obstruction. In some patients a pseudobulbar palsy will be apparent clinically. Sometimes only neuromuscular dysfunction will be revealed on Ba swallow—e.g. corkscrew oesophagus.

Peptic ulceration

Although acid secretion tends to fall with age, the frequency of peptic ulceration seems to rise. This appears to be true for lesions in the three common sites of oesophagus, stomach and duodenum.

OESOPHAGITIS

For this to occur, with or without actual ulceration, definite acid reflux is required. Of patients with a known hiatus hernia, about a quarter are aged over 70 years. However, as such series are based on the presence of symptoms, they do not give a true incidence of the lesion, as it is thought that about a quarter of all hiatus herniae are asymptomatic. Also symptoms of reflux may occur without confirmation on radiological examination in about two-thirds of patients.

It is not only where the hernia is of the sliding type or a combination of sliding and rolling that acid can reach the oesophageal mucosa and cause oesophagitis and ulceration. The symptoms of lower chest/upper abdominal discomfort and burning often so poorly described by geriatric patients, make the differentiation between oesophageal and cardiac pain extremely difficult. Many elderly patients suffer symptoms from both sources. Others experience no pain, but simply present with persistent vomiting which is not always related to stooping or lying flat.

Elderly patients particularly at risk from developing oesophagitis are the obese, those with structural pyloric stenosis and those with functional pyloric spasm and gastric stasis secondary to anticholinergic drugs. The use of anti-inflammatory drugs increases symptoms in patients known to have a hiatus hernia. Chronic bleeding leading to iron deficiency anaemia is a very common problem.

Another major complication is oesophageal stenosis with the risk of inhalation, necessitating recurrent oesophageal dilatation.

In uncomplicated cases, treatment is basically the same as in other age groups.

GASTRIC ULCERATION

Like so many conditions in old age, peptic ulceration of the stomach is often silent. The incidence of the condition can therefore only be assessed from post-mortem material, but such patients are obviously a specially selected group. However, from such a series it would seem that gastric ulceration increases with age (an incidence of 5·2 per cent over 65 years of age, 8·5 per cent over 70 years), and reaches approximately the same incidence as duodenal ulceration, and affects men and women almost equally when they are old. Giant ulcers are more common in old age but may heal even in spite of their size.

It is lack of symptoms, rather than any special features which distinguishes presentation in old age. The patient may only offer non-specific complaints such as loss of appetite or vomiting. Bleeding, if slow, may also go unnoticed, even when the haemoglobin falls to very low levels, especially if the patient is incapacitated by other conditions. It is, however, in just this situation that the correction of the anaemia becomes more important than in the young, if a cascade of complications and rapid breakdown in health is to be avoided. Massive sudden haemorrhage is as always, dramatic, but in old age a rapid decision concerning surgery must be made. Because the patient is generally frail, there is a natural reluctance to resort to surgery. Unfortunately, such patients cannot be kept waiting, and if the bleeding is not quickly stopped, a breakdown in another system, such as cerebral-blood flow or coronary flow, may intervene. Death may therefore occur for a variety of reasons, and a third of all ulcer deaths occur in the elderly. Some patients may survive their bleed, but acquire a stroke or other complication during their acute illness. For successful management, a quick decision is obviously needed, but based on full information, as the presence of another serious pathology such as severe established dementia, must also be taken into account. The surgical treatment of perforation in the elderly should be decided with the same care and speed.

Extra skill is also needed for the medical treatment of the less dramatic symptoms. Traditional bed-rest is potentially dangerous and may result in permanent loss of mobility. Antacids should be monitored and titrated to avoid upsetting or worsening the patient's bowel habit. Cimetadine (an H_2 receptor antagonist) does not appear to have any special problems when used in elderly subjects.

Barium meal examination remains the most common form of investigation for the diagnosis and follow-up of gastric ulcers. Fibre-optic gastroscopy is fortunately becoming more readily available, and is a most suitable form of investigation for the elderly, well tolerated and may provide more information than radiology.

DUODENAL ULCERATION

Men retain their numerical supremacy for this condition, even in old age, but the symptoms tend to be less dramatic in the elderly than in the young. The statements made above for the investigation and surgical treatment of gastric ulceration and its complications, apply equally well to lesions in the duodenum. Cimetadine offers a safe and effective form of treatment for all ages. Mild sedatives and antispasmodics, which are of doubtful value in young patients, have real risks in the elderly. Even mild sedation may cause confusion. Antispasmodics will also have anticholinergic effects on the eye, bladder and large bowel, with the risk of producing glaucoma, retention and constipation.

Pyloric stenosis whether due to ulceration or malignancy, is less well tolerated in the elderly. As there is often concurrent renal impairment, any prolonged vomiting will rapidly result in dehydration and electrolyte imbalance. Treatment will have to be surgical, but only after correction of any biochemical or haematological abnormalities.

Ischaemic bowel disease

Ischaemic bowel disease in the elderly may be acute or chronic, and affect either the small or large bowel. Most patients will have evidence of generalized vascular disease, due to widespread atheromatous changes, especially in diabetics. A recent series suggests that this condition may account for just under 1 per cent of acute admissions to a geriatric unit. The prognosis is usually gloomy, and recovery in this age group, rare.

The mechanism of occlusion may be embolic or thrombotic. However, in many instances discovered at post-mortem, the main vessels will be found to be patent. In such cases, changes in the microcirculation of the gut are thought to be responsible, and actual occlusion may not occur, but damage can result from haemodynamic changes secondary to hypotension, caused by some distant pathology.

ACUTE MESENTERIC OCCLUSION

This is the variety of ischaemic bowel disease most likely to be embolic in origin. The responsible embolus may arise from a mural thrombus after myocardial infarction, from a fibrillating atrium, or from infected valves in subacute bacterial endocarditis. However, not all acute episodes are embolic. The onset is usually dramatic with sudden abdominal pain, blood loss, ileus, and later, peritonitis and hypovolaemia as fluid is lost into the gut lumen. The severity of the symptoms will depend on the size of the embolus and the extent of the resulting vascular shutdown. In mild cases, spontaneous resolution may occur, and treatment is directed at the source of the embolus. Where the damage is more extensive, surgical resection of the infarcted length of bowel will be necessary to preserve life.

CHRONIC MESENTERIC OCCLUSION

This condition is sometimes known as abdominal angina. As with the cardiac variety, symptoms occur when extra demands are made. The patient therefore complains of pain after eating; the larger the meal, the more severe the pain. The pain is usually constant and situated centrally in the abdomen. Because of the association of pain and eating, the patient's appetite becomes poor, and weight loss follows. In addition, the bowel ischaemia may lead to atrophic changes in the small bowel mucosa and the presence of malabsorption may also play a part in causing weight loss.

As the underlying vascular disease is usually widespread, the only form of treatment is symptomatic relief, which can be gained by taking small, frequent meals. Definite confirmation of the diagnosis is difficult and can only really be obtained by arteriography. Because of the diffuse nature of the vascular changes, the possibility of surgical correction is rare, and such investigation can therefore rarely be justified in old age.

ACUTE ON CHRONIC MESENTERIC OCCLUSION

The chronic condition described above may continue for many years and twenty years of symptoms have been recorded. If malabsorption does not occur, the threat to life is small. There is, however, in these patients, the risk that the narrowed vessels will become completely blocked. When this occurs, the resulting damage is often extensive, as the collateral vessels are usually poor. Considerable lengths of bowel will then become necrotic and the picture of acute mesenteric occlusion will then be superimposed on the long-standing chronic history.

ISCHAEMIC COLITIS

A background of generalized vascular disease usually sets the scene for this condition. It should therefore not be surprising that this most commonly affects the elderly. Areas of the large bowel most at risk are those where the major supply vessels anastamose and the blood supply is precarious. The region of the splenic flexure is most frequently affected. The clinical picture consists of abdominal pain, usually left sided, with diarrhoea, which may be blood-stained. An early barium enema may show evidence of ulceration and mucosal swelling, with the typical thumbprinting sign, but this stage can easily be missed.

If the resulting ischaemic area is small and superficial, complete resolution may occur spontaneously. Fibrous constriction may, however, remain as a permanent scar and cause obstruction later.

Treatment will range from symptomatic measures in mild cases, to drip and suck and transfusion in moderate episodes. Only when the ischaemic lesions are more extensive, with a long section of colon becoming gangrenous, will surgical resection be needed. Symptoms in such patients are similar to above, but more dramatic, and the development of peritonitis is a serious prognostic sign, indicating the necessity for surgical treatment.

Inflammatory bowel disease

Crohn's disease and ulcerative colitis are usually thought of as diseases of the young or middle aged. Evidence that these conditions do, however, occur in the elderly, is gradually accumulating. The differentiation between the two conditions does, unfortunately, become even more difficult in the elderly. In old age, Crohn's disease more often affects the large bowel, and biopsy by sigmoidoscopy or colonoscopy may be the only sure way of making a definite diagnosis. Once the diagnosis is established, the management is similar to that of younger patients. More careful supervision will be required in the elderly, as even minor degrees of anaemia or electrolyte imbalance will be poorly tolerated.

Patients with long-standing ulcerative colitis who have retained the whole or part of their colon and survived into old age, also need extra careful follow-up because of the high risk of carcinomatous change.

Degenerative gut disease

The topics to be discussed under this heading are diverticular disease of the large and small bowel, and atrophic gastritis. The causes of all are speculative. The first and third conditions are common in old age, and the second offers simple therapeutic possibilities.

LARGE BOWEL DIVERTICULAR DISEASE

This is a disease of Western society and among Europeans over the age of 80, there is a 50 per cent incidence on radiology. A highly refined low-residue diet is held responsible for the changes which occur in the colon. It is thought that the extra muscle power, and increased colonic motility required for the passage of low bulk stools, results in stretching and blow-outs of the gut wall at weak points. Common symptoms are colicy abdominal pain and alternating diarrhoea and constipation. These diverticula are then liable to colonization by abnormal bacteria, abscess formation, scarring, perforation and bleeding.

If any of the above complications give rise to severe symptoms, or if there is doubt as to whether diverticular disease or malignancy is responsible, then surgical treatment will be required if the patient is otherwise sufficiently fit. In milder cases, dietary modifications with an increase in residue will be enough. However, it is often very difficult to persuade the elderly to make drastic changes in their diet at the age of 80, and wholemeal bread and bran are often unacceptable. In such cases, it is often kinder and more realistic to accept that it is too late to really effect change, but symptomatic relief may be achieved with bulk laxatives, such as Celevac. Anti-spasmodic preparations should generally be avoided in the elderly, because of their anticholinergic side effects.

Large bowel diverticular disease may not only be responsible for bowel symptoms in the elderly, but may also cause acute toxic states, when diverticulitis occurs. This condition may sometimes account for the worrying combination of a low haemoglobin and high ESR often found in geriatric medicine. Because of the very common finding of diverticulosis, it must not always be assumed that it is the cause for the symptoms under investigation.

SMALL BOWEL DIVERTICULAR DISEASE

Although not as common as large bowel diverticula, the incidence is thought to increase with age and to reach levels of 10–20 per cent in the geriatric age range. The duodenum, especially the second part, is more frequently affected than the jejunum.

It is only during the last ten or so years that small bowel diverticula have been thought to be of any significance. Colonization of the pouches by abnormal bacteria may well be the change which makes these lesions potentially troublesome. Such bacteria may deconjugate bile salts, and interfere with fat absorption and the absorption of fat soluble vitamins. Steatorrhoea and osteomalacia are therefore possible modes of presentation. Ulceration of the diverticula may result in blood loss and iron deficiency anaemia, and bacteria present may consume the dietary content of vitamin B_{12} and produce a macrocytic anaemia.

Small bowel diverticula are usually only actively considered if diarrhoea, steatorrhoea or malabsorption is found. Most are found by chance on barium meal carried out for the investigation of dyspepsia. If found and thought to be causing complications, the simplest method of treatment is with a course of broad-spectrum antibiotic such as tetracycline. Follow-up will be required to detect and treat any evidence of recurrence. Surgical removal is another possibility, but rarely required.

ATROPHIC GASTRITIS

Gastric acid secretion falls with age, and present evidence suggests that this is due to a rising incidence of atrophic change. Postulated mechanisms are ageing itself, ischaemia and auto-immune disease. Although some victims will experience dyspeptic symptoms, including nausea and vomiting, the main concern is, however, the risk of pernicious anaemia and malignant change. Treatment is rarely required, unless vitamin B_{12} deficiency is demonstrated; metoclopramide (Maxolon 10 mg thrice daily) may bring symptomatic relief, but carries the risk of producing extra-pyramidal spasticity.

Neoplastic bowel disease

Malignancies of the alimentary tract occur predominantly in the elderly, their incidence clearly rising with age. The elderly are, however, more likely to be disabled due to additional pathology, and investigation is therefore often more difficult. Nevertheless, wherever possible, an accurate diagnosis should be made, as the best patient management will depend on such information. In many cases, the aim should be humane care rather than attempted heroic cure. The care, in some instances, will include palliative radiotherapy or surgery for relief of symptoms.

Certain malignancies are associated with particular risk factors—

(a) *Carcinoma of the stomach*—pernicious anaemia or atrophic gastritis; long-term survivors from previous partial gastrectomy, especially for gastric ulcers.

(b) *Carcinoma of the pancreas*—diabetics.

(c) *Carcinoma of the gall-bladder*—gall-stones.

(d) *Carcinoma of the large bowel*—ulcerative colitis.

For surgical treatments see Chapter 19.

Iatrogenic bowel disease

Sadly, much of gastrointestinal disease in old age is man-made. In some instances, the disease is an unfortunate side-effect of an essential operation carried out many years previously, and often forgotten by the patient. Other cases, unhappily, are the result of misguided advice or therapeutic activity.

Constipation—see Chapter 11.

Complications of abdominal surgery

Here, the success of the original operation has enabled the patient to live long enough to develop permanent structural changes or to develop various deficiency states.

POST-GASTRECTOMY DEFICIENCIES

These are most common in those who underwent a Polya gastrectomy with the production of a blind loop, exposing the patient to the potential risk of steatorrhoea. The responsible mechanism is the deconjugation of bile salts by abnormal bacterial colonization of the blind loop. Vitamin D absorption is then impaired as it is fat soluble, and osteo-malacia may result. Many post-gastrectomy patients are also at risk from developing a vitamin B_{12} deficiency megaloblastic anaemia, due to removal of the intrinsic factor producing area of the stomach, or due to associated atrophic changes. Iron absorption is defective in these patients, and chronic iron deficiency anaemia is especially likely in those patients who had poor iron stores at the time of their operation.

POST-OPERATIVE STRICTURES

If very tight, there is always the risk of obstruction, which will increase as bowel motility reduces with age. Bacterial changes may also occur proximal to the lesion, and if so, small bowel steatorrhoea and mal-absorption may result.

ADHESIONS

These seem a less common cause for late post-operative complications than in the young or middle-aged. However, such lesions may form the basis for an episode of obstruction. A volvulus may also occur due to their presence. Such twisting and dilatation of a loop of large bowel occurs from time to time in aged patients. If diagnosed early, and simply by a straight X-ray of the abdomen, it can sometimes be easily relieved by the passage of a sigmoidoscope or flatus tube. Recurrent, large bowel volvulus sometimes occurs spontaneously in institutionalized old people. Surgical intervention may be required after good pre-operative preparation.

LOSS OF THE TERMINAL ILEUM

The value of the terminal ileum is often overlooked. It is, however, essential for vitamin B_{12} absorption, and for the entero-hepatic circulation of bile salts, and therefore for efficient fat absorption. It is also a region at surgical risk. A patient found to have a caecal carcinoma may also have the terminal ileum removed. This is a disease which carries a favourable prognosis if detected early. Patients, therefore, survive sufficiently long to develop malabsorption of B_{12} and fat. The same area may also be removed with an appendix abscess or in patients with Crohn's disease. Any of these conditions may arise in old age, and long-term follow-up is required.

Complications of dietary advice

We sometimes accuse our patients of not listening to our words of wisdom, but in some instances, patients adhere too strictly to the advice given. This situation is particularly dangerous when doctors are over-dogmatic, and correction of instructions later found to be harmful can be extremely difficult.

ROUGHAGE

If any doctor has any doubt about the fallibility of his profession, he needs only to direct his attention to the topic of dietary advice given to patients with large-bowel diverticular disease. Until quite recently, the patients were instructed to take a low-residue diet, and many have carefully followed the instructions given. Current thought is that such a diet is detrimental, and may even have caused the condition in the first place. If true, these patients have obviously been worsened by their medical attendants.

FAT-FREE DIETS

These have often been advised for middle-aged ladies with a history of gall-stones, and have, on occasions, been so carefully adhered to that deficiency diseases have resulted. Such a diet makes the absorption of fat-soluble vitamins difficult, and patients have been known to develop osteomalacia.

GASTRIC DIETS

Although it is now unfashionable to give strict advice about dietary content to patients with peptic ulcer, this has not always been the practice. Many geriatric patients in their youth were advised to maintain a fish/chicken/milk diet for the sake of their ulcers. Some were trusting enough to have kept to this diet for the rest of their lives, and take a diet deficient especially in vitamin C.

The intestinal complications of drug therapy

The adverse effects of drugs is a recurrent theme in geriatric medicine. The gastrointestinal tract is certainly no exception.

GASTRITIS

Anorexia and epigastric discomfort follow the taking of many pharmaceutical preparations. The elderly, because of the frequency of arthritis, and other painful conditions, consume large quantities of anti-inflammatory analgesics. In many instances, gastric irritation will cause considerable discomfort. Bleeding may also occur, and if acute, it may well prove fatal, if chronic it may severely limit activity, as the resulting iron deficiency anaemia worsens. Oral steroids, in addition to their effect on many other systems, will have the same gastric disadvantages as the anti-inflammatory analgesics.

Digoxin and similar preparations can cause such severe anorexia, nausea and vomiting and weight loss as to mimic gastric carcinoma.

L-dopa is another potent cause of nausea and vomiting. Whether this complication is due to a central or local effect is not yet clearly decided. Results from the combination tablets of L-dopa with a decarboxylase inhibitor suggests that local effects may be of importance.

DIARRHOEA

The use of broad spectrum antibiotics is perhaps the commonest iatrogenic cause of diarrhoea, at least as far as medically prescribed treatment is concerned. Purgative abuse in old age, however, causes much self-inflicted diarrhoea. The over-enthusiastic treatment of myxoedema with thyroxine can also lead to excessive looseness of the bowels. Digoxin may cause this symptom, by its effect on the bowel distal to the stomach, and the diarrhoea may be bloody.

CONSTIPATION

As so many elderly patients already have a tendency to be costive, an awareness of drugs likely to make this symptom more troublesome is essential in geriatric practice. Analgesics, particularly those containing codeine and its derivatives are frequent culprits.

Tricyclic antidepressants and anticholinergic drugs, such as those used in the treatment of parkinsonism can also make a slow bowel worse. In such patients, antacids with aluminium salts are also best avoided. Dehydration due to excessive diuretic administration can also lead to progressive constipation.

JAUNDICE

Drug-induced jaundice is a very important form of painless jaundice in old age. Many drugs can be responsible, but those of the phenothiazine group are most commonly implicated.

Disease of the gall-bladder, liver and pancreas

Disorders of any of these organs are not uncommon in old age. Presentation and management will, in many instances, be the same as in younger subjects. Short notes will therefore only be given to emphasize special points relevant to elderly patients.

Gall-bladder

In old age, the differentiation between ischaemic heart pain, oesophageal pain and gall-bladder disease becomes even more difficult. In many cases, there will be evidence implicating more than one of these sites. Furthermore, the finding of gall-stones does not mean that they are responsible for symptoms. Nevertheless, it has to be accepted that the longer stones are present, the more likely they are to produce symptoms. This argues in favour of the prophylactic removal of stones in an otherwise well, elderly patient. It is not, however, an easy decision, and most surgeons prefer to wait until symptoms arise.

Where the stones are of the cholesterol type, and without evidence of calcification, there is an alternative. If therapeutic doses of bile salts (Chenodeoxycholic acid) are given, cholesterol metabolism can be altered so that the stones 'dissolve'. Treatment needs to be continued for about six months, and so far seems safe and trouble-free, but diarrhoea can be a problem.

Liver disease

Carcinomatosis, drug-induced jaundice and hepatic congestion in heart failure, are the most common liver disorders. Cirrhosis is increasing in the United Kingdom, and occurs in the very old. It is not always cryptogenic but is sometimes alcoholic in origin. Often it is symptomless; the only clue in life may be splenomegaly, the result of portal hypertension. Biochemical changes may also be minimal, and often no more dramatic than the reduced albumin which is so frequently found in geriatric patients.

Pancreatic disease

Pancreatitis becomes a more serious disease with increasing age. Those elderly patients who become shocked, have a very poor prognosis as they are less well able to compensate for the reduction in blood volume. Silent pancreatitis becomes more common in the elderly, and is frequently only diagnosed at post-mortem. It is assumed that ischaemia is a common aetiological factor in cases of pancreatitis in old age, but there is little in the way of conclusive evidence. Hypothermia is a common cause of pancreatitis in this age group.

Chronic pancreatitis and early carcinoma of the pancreas are always difficult diagnoses to confirm. Even more difficulties are encountered when the patient is elderly. In carcinoma of the pancreas, intensive and distressful investigation can therefore rarely be justified. Symptomatic treatment whilst the disease takes its natural course is often the kindest form of management because the results of surgical treatment in carcinoma of the pancreas are poor. In chronic pancreatitis enzyme replacement therapy is worth trying.

Investigation of the alimentary tract in old age

It is essential in geriatric medicine to temper scientific expertise and curiosity with humanity and humility. When investigations are planned for the diagnosis of gut symptoms in old age, the ability of the patient to co-operate and the value of the information to be gained must be carefully balanced against the risks and distress which might be inflicted.

UPPER GASTRO-INTESTINAL INVESTIGATIONS

Tests which may be very helpful are the barium swallow and meal, fibre-optic gastroscopy and isotope investigations for vitamin B_{12} absorption. Tests of acid secretion and pancreatic function are all possible, but make considerable demands on the patient, and usually contribute little to the management in the elderly.

Barium studies of the oesophasgus, stomach and duodenum can be easily performed in even very ill and frail patients. Although the quality of films obtained is not as good as in younger subjects, valuable information can be gathered which will significantly affect the patient's management, and that of her relatives.

Cineradiography can also be useful in assessing elderly patients with the common symptom of dysphagia. Neuromuscular inco-ordination is often successfully demonstrated as the only abnormality.

If further confirmation is required of dubious X-ray findings, then gastroscopy may provide the complete answer. With the introduction of flexible fibre-optic instruments, the dangers of the earlier rigid instruments have been abolished. When the patient has been carefully premedicated, the procedure can be both speedy and without distress. In addition to direct visualization, histological evidence can also be obtained in many instances. In the hands of an experienced operator, all areas of the oesophagus, stomach and duodenum can be examined with ease. Skilled endoscopists can even enter the pancreatic duct and gain information about possible obstructive lesions.

The only commonly performed test of absorption involving the upper gastrointestinal tract, is the measurement of vitamin B_{12}, and in particular, evaluation of the availability of gastric intrinsic factor. The commercially prepared double isotope packs, with half the labelled vitamin B_{12} bound to intrinsic factor, is the most convenient. The most valuable advantage of this system is that a complete 24-hour sample of urine is not required for the differentiation of a gastric from a terminal ileal defect. As the accuracy of 24-hour collections in old age is often very poor, and as the majority of cases of vitamin B_{12} deficiency are due to gastric lesions, the double isotope will often give a complete and easy confirmation of the diagnosis of Addisonian pernicious anaemia. It is the ratio of the isotopes recovered from the urine which helps in the differentiation of pernicious anaemia from the other causes of B_{12} malabsorption.

SMALL BOWEL TESTS

These are predominantly carried out to confirm or exclude malabsorption. A follow through barium meal in the elderly will often be very time-consuming for the radiologist, due to slow transit, and very tiring to an old frail patient. Such an examination should not therefore be requested lightly, but only if there is true clinical or laboratory evidence to suggest malabsorption—(i.e. reduced red-cell folate, low serum albumin, low serum iron and biochemical evidence of osteomalacia—not necessarily all of these together, but at least two). The most likely valuable finding is identification of small bowel diverticula.

Laboratory function tests for malabsorption are usually of little use in old age, because of difficulties in obtaining complete and accurate collections of urine and faeces. Also, most tests are dependent on all other systems, especially the kidneys, being in perfect working order, and this is obviously not the case in many geriatric patients.

The standard xylose test is unreliable because of concurrent renal impairment. However, if the results of urinary excretion after both oral and intravenous loading with xylose are compared, relevant conclusions can be drawn about small bowel function even when severe renal impairment is present. The ratio of 5-hour urinary excretion after 25 G of xylose orally to the 5-hour excretion after 5 G intravenously is usually greater than 1·8:1 in fasting normal subjects.

Small bowel biopsies are rarely of much use in the management of geriatric patients. Minor variations from normal are very common, but the significance of this finding is unknown. Even when the grossly atrophic appearances of coeliac disease are found, it is not possible to justify a strict gluten-free diet. If bowel symptoms are present, they can usually be relieved symptomatically, and vitamin deficiencies can easily be corrected. The prevention of the long-term risk of carcinomatous change is irrelevant in this context.

LARGE BOWEL INVESTIGATIONS

Although barium swallows and meals can be carried out in even demented patients, the situation concerning barium enemata is quite different. Full and prolonged co-operation is required, and will not be available from a distressed patient unable to understand the reasons and necessity for such a socially unacceptable procedure. When contrast studies of the large bowel are thought to be necessary, the usual preliminary sequence of rectal examination and sigmoidoscopy should of course be followed. The use of the fibre-optic colonoscope may provide geriatric medicine with a very valuable tool for investigating this region of the bowel, which so often in old age is full of pathology. There may, however, be considerable problems in bowel preparation before colonoscopic examination in the very old. The essential large bowel preparation makes both these investigations inpatient procedures.

CHAPTER 16 · ENDOCRINE, METABOLIC AND RENAL DISORDERS

> I have often been credibly told
> That when people are awfully old,
> Though cigars are a curse
> And strong waters are worse,
> There is nothing as fatal as cold.

> *Obiter Dicta*
> from 'Selected Cautionary Verses',
> by HILAIRE BELLOC

In the main, these diseases are discussed fully in works on general medicine, so that only those conditions occurring particularly frequently, or presenting distinctive features in elderly persons, will be mentioned here.

Diabetes mellitus

Incidence and definition

Diabetes mellitus is an extremely common disease in all ages. Although it is often detected as an incidental finding in the elderly, it heightens the susceptibility to infection and may thus lead to overt ill health. The specific complications of the disease are more serious, and they affect the peripheral nerves, the arteries, the kidneys, and the eyes: some of these complications have indeed been described as an acceleration of the normal ageing process.

There seems to be a steady decline in glucose tolerance with increasing age, and in a large-scale population survey in Bedford it was found that the incidence of abnormal glucose tolerance tests among subjects aged seventy or more was greater than 50 per cent. The definition of a diabetic curve, at best arbitrary, thus becomes almost meaningless in old age, and it is now recognized that every gradation exists between unequivocally pathological hyperglycaemia on the one hand, and unequivocally normal glucose tolerance on the other (Table 16.1). All intermediate values represent a state of 'impaired glucose tolerance', and very many elderly subjects come into this category, which carries a risk of complications.

Table 16.1 Diagnostic criteria using 75 g oral glucose load
(Source: WHO 1980)

		Glucose concentration (mmol/l)		
		Venous blood	Capillary blood	Venous plasma
Diabetes mellitus	Fasting and/or 2 h after load	≥7 ≥10	≥7 ≥11	≥8 (2 occasions) ≥11 (140 mg in USA)
Impaired glucose tolerance	Fasting *and* 2 h after load	<7 7-10	<7 8-11	<8 8-11
Diabetes excluded	Fasting			<6 (115 mg% in USA)

The classical symptoms are polyuria due to osmotic diuresis, and thirst due to the resulting dehydration. A habitual jug of water on the bedside table which has been half emptied by morning is strongly suggestive, and weight loss and pruritus vulvae should also arouse suspicion. Fortunately it is seldom necessary to proceed to a full glucose tolerance test, as a random blood sugar of 10 mmol/l (180 mg/100 ml) or more is to all intents and purposes diagnostic.

Among the elderly, it is unusual to find an underlying cause for diabetes, although certain drugs may precipitate, unmask, or aggravate the condition. These include the corticosteroids, and also diuretics of the benzothiadiazine group, which appear to inhibit directly insulin secretion by the islet cells.

Diabetics in geriatric practice can be divided into the following categories:

1 Patients diagnosed earlier in life
  (a) The young, insulin-dependent diabetic, of 'juvenile-onset' type. Those who reach old age should by then know far more about their own disease than any doctor, and it takes a brave man to suggest any alteration in regime.
  (b) The middle-aged who contracted the 'maturity onset' non-insulin dependent form of the disease. These subjects may have been satisfactorily controlled by dietary restriction of calories and carbohydrates, or they may have been stabilized on one of the oral hypoglycaemic drugs.
2 Patients diagnosed in old age
  (a) Chemical diabetics, picked up on a chance finding of glycosuria, who may need no special dietary or other restriction.

(b) Those who are grossly overweight and who are best managed by an attempt at weight reduction.

(c) Patients who require drug therapy because they still have glycosuria and marked hyperglycaemia even when the calorie and carbohydrate intake has been sharply curtailed in an effort to lose weight—and patients who were not significantly over-weight in the first place. Occasionally, fulminant diabetes of the 'juvenile-onset' type presents in old age, when insulin will be imperative just as it is in the young.

Treatment

The first principle in the management of diabetes is the education of the patient, and the second is the control of the diet. It must be confessed that both these measures are often unsatisfactory and some sort of compromise is the only realistic aim. Perfect control is in any case unnecessary, as a fairly short-term view can be taken.

The same limitations apply to drug treatment, and it is over-ambitious to try to eliminate glycosuria. The renal threshold is very variable in this age group, so that blood sugars are the only reliable guidelines to control. Over-treatment is far more dangerous than under-treatment, and the hazards of hypoglycaemia must be avoided, as confusion, coma, and possibly permanent neurological damage can ensue. Hypoglycaemia is often atypical in its presentation in elderly people. It is therefore safer to allow some glycosuria to persist.

There are two groups of oral drugs available for the treatment of diabetes:

I SULPHONYLUREAS

These compounds, including the closely related sulphapyrimidine glymidine, stimulate insulin production by the pancreatic beta cells (Table 16.2). Side effects include flushing with alcohol, and severe and

Table 16.2. Sulphonylureas and related drugs

Proper name	Trade name	Daily dose (mg)	Number of doses
Tolbutamide	Rastinon	500–2000	2–3
Chlorpropamide	Diabinese	100–375	1
Acetohexamide	Dimelor	250–1500	1–3
Tolazamide	Tolanase	100–750	1–2
Glymidine	Gondafon	500–2000	Usually 1
Glibenclamide	Daonil	2·5–20	1
Glipizide	Glibenese	2·5–30	Initially 1
Glibornuride	Glutril	12·5–75	Usually 1

insidious hypoglycaemia, both associated especially with chlorpropamide which has a long duration of action. Tolbutamide is therefore favoured and the newer agents seem to offer no particular advantage over it. A report from the USA that these drugs might lead to an increase in cardiovascular deaths has not carried sufficient conviction in this country to curtail their use.

2 BIGUANIDES

Phenformin is especially liable to cause lactic acidosis and is now seldom used. Metformin ('Glucophage') 1 g twice or thrice daily may be given in addition to one of the sulphonylureas if adequate control is not achieved at maximal dosage but it is hoped to avoid having recourse to insulin. The usefulness of the biguanides is restricted by their tendency to cause gastrointestinal intolerance, lactic acidosis, and folic acid and vitamin B12 deficiency.

Hyperosmolar non-ketoacidotic crisis

This complication seems to be confined to middle-aged and elderly patients with maturity-onset diabetes. Many of these patients have not previously been recognized as being diabetic, and initially present with this crisis, which may be of gradual or sudden onset. The clinical picture is of increasing weakness, drowsiness, confusion and coma, associated with an osmotic diuresis which leads to profound dehydration. The resulting thirst is occasionally slaked with Lucozade which will exacerbate the situation. There is, however, no acidosis and therefore no air-hunger. Hypotension is often profound. Biochemical disturbances generally include extreme hyperglycaemia and hypernatraemia. The sheet-anchors of treatment are insulin and intravenous half-normal saline. The insulin is given intramuscularly 20 units stat followed by 5 units every hour until the blood sugar level falls to 14 mmol/l (250 mg/100 ml). Then a change is made to subcutaneous insulin on a sliding scale related to the urinary glucose level (six-hourly injections: 20–30 units if urine sugar 2 per cent, 16 units if 1 per cent, 6–12 units if under 1 per cent). The saline, which may be isotonic if the serum sodium is under 155 mmol/l, is run in under central venous pressure monitoring. Some authorities recommend heparinization because of the high risk of widespread intravascular thrombosis. The mortality remains high, but those who do recover can often be managed perfectly satisfactorily thereafter by means of diet and oral hypoglycaemic drugs.

Other diabetic crises

Diabetic ketoacidosis occurs in elderly diabetics just as in other age groups, and is treated along similar lines. It carries a higher mortality (over 50 per cent).

Hypoglycaemia is especially hazardous since it may produce permanent neurological deficits, particularly intellectual, and it may result from the injudicious use of insulin or the sulphonylureas.

The thyroid gland

Next to diabetes, thyroid disorders are the most common endocrine diseases to affect old people. Disorders of thyroid function are often difficult to diagnose, but they are among the conditions in this age group which are usually very rewarding to treat. Geriatrics is a predominantly 'female' specialty, and thyroid disease favours the female sex at all ages, but old men are not uncommonly affected. Overactivity and under-activity of the gland occur with approximately equal frequency.

Thyrotoxicosis

The characteristic features of heat intolerance, diffuse goitre, exophthalmos, hot, sweaty, trembling hands, and a high cardiac output, are usually inconspicuous or lacking in older subjects, when the disorder more often presents as hidden thyrotoxicosis. The eye signs which so often attract medical attention in the young are seldom obvious in the elderly. Although there is usually no true exophthalmos or lid retraction, the eyes do give a rather bright and staring expression. This, in conjunction with the hollow cheeks and cachectic appearance, results in confusion with other wasting diseases. Typical Graves' disease does sometimes occur, even in old age; but hyperthyroidism in the old is usually of the secondary type, complicating a pre-existing nodular gland. This may be large and obvious, but usually it is small and difficult to detect, especially if it is retrosternal. The term 'masked' thyrotoxicosis is more properly reserved for a monosystemic presentation, usually cardiac. In any event, the clinical picture is likely to be non-specific, and may include any combination of the following manifestations:

I CARDIAC

Cardiac failure of obscure origin should arouse suspicion, especially if precipitated by a supraventricular tachyarrhythmia. Atrial fibrillation is the most common of these, and the ventricular rate may be resistant to control with digoxin but often responds better to the beta-adrenergic blocking drugs.

2 WEIGHT LOSS

This highly significant symptom may go completely unnoticed in the elderly, or it may be regarded as natural, or concealed by fluid retention. It may also be produced by many other conditions.

3 GASTROINTESTINAL

Diarrhoea in thyrotoxicosis is probably due to intestinal hurry. It may be associated with anorexia, nausea, vomiting, and abdominal pain, and closely mimic a gastrointestinal neoplasm.

4 NEUROMUSCULAR

The presenting feature may be muscular weakness and wasting, which may amount to a true myopathy, mainly affecting the limb girdle musculature.

5 PSYCHIATRIC

As with so many diseases in old age, the rapid onset of confusion or psychosis is often the psychiatric tip of an organic iceberg.

6 APATHETIC THYROTOXICOSIS

There is a small group of hyperthyroid subjects in whom apathy, depression, and lethargy predominate, and who may progress, in the absence of appropriate treatment, to coma and death. The skin is dry and cool. There is marked muscle wasting or myopathy, and ptosis occurs rather than exophthalmos. Tremor is absent, and the disease is sometimes so atypical that hypothyroidism may be suspected, but atrial fibrillation and profound weight loss should indicate the true state of affairs.

Diagnosis

The diagnosis depends on a high index of suspicion, and requires laboratory confirmation. At the time of writing, the serum thyroxine in conjunction with the free thyroxine index appears to be the most reliable investigation. Ideally, radioimmunoassay of serum triiodothyronine (T3) should be requested as well in order to pick up the occasional patient with T3-toxicosis.

Treatment

When the diagnosis is not in doubt and in the absence of pressure symptoms from a goitre, irradiation with I^{131} or I^{125} is recommended for the elderly because of its ease and simplicity. However, this form of treatment is undeniably something of a hit-and-miss affair, even when the dose is related to the size of the gland, as some 25 per cent of patients require a second dose, and about 50 per cent are hypothyroid ten years later. The insidious and often late onset of this hypothyroidism necessitates life-long observation. Another characteristic of treatment with radio-iodine is that it takes two or three months to become effective, so that, if rapid control is required, for instance because of heart failure, it is worthwhile using antithyroid drug therapy until control is achieved. Carbimazole is the agent of choice, and it is withdrawn for two or three days before and after I^{131} administration, then gradually reduced in dose. The initial dose is 10 to 15 mg eight hourly. The other advantage of drug treatment is that it can be used as a therapeutic trial, and the response to treatment may confirm the diagnosis when physical signs and biochemical investigations have been inconclusive. Rapid symptomatic relief may be achieved by the non-specific use of beta-blockers to suppress end-organ response.

Hypothyroidism

Florid myxoedema is the easiest of all conditions to recognize—for everyone except the family doctor! Its onset and progression are so insidious that anyone who sees the patient regularly is in the worst possible position to appreciate what is at once apparent to the stranger. The patient is for the same reason unlikely to seek advice, and in any case becomes too befuddled to do so. The family either fail to notice the changes wrought by the illness, or accept the gradual slowing down of all bodily and mental functions as part of the natural ageing process. Until recently the diagnosis of hypothyroidism was an easy one. It is becoming less so now that it is realized that hypothyroidism is not an all-or-none phenomenon but that earlier stages of diminished reserve and subclinical hypothyroidism can be identified. Pre-myxoedema may carry an increased risk of coronary artery disease, and can be demonstrated by finding a raised level of circulating thyroid stimulating hormone (TSH).

Aetiology

There are many uncommon causes of hypothyroidism, but only three types which are important in the elderly.

I AUTO-IMMUNE

It is now clear that the majority of cases of so-called idiopathic myxo-edema are in fact of auto-immune origin, and there is an association with other disorders of similar aetiology such as pernicious anaemia. There seems to be an overlap of both clinical and serological manifestations among the chronic organ-specific diseases, which also include idiopathic Addison's disease and some forms of chronic hepatitis and diabetes mellitus. Vitiligo shows a highly significant association with this group of diseases although the precise causation of the vitiligo remains far from clear.

2 IATROGENIC

Before effective treatment became available for thyrotoxicosis, a natural remission occurred in some 30 per cent of patients, and this was sometimes followed by the development of myxoedema. This may have been in the group of patients in whom the thyrotoxicosis represented the early phase of Hashimoto's disease. Hypothyroidism may likewise follow the successful treatment of hyperthyroidism. Attention has already been drawn to the magnitude of the risk after irradiation, but it should be trivial with properly supervised drug therapy. It is now becoming clear that thyroidectomy carries a high risk of this complication, perhaps 10–20 per cent. It may occur within a year due to the extirpation of too much thyroid tissue. Sometimes hypothyroidism develops several years after surgery due to slow progression of the auto-immune process. Raised TSH levels will indicate those at high risk of becoming hypothyroid following treatment with I^{131} or operation.

3 SECONDARY

Hypothyroidism secondary to hypopituitarism is occasionally seen. The appearance is more often of someone who is pale, and hairless rather than puffy with mucinous oedema. Hypopituitarism is a well-recognized complication of postpartum haemorrhage, and a history of inability to breast-feed and the failure of the menses to recommence following childbirth is particularly suggestive. However, the disorder may present in old age due to pituitary destruction by a slowly growing lesion such as a craniopharyngioma. Hypopituitarism is often initially selective, and the term panhypopituitarism should be reserved for patients whose secretion of gonadotrophic, adrenocorticotrophic, thyrotrophic and growth hormones have all been shown to be defective.

Clinical features

The clinical picture of classical myxoedema needs no description here, but there is the occasional atypical presentation. Coma or hypothermia are examples, although myxoedema is only a rare cause of either. Other neurological manifestations include cerebellar ataxia and psychiatric disturbance—the so-called 'myxoedema madness'. Pain and tingling in the hand, due to carpal tunnel syndrome, occasionally stimulates the patient to seek advice. Pericardial and other serous effusions are uncommon but serious complications which may be responsible for referral to hospital. In younger patients, one of the most useful pointers to this disease is the delayed relaxation of the tendon reflexes, which can be recorded graphically. Unfortunately, in the elderly, frequent loss of reflexes, coarse somatic tremor, and oedematous extremities combine to militate against the successful recording of the reflexes.

Treatment

Replacement therapy has to be instituted extremely slowly because of the danger of cardiac arrest. Some clinicians are hesitant to institute treatment in the presence of severe angina. However, the angina may be the result of the hypothyroidism, and it often improves with treatment of the underlying disease, although even more caution than usual must be exercised.

The starting dose of thyroxine is 50 micrograms daily, and it is increased by 50 micrograms at intervals of two weeks until a maintenance dose of 150–250 micrograms daily is reached. The transformation in the appearance and health of the patient is one of the most gratifying experiences in geriatric medicine.

The pituitary and adrenal glands

1 **Hypopituitarism** is uncommon in old age, but the pituitary may be destroyed by metastases or auto-immune hypophysitis in addition to the conditions already referred to. Although always mentioned among the causes of coma, it must be regarded as an exceedingly rare one.

2 **Cushing's syndrome** is usually iatrogenic in this age group. Prolonged corticosteroid administration in doses greater than the equivalent physiological secretion of cortisol inevitably results in the well-known side-effects, among which osteoporosis is likely to be particularly painful. Sudden withdrawal must never be attempted but if there is no clinical indication for continuing the drug a gradual

reduction in dosage should be contemplated. It may then be possible to withdraw the drug altogether even after many years of treatment. Unfortunately there is no simple way of testing the integrity of the entire hypothalamus-pituitary-adrenal axis because insulin-induced hypoglycaemia is particularly hazardous in elderly patients.

The other form of Cushing's syndrome encountered in geriatric practice is the biochemical variety which occasionally complicates oat-cell carcinoma of the bronchus. These patients seldom survive long enough to develop the characteristic physical appearance and the clinical picture is usually dominated by the biochemical disturbances, particularly hypokalaemic alkalosis. Profound muscle weakness will be the main extra-pulmonary symptom.

3 **Addison's disease** is very uncommon at any age, but is occasionally encountered among the very old. It may complicate tuberculosis, or carcinomatosis, but it is much more likely to be due to adrenal atrophy. Adreno-cortical insufficiency much more commonly results from the injudicious withdrawal of steroid therapy.

Hypothermia

Although not usually an endocrine disorder, hypothermia can be conveniently considered here. Accidental hypothermia has recently received increasing publicity, and the old are especially vulnerable. Indeed, among younger and fitter subjects, it is virtually confined to those who court exposure to sea or snow—including 'wet walkers on windy uplands'.

Definition

Accidental hypothermia is said to occur if the temperature of the body core is unintentionally allowed to fall below 35°C.

Diagnosis

This requires a high index of suspicion. If the oral temperature is low or the patient's abdomen cold to the touch, then the rectal temperature must be taken over a period of five minutes, using a thermometer registering down as far as 25°C.

Aetiology

The predominant factors in the causation of hypothermia are a low environmental temperature and defective thermoregulation. The old tend to be too poor to maintain the temperature of the external environment and too inefficient homoeostatically to maintain the temperature of the internal environment. In a national survey 75 per cent of the sample of elderly people's houses had living-room temperatures at or below 18·3°C and 90 per cent were below 21°C, even in the absence of unduly severe weather. The main reasons why the old are so vulnerable to accidental hypothermia can be summarized as follows:

Poverty and high fuel costs

Habits—open bedroom windows, unaccustomed to adequate heating

Unawareness of cold—do not wrap up, move about, close windows, light fire

Autonomic failure—inability to increase heat production by shivering
          —inability to decrease heat loss by cutaneous vasoconstriction

Medical factors—strokes and falls resulting in the victim lying helpless on the ground all night
      —drugs: in particular, phenothiazines, barbiturates, alcohol
      —infrequently, complicating myxoedema.

Incidence

This remains a matter of conjecture, but there are some 400 to 500 deaths annually attributable to hypothermia, mainly among the old. Many more must go unrecorded. According to one estimate, there were no fewer than 9,000 hospital admissions due to this condition during three winter months in the United Kingdom.

Clinical features

Between 35 and 30°C the mortality is about 33 per cent, but below 30° the mortality rises to 70 per cent. Below 32° there is usually some clouding of consciousness, and early signs are sluggishness of movement, thought and speech. All these patients therefore give a strong impression of hypothyroidism. Rigidity of the limbs, oliguria, bradycardia, and hypotension are commonly found. The electro-cardiogram characteristically shows 'J' waves at the junction of the QRS complex and the S-T segment. Vomiting may occur, and pancreatitis is a complication more often detected at autopsy than during life. Hypoglycaemia occasionally develops, particularly during rewarming, and it is important to be alert to this possibility.

Management

1 WARMING

This is the sheet-anchor of treatment but also one of the greatest sources of danger. In the presence of hypotension despite marked cutaneous vasoconstriction, rapid warming is likely to produce vasodilation with a catastrophic further drop in the blood pressure. However, below 30° the danger of ventricular fibrillation is so high anyway that some authorities feel that the risks of rapid rewarming are justified in the presence of profound hypothermia.

Normally, therefore, the aim is to rewarm at the rate of $\frac{1}{2}$ to 1°C hourly, while carefully monitoring the blood pressure. This is best achieved by wrapping the patient in a metallized reflective blanket and nursing her in a room at about 25°. An indwelling rectal probe is used for continuous core temperature observation. If the blood pressure falls, the patient is temporarily recooled.

2 SUPPORTIVE

Fluids are given intravenously only if there is clinical evidence of dehydration. Intubation and instrumentation are in general avoided as far as possible because of the danger of provoking ventricular fibrillation. Oxygen is usually given. Cardiac monitoring is useful because dysrhythmia are very common.

3 MEDICATION

Most centres recommend the administration of intravenous hydrocortisone in large doses on the grounds that this measure is at least likely to be harmless, even though there is no evidence that it is of great benefit. Tri-iodothyronine is a dangerous drug and should not be given in the absence of convincing evidence of hypothyroidism—which is very hard to come by in this situation. A broad spectrum antibiotic should be given prophylactically.

Prevention

Elderly people not fortunate enough to live in centrally heated accommodation should be encouraged to install some form of effective, safe heating such as convector heaters or night storage heaters, for which an allowance from the DHSS may be available. Adequate and sensible clothing is also very important. Half of the body's heat loss is from the head, so the night-caps of a bygone era had a sound scientific basis. The wearing of headgear, bedsocks, mittens and long underwear should be encouraged, and a low voltage electric overblanket is both safe and effective.

Effects of heat

The defective homoeostasis which renders the aged vulnerable to a cold external environment renders them equally ineffectual at adapting to the opposite extreme. Although it might be supposed that this would present a fairly minor problem in the UK, it is well documented that mortality rates in this age group soar during heat waves. In other countries, notably the USA, reports of heat stroke in the elderly have appeared. Body temperatures in this condition range from 40 to 43·3 °C. In the young, heat illness follows physical exertion, but in the old, very hot weather alone is a sufficient cause.

Renal disease

The two most important factors likely to cause damage to the kidneys in old age are infection and back pressure due to obstruction. These two factors result in pyelonephritis and obstructive nephropathy respectively, and the two are frequently associated. Other kidney disorders occur from time to time, but are commoner in earlier life. An exception is perhaps **renal amyloidosis** which should be considered when routine testing reveals heavy proteinuria. The underlying disorders (myelomatosis, rheumatoid disease, chronic pressure sores) are commonly encountered.

Whatever the underlying disease, renal function in the old is especially susceptible to impairment through pre-renal factors. Dehydration in particular is likely to precipitate renal failure, as tubular function diminishes with age, and the ageing kidney is less able to concentrate the urine in response to fluid deprivation. There is also a reduction in the glomerular filtration rate in late life, and a creatinine clearance of 50 ml per minute in the ninth decade is perfectly compatible with a normal blood urea and does not then indicate renal disease. It is likely that there is a fall-off in the number of functioning nephrons.

There is also some evidence that osmoreceptor function becomes impaired in many elderly people, who are thus less likely to respond to an increase in plasma osmolality by increasing their fluid intake. Because they are unlikely to complain of thirst, it behoves nursing and medical staff responsible for the care of the old and immobile to try to encourage an intake of 1·5 to 2 litres a day. The elderly are also susceptible to arterial hypotension due to cardiogenic, bacterial, or oligaemic shock and these conditions are also likely to lead to pre-renal uraemia (Table 16.3).

Table 16.3. Differential diagnosis of oliguria (urine output under 400 ml/24 hours)

	Pre-renal ('Incipient' renal failure)	Established acute renal failure	Post-renal
Clinical features	Dry. BP ↓ . CVP ↓	Fluid overload likely to develop	Bladder may be ↑ . If in doubt, catheterize to exclude low obstruction and arrange urography to exclude high obstruction (pyelogram may be delayed 12–14 hours)
Urine protein	±	+ +	
Serum K	Often normal	↑	
Urine: plasma osmolality	>1·5:1	<1·1:1	
Urine: plasma urea	>10:1	<10:1	
Urine Na mmol/l	<20	>40	
Response to i.v. saline/dextran/ plasma or mannitol 10% 150 ml and/or frusemide 80 mg	Output increases to 40 ml/hour	Little or no increase in output: CVP ↑	

Pyelonephritis

Pyelonephritis is generally caused by ascending infection from the lower urinary tract, and it not uncommonly progresses to death in chronic renal failure. At post-mortem, the kidneys are typically small and scarred with focal inflammation and interstitial fibrosis. Neurological disorders of the bladder, catheterization, bladder neck obstruction, and diabetes mellitus are among the predisposing factors. In its most acute and severe form, there may be fever, rigors, loin pain and dysuria or haematuria: very often, however, the disease presents in the undramatic, rather non-specific way so typical in geriatric medicine, and confusion and incontinence should arouse suspicion.

The commonest causative organism is E. coli, but proteus, pseudomonas, staphylococci, and streptococci are also common pathogens in the urinary tract. To establish the diagnosis, it is necessary to examine a fresh mid-stream urine specimen, which will contain protein, pus cells, and organisms in numbers exceeding 100,000 per ml. Counts between 10,000 and 100,000 or mixed growths may be due to contamination and should be repeated.

The treatment is to maintain a high fluid intake and to give the appropriate chemotherapeutic agent. The sulphonamides are often effective against coliform bacilli, but amoxycillin or ampicillin, septrin, or nalidixic acid may be used. Tetracycline, despite its wide range of activity, is probably best avoided because of its notorious liability to drastically impair renal function, although doxycycline is safe in renal failure. Nitrofurantoin should not be prescribed for patients with renal failure because of the enhanced risk of peripheral neuropathy. It may also cause liver damage and more rarely, pulmonary alveolitis. The drug is, in any case, poorly excreted in the urine and seldom reaches concentrations sufficient to inhibit bacterial growth.

One complication which may arise with dramatic suddenness is **Gram negative septicaemia,** which may lead to bacteraemic shock. As the name implies, this is associated with profound circulatory collapse, and intravenous fluids and large doses of intravenous hydrocortisone should be given in addition to parenteral antibiotics.

Obstructive nephropathy

Urinary tract obstruction most commonly affects the male, due to benign or malignant enlargement of the prostate. Men are also liable to urethral strictures and women to pelvic tumours, but in both sexes, the cause may be neurogenic. At the ureteric level, stones and tumours can give rise to unilateral obstruction, affecting the ipsilateral kidney. A rare disease which causes bilateral ureteric obstruction is retroperitoneal fibrosis. This is a disease of the middle aged and elderly, and although usually idiopathic, there is evidence that it may be associated with the administration of certain beta adrenoreceptor blocking drugs. The condition leads to oliguric renal failure or hydronephrosis.

Whatever the cause, the effect of ureteric obstruction is to cause the kidney to enlarge, due to dilatation of the pelvis and calyces, and eventually there is destruction of the parenchyma. A hydronephrosis is likely to become infected and progress to pyonephrosis.

Pain in the loin is a classical but infrequent complaint, and when the obstructing lesion is low enough to cause bilateral renal involvement, these patients may not even complain of urinary symptoms. On questioning, a history suggestive of retention with overflow may be forthcoming. Sometimes, however, the presentation is in chronic renal failure, often with a degree of uraemia and polyuria leading to dehydration. Palpation of the bladder is thus a very important aspect of the examination of the abdomen.

It is very important to remember the possibility of obstructive nephropathy in patients with evidence of renal disease because of the therapeutic implications. Even after three or four months of unilateral ureteric occlusion, surgical relief of the obstruction is likely to lead to an improvement in renal function.

Analgesic nephropathy

Although it is by no means confined to old age, a mention must be made of the chronic interstitial nephritis which occurs in association with the long-term consumption of analgesics, especially those containing phenacetin. Many elderly people do take large quantities of analgesics, often purchased over the counter, because of the ills that ageing flesh is heir to, such as spondylosis, osteoporosis, and rheumatoid or osteo-arthritis. The pathological changes are papillary necrosis and later renal scarring with interstitial fibrosis, glomerular hyalinization, and severe tubular atrophy.

The clinical features are often indistinguishable from those of chronic pyelonephritis, and include polyuria, polydipsia and nocturia. Ureteric colic and haematuria are frequent, but proteinuria is absent or slight. Sterile pyuria in particular should nowadays lead the clinician to suspect this condition before he thinks of renal tuberculosis. The presence of dyspepsia or hypochromic anaemia may be additional pointers to a history of analgesic abuse, which is seldom volunteered.

The importance of recognition of this disease is the favourable response to withdrawal of the causative agent, which generally leads to some improvement in renal function. The consequence of continued ingestion, however, will be progression to renal failure.

Disturbances of fluid and electrolyte balance

Retention and depletion of salt and water

Oedema is a commonplace finding in geriatric practice, and its causes have been discussed (Table 14.1). It often, but not automatically, requires treatment with diuretics and occasionally mild restriction of salt intake.

Dehydration implies salt and water depletion more often than predominant salt loss or predominant water loss (Table 16.4). As has been stressed, old people are prone to dehydration, and the assessment of tissue turgor should be part of the routine examination. Persuading your patient to eat and drink plenty is another matter!

Hyponatraemia

This is a frequent biochemical abnormality among elderly patients admitted to hospital. It sometimes reflects the severity of the illness, especially in the presence of dehydration: severe cardiac failure and

Table 16.4. Causes and features of salt and water depletion

	Mixed	Mainly water	Mainly salt
Causes	G.I. loss 　Diarrhoea 　Vomiting 　Obstruction 　Fistula Urine loss 　Diuretics 　Diabetes mellitus 　Addison's disease 　Chronic renal 　　failure 　Hypercalcaemia Sweating 　Heat exhaustion	Failure to drink 　Not thirsty 　Immobile 　Depressed 　Demented 　Nauseated 　Self-neglect 　Wish to postpone 　　micturition 　Coma Unable to swallow 　Oesophageal stricture 　Pseudobulbar palsy Urine loss 　Diabetes insipidus	Salt and water loss replaced by water
Features	Compartment mainly affected ≡ ECF. Hence: Confusion Weakness Loss of tissue 　turgor Postural 　hypotension Tachycardia Relative 　polycythaemia	Compartment mainly affected ≡ICF thus protecting ECF in fit subjects. Hence: Confusion Weakness Thirst Drowsiness	Compartment mainly affected ≡ECF

diuretic therapy are other causes, and Addison's disease turns up from time to time.

The other basis for this finding which should be remembered is **inappropriate secretion of antidiuretic hormone** (ADH) which leads to dilutional hyponatraemia and should be suspected if urine osmolality exceeds that of the plasma. The intracellular overhydration may culminate in confusion, convulsions, and coma, which should be treated with intravenous hypertonic saline. Originally described as a complication of oat cell bronchogenic carcinoma, it also occurs in association with pneumonia, pulmonary tuberculosis, islet cell carcinoma of the pancreas, hypothyroidism, and various diseases of the central nervous system including infections, metastatic tumours and strokes: certain drugs are known to stimulate ADH production, including chlorpropamide and indomethacin. The diagnosis is supported by failure to excrete a water load. Water restriction or demethylchlortetracycline (which blocks the action of ADH on the distal tubule) are helpful in the management, if the underlying cause cannot be corrected.

Potassium

Hyperkalaemia, though exceedingly dangerous, is seldom seen except as a complication of renal failure or of treatment with potassium-sparing diuretics.

Hypokalaemia is a specific disturbance of electrolyte balance requiring special consideration. Potassium depletion is frequently encountered in geriatric practice, and the following causes should be borne in mind (and are compounded by poor renal conservation):

Vomiting
Diarrhoea (including (a) purgative abuse and (b) villous adenoma of rectum with leakage of mucus)
Diuretic therapy
Carbenoxolone therapy
Cushing's syndrome (especially due to carcinoma of bronchus)
Dietary deficiency—rare except in the elderly

The principal effect of hypokalaemia is profound weakness of skeletal muscle which may lead to immobility, and which is associated with sluggish or absent deep tendon reflexes. Hypokalaemia is also important because it enhances myocardial sensitivity to digitalis and thereby increases the likelihood of toxicity and dangerous arrhythmia. Potassium deficiency is treated (or, preferably, prevented) by giving one of the many available preparations of potassium salts. The chloride is more effective than an organic compound, particularly if there is a tendency to hypochloraemic alkalosis. Potassium chloride is unpleasant to take and may cause dyspepsia, and enteric coated tablets can cause intestinal ulceration. It is therefore usually given in a slow release form such as potassium chloride slow tablets ('Slow-K') (8 mmol potassium each) or as potassium chloride effervescent tablets ('Sando-K') (12 mmol potassium each). The daily dose should be 24–48 mmol.

CHAPTER 17 · BLOOD DISORDERS AND
MALIGNANT DISEASE

Other things are all very well in their way, but give me
blood!

Mr Waterbrook in *David Copperfield*
by CHARLES DICKENS, 1812–1870

Causes and frequency of anaemia

Anaemia is common in the elderly, but it is not part of the ageing process
as was once believed. Many studies on 'run of the mill' admissions to
departments of geriatric medicine have shown an incidence of 30–40 per
cent using 12 g/dl as the lower limit of normal. However, fit old people
have a normal blood picture. A study of healthy old people, living in
their own homes in Cambridge, found mean levels for haemoglobin of
14 g/dl for males and 13 g/dl for females. These figures compare very
well with the WHO (1968) suggested minimum 'normal' levels for
adults of not less than 13 g/dl for men and not less than 12 g/dl for
women. Individual people vary in their normal level of haemoglobin,
but in clinical practice anything below 12 g/dl should be regarded as
anaemia.

Anaemia is important in the elderly for a number of reasons:

1   It is a common disorder.
2   It is easily overlooked, being notoriously difficult to diagnose on
inspection.
3   It is frequently due to previously unsuspected underlying disease.
4   It may have grave effects, especially in conjunction with atherosclerosis affecting brain, heart, kidneys and limbs.
5   It may tip the balance against a frail old person who was previously
able to cope.
6   Correction of the anaemia is usually simple and cheap. Thus the
careful diagnosis and treatment of anaemia, with the investigation and
correction of any underlying pathology, is one of the more interesting
and encouraging aspects of geriatric medicine.

Iron deficiency is central to the vast majority of anaemias in the elderly
but lack of the other haematinic factors is also common and often there

is considerable overlap between the different types (Fig. 17.1). Further-more many more patients can be shown to have iron deficiency without anaemia (sideropenia sine anaemia) than have actual anaemia. In a

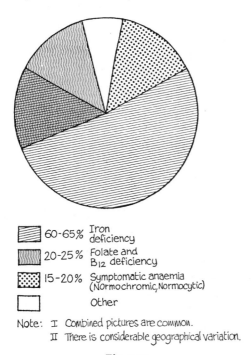

60-65% Iron deficiency

20-25% Folate and B_{12} deficiency

15-20% Symptomatic anaemia (Normochromic, Normocytic)

Other

Note: I Combined pictures are common.
      II There is considerable geographical variation.

Fig. 17.1

study of more than 400 admissions to the Cambridge geriatric depart-ment, twice as many patients had iron deficiency with a normal haemo-globin as had iron deficiency with anaemia (haemoglobin less than 12 g/dl). In 73 per cent of the patients in this series the marrow iron stores were low and in 48 per cent the marrow contained no or practically no iron. These cases of sideropenia sine anaemia should be regarded as cases of latent iron deficiency anaemia and be investigated and

Table 17.1 Types of anaemia

Hypochromic
Megaloblastic
Normochromic, normocytic
Aplastic, leukoerythroblastic

These types often co-exist

K

treated in the same way as if they were already anaemic. Left untreated, hypochromic anaemia will develop over the ensuing months.

The main causes of anaemia may be classified under two basic headings (Table 17.2).

Table 17.2. Causes of anaemia

1 Failure of RBC production
Lack of haematinic factors
Marrow depression or destruction
2 Excess blood loss
Bleeding
Haemolysis

Multiple factors are often present in an individual case.

Malabsorption of haematinics

Iron and folate are absorbed in the upper small gut; vitamin B_{12} in the terminal ileum. Atrophic gastritis increases with age and the secretion of intrinsic factor (essential to the absorption of vitamin B_{12}) falls. Anatomical abnormalities of the small gut—especially duodenal and jejunal diverticula which are not uncommon in the elderly—may lead to malabsorption of iron, folate and B_{12} (see Chapter 15). Malabsorption may also be due to previous surgery especially partial gastrectomy.

Dietary deficiencies

The body's minimum daily requirements of the three essential haematinics are of the order: iron—1 mg, folate—50 μg and B_{12}—2 μg. (Fig. 3.2) Normally, there is no difficulty in absorbing these quantities from the gut, and an ordinary mixed European type diet gives all of them in ample amounts. Fresh fruit and vegetables provide, in addition, plentiful vitamin C which aids iron absorption and erythropoiesis. However, meat, fruit and vegetables are expensive to buy in the UK. They are also perishable and mostly need a certain amount of preparation. Thus poverty, apathy, mental confusion or physical disability might well lead to dietary deficiency. Strict vegans (in youth) seem to manage surprisingly well on miniscule amounts of B_{12}, but the vegan lifestyle is less easy to maintain satisfactorily in old age, because of the effects of other adverse factors such as occult haemorrhage, malabsorption, systemic diseases and the drugs used to treat them. In younger folk the body combats deficiencies of haematinics (and other substances) by enhanced absorption. In old age this compensatory mechanism, increasingly, fails.

Underlying diseases

MALIGNANT DISEASE

Often the patient with cancer feels so unwell that she has no desire to eat and so there is a primary lack of intake of the essential haematinics. This may have existed for months before medical help is sought. Chemotherapy and radiotherapy may impair haemopoiesis and also (initially at least) add to the malaise and anorexia. In cancer of the gut, occult blood loss is common. Apart from bleeding, malignant disease may produce a normochromic normocytic anaemia due to impaired utilization of iron and depression of marrow activity even without actual marrow infiltration. Additionally there may be small bowel mucosal changes leading to malabsorption. Excess haemolysis also occurs very frequently in malignant disease. Marrow infiltration is seen with many malignancies, especially in prostatic carcinoma, and this produces a leucoerythroblastic anaemia.

RENAL DISEASE

Anaemia occurs in renal disease with progressive renal failure. It is usually normochromic and normocytic but often with iron deficiency. Multiple factors are involved, including lack of a satisfactory food intake as in any serious illness. Blood loss occurs due to the haemorrhagic tendency seen in uraemia, there may be a mild degree of haemolysis and there will be increasing marrow failure as the uraemia worsens. This latter factor becomes dominant in later stages. If the blood urea is persistently raised to greater than 25 mmol/l (150 mg/100 ml) anaemia is likely to occur. The serum iron falls but the total iron binding capacity is often raised. Iron utilization by the marrow is decreased. The anaemia of chronic renal failure does not respond satisfactorily to treatment with haematinics. Repeated blood transfusions are sometimes used to maintain the haemoglobin in the 8·5 to 10 g range. However, it may cause rapid worsening of the renal failure due to the parenteral protein load.

RHEUMATOID DISEASE

Rheumatoid disease is common in the elderly (see Chapter 9) and it is frequently associated with anaemia. A hypochromic normocytic blood picture is most often seen. The MCHC is usually low (less than 30 g/dl) but the MCV is normal (75–95 fl or cubic microns). The serum iron is low. Often the anaemia is due to multiple factors: e.g. blood loss (antirheumatic drugs), interference with iron metabolism and the presence of folate and vitamin B_{12} deficiency. Megaloblastic erythropoiesis is often seen on examination of the marrow smear. Low folate values in serum and red cell may be due to poor diet or possibly increased utilization by the rapidly proliferating synovial cells. Vitamin B_{12} deficiency is probably no more common than in other ill old people although an increase in incidence might be anticipated as in certain other autoimmune diseases.

The complications of rheumatoid disease increase the likelihood of anaemia. For example pyarthrosis, vasculitis and amyloidosis especially with renal failure. Renal failure may also occur due to prolonged analgesic ingestion (see also Chapter 16).

HYPOTHYROIDISM

A macrocytic anaemia may be seen in up to 60 per cent of cases. It is usually mild and is never megaloblastic unless there is associated vitamin B_{12} deficiency. Coexisting iron deficiency is not uncommon. The anaemia of hypothyroidism responds slowly to treatment with thyroxine. Pernicious anaemia occurs in about 10 per cent of cases of hypothyroidism and autoimmune mechanisms probably explain this association.

SCURVY

A macrocytic normoblastic type of anaemia is also seen in scurvy and protein deficiency. As with the macrocytic anaemia of hypothyroidism, it is important to differentiate this type of anaemia from the megaloblastic anaemias. The anaemia responds to ascorbic acid.

Blood loss

This is mostly from the gastrointestinal tract (Table 17.3). It is often intermittent and therefore may easily be missed on faecal occult blood (FOB) tests. Furthermore, the importance of a chronic minor loss must be stressed as liable to produce anaemia, especially if it is combined with other factors. Each factor existing alone would be insufficient to produce anaemia but together anaemia results. Multifactorial causation of anaemia is common in the elderly; for example minor blood loss from the gut, together with a minor degree of malabsorption, in the presence of a relatively quiescent systemic disease such as rheumatoid arthritis, in a patient taking an inadequate diet. Bleeding due to the causes listed in Table 17.3 is usually chronic, intermittent and occult, but brisk bleeds may occur with haematemesis and/or melaena. Bleeding from haemorrhoids and rectal prolapse will usually be self-evident. Blood loss from other sites may be important; especially pressure sores, leg ulcers and the urogenital tract.

Table 17.3. Blood loss from gut

Drugs especially antirheumatic
Hiatus hernia
Haemorrhoids
Gastroduodenal ulcer
Diverticula of colon or duodenum
Carcinoma of stomach, colon or rectum

Investigation of anaemia

A detailed history and a full clinical examination is required. Particular attention must be paid to symptoms referable to the gut and the drugs consumed, especially analgesics and anti-inflammatory agents. Most cases of anaemia will be diagnosed in the course of the routine work-up. However, the appearance of pallor is a poor guide, and angular stomatitis is more often due to overclosure of the mouth due to inadequate dentures, than to the presence of multiple vitamin B deficiencies. All patients need some routine haematological investigations e.g. haemoglobin, PCV, MCV, MCHC and an examination of the blood film. The blood urea level should also be estimated. Since the cause of the anaemia will usually be iron deficiency, often with other deficiencies, it will be important to look for a source of blood loss and the stool should be tested for this. Evidence of malignant disease must be sought by palpation of the neck, axillae and groins for enlarged lymph nodes. Palpation of the breasts and abdomen followed by vaginal and rectal examination will be required. Particular attention should be paid to evidence of previous abdominal surgery. It is remarkable how often patients forget that they have undergone (often major) surgery and the majority have only the vaguest notion of what the actual surgical procedure was.

Estimation of serum iron, the total iron binding capacity, serum B_{12} and folate levels may be required in certain cases. In some geriatric departments all of these are performed on every case of anaemia because multiple deficiencies of the three major haematinics are so common. A peripheral blood picture of iron deficiency may be due to lack of utilization of iron rather than to a total lack of iron stores.

Examination of a **sternal marrow smear** should be carried out whenever there is doubt about the diagnosis or if the response to treatment is unsatisfactory. This procedure tends to be neglected in the elderly, yet it is generally well tolerated and often very helpful in establishing the diagnosis. In particular it will show the type of erythro-poiesis—an important point if there is evidence of macrocytosis in the peripheral blood, even in the absence of anaemia. With suitable staining of the marrow film, an assessment of the body iron stores can be made. Abnormal cell types suggesting a diagnosis of myelomatosis or leukaemia may be seen. To establish the diagnosis of myelofibrosis it is necessary to study the marrow architecture and an iliac crest biopsy is required.

The erythrocyte sedimentation rate (ESR)

The normal ESR in younger folk is up to 5 mm/h Westergren in males and up to 10–15 mm/h in females. High levels are commonly observed in the elderly, so that many physicians would regard up to 20 for males and 30 for females as normal for geriatric practice. Yet these values almost certainly include some abnormally raised values due to sub-clinical disease—chronic gastritis, diverticular disease, urinary infection or whatever. Thus for one patient the ESR is regarded as elevated at 30 because the treatment of a recognized disease subsequently causes the level to drop to say 12. But for another patient with no recognizable disease an ESR of 30 is labelled 'normal' although at autopsy an unsuspected disease such as carcinoma of the caecum, cholecystitis, pyelonephritis, infected arthritis or pyometria is found! 'Silent' (but oft-times not quite) pathology is an ever-present probability in the aged.

A raised ESR must suggest the possibility of some underlying disease but it gives no clue to the precise diagnosis. A very low ESR (say 1) due to increased blood viscosity is seen in polycythaemia. A grossly elevated level (80 mm and more) suggests collagen disease, arteritis, myelomatosis, serious infection or malignant disease.

Plasma proteins

As with the ESR the plasma protein patterns are often markedly abnormal for a whole variety of common reasons. Frequently the albumen level is low, and one or more globulin fractions are raised. Factors influencing the plasma proteins are, malnutrition, infection, malignancy and immobility as the result of any serious disease. Evidently routine fractionation of the plasma proteins is of little value in geriatrics but electrophoresis and immunophoresis are of importance in a few selected cases as for example in the search for gammopathy associated with myelomatosis.

Types of anaemia

Brief descriptions of the common types of anaemia seen in the elderly are given separately below. However it must be emphasized that combined pictures are often seen. This does not mean that blunderbuss therapy is indicated, but it does mean that a careful investigation is required in each case, and that response to treatment must be followed to ensure that success is achieved.

Hypochromic anaemia

Hypochromic anaemia is usually, but not invariably, due to iron deficiency. Some cases will be seen with plentiful iron stores, but in these patients, iron utilization is impaired due to the presence of some other disease, for example malignancy or rheumatoid arthritis.

Iron deficiency anaemia is usually an insidious process so that the anaemia may be well advanced before the patient seeks help. More often it is diagnosed incidentally, when some other medical problem brings the patient to the doctor. In these latter cases there are no diagnostic clinical signs. In the long-standing severe cases there will be obvious pallor, swelling of the ankles and the well-known Plummer-Vinson syndrome may be in evidence: smooth tongue, spoonshaped nails and dysphagia. A fine mucosal fold may develop across the upper end of the oesophagus in the late stages. It is readily dilated by bouginage and the whole syndrome responds satisfactorily to treatment of the iron deficiency. It must be emphasized that sideropenia is a rather rare cause of dysphagia in anaemic old people. Cancer of the oesophagus, benign stricture following oesophagitis or a neurological lesion are much more common. The main causes of the iron deficiency have already been mentioned; blood loss, malabsorption and malnutrition. Anaemia due to blood loss occurs when the body's iron reserves (normally 1,000–1,500 mg) have been exhausted.

The blood picture will show hypochromia and the MCHC and MCV will be low (below 32 g/dl and 70 fl or cubic microns respectively). The serum iron level will be low and the total iron binding capacity (TIBC) raised. However, there is peculiar difficulty in the interpretation of these data. Certainly serum iron levels should only be interpreted in the light of the TIBC level. The approximate normal range for serum iron is 11–32 μmol/l (60–180 μg/100 ml) and for TIBC 45–72 μmol/l (250–400 μg/100 ml). A percentage saturation of less than 16 is usually taken as a good index of iron deficiency anaemia. In the majority of cases of iron deficiency anaemia routine estimation of the serum iron and TIBC is unnecessary. The clinical picture together with the peripheral blood examination will suffice. The response to treatment will usually give adequate confirmation of the diagnosis.

In patients of Mediterranean or South East Asian stock, the presence of mild chronic hypochromic anaemia not responding to iron and not otherwise accounted for should raise the possibility of thalassaemia minor.

TREATMENT OF IRON DEFICIENCY ANAEMIA

The treatment of iron deficiency anaemia, consists of the identification and correction of its cause, together with the administration of sufficient iron to bring the haemoglobin level up to normal (this usually takes two to three months) and to replenish the body stores. This means the continuation of oral iron for at least six months after correction of the anaemia. Numerous preparations of oral iron are available. The standard (and cheapest) is ferrous sulphate 200 mg tablets BP. Each tablet contains 63 mg elemental iron. The usual dose is one tablet thrice daily. If gastric intolerance occurs, fewer tablets are given initially or an alternative preparation is tried. E.g. ferrous gluconate 300 mg tablets, each containing 36 mg elemental iron, in a dose of 1–2 tablets thrice daily.

Table 17.4. Failure to respond to oral iron

Not taking tablets
Persistent blood loss
Wrong diagnosis
Chronic infection
Malignancy
Renal failure
Malabsorption

Failure to respond to oral iron usually means that the patient is not taking the tablets as prescribed, that persistent blood loss outstrips the haemopoietic capabilities or that the original diagnosis was wrong. Less often the (possibly relative) lack of response will be due to underlying malignancy, chronic infection or renal disease. Rarely will the gut be incapable of absorbing the iron.

From time to time there is enthusiasm for the use of adjuvant substances to promote the absorption and utilization of oral iron. Dilute hydrochloric acid, ascorbic acid and succinic acid have all been used to enhance absorption. In practice they are not generally used.

PARENTERAL IRON

If the diagnosis of iron deficiency is not in doubt, and if there is no response to oral therapy or if for some reason the oral route cannot be used, then parenteral iron is indicated. Parenteral iron must never be given concurrently with oral iron because this greatly increases the likelihood of toxicity. Repeated intramuscular (IM) or repeated intravenous injections of iron are much less often used although the former still has a place especially in general practice. The doctor should consult the manufacturer's literature for details of usage. The IM injection is to be given deep into the muscle of the outer aspect of the thigh or into the upper outer quadrant of the buttock.

Total dose infusion (TDI) intravenously, using iron dextran (Imferon), has its advocates in geriatric practice. The advantages are obvious. The total iron deficit can be made good in a matter of hours, possibly in the day hospital. The doctor is spared the problem of securing regular medication over the period of a year for a possibly forgetful old lady living alone, and the patient is spared the necessity of consuming any number of tablets, upwards from 1,000, over the same period. Furthermore the alternative of ten to twenty intramuscular injections, over a period of two to three months, may carry little appeal to the patient, especially when muscle bulk is minimal.

However attractive the proposition the authors adopt a cautious use of TDI. Reports to date show it to be generally safe, but it is potentially dangerous, and there have been some alarming reactions similar to those described for IV iron. TDI is not to be used if there is a history of allergy, previous toxic reaction to iron, or lack of close medical and nursing supervision.

Blood transfusion is not usually essential in the treatment of anaemia in the elderly, but it is commonly employed to prepare quickly an anaemic patient for surgery or special investigations e.g. barium studies.

Transfusion is also used to maintain the haemoglobin level in patients with an aplastic marrow and in patients with chronic blood loss which cannot be eradicated and which outstrips the haemopoietic capacity of the marrow. It is best avoided in severe chronic anaemia, because the risk of heart failure is high. In this situation, packed cells should be used, and frusemide given to help avoid circulatory overload.

SIDEROBLASTIC ANAEMIA

Acquired secondary sideroblastic anaemia may be seen in the elderly but the primary form is very rare. There is plenty of iron available in the serum and marrow, and the erythroblasts are loaded with iron (hence the name sideroblasts), but impaired utilization results in a blood picture of chronic iron deficiency anaemia. As might be expected, there is no response to medicinal iron. Secondary acquired sideroblastic anaemia appears to be induced by other diseases or occasionally drugs. Thus it may be seen in association with malignant disease including myelomatosis, rheumatoid arthritis, malabsorption and myxoedema and following the use of antituberculous drugs, phenacetin, paracetamol and chloramphenicol. Treatment should be directed at the underlying cause.

Megaloblastic anaemia

The megaloblastic anaemias are due to a deficiency of vitamin B_{12} or folic acid. The marrow appearances are identical in showing the presence of abnormally large nucleated red-cell precursors or megaloblasts. In the UK, the megaloblastic anaemias are nothing like so common as iron deficiency anaemia, but they do occur more frequently in older patients than in the young and quite often there is overlap with other types of anaemia. Furthermore, the megaloblastic change may go unrecognized when it occurs without anaemia, or with a peripheral blood picture of iron deficiency anaemia or with a normocytic anaemia. As mentioned earlier it is for this reason that some geriatric units now undertake routine vitamin B_{12} and folate assays. Using this approach, one reported series with haemoglobin levels below 10 g/dl, showed that 67 per cent were iron deficient, and about one-half were megaloblastic with the combined picture present in about one-third representing a considerable overlap. This is a very much higher proportion of megaloblastic change than has been reported in other series. However the main thesis is generally accepted, that megaloblastic change is to be considered as a possibility in almost any anaemic old person. Presumably the incidence varies in different geographical locations and in different socioeconomic groups. A study in the Cambridge geriatric department showed that less than 3 per cent of all admissions had megaloblastic marrows (14 out of 400 patients and 5 of the 14 had a haemoglobin above 12 g/dl). On careful investigation all proved to be cases of pernicious anaemia.

The 'normal range' for serum vitamin B_{12} is 140–750 ng/l (pg/ml) and for folate 3–20 μg/l (3–20 ng/ml). The actual ranges will vary somewhat with the locality and with the laboratory technique used. Low values of both are commonly found in the elderly. The estimation of red-cell folate (normally greater than 150 μg/l), provides a more accurate indication of the state of the body stores, but in pernicious anaemia the red-cell folate may be low when the serum level is normal or raised.

VITAMIN B$_{12}$ DEFICIENCY

Addisonian pernicious anaemia (PA) is the commonest cause of vitamin B$_{12}$ deficiency. Other causes are gastrectomy, bacterial colonization of anatomical lesions in the gut (diverticula and stricture), ileal resection and more general malabsorption states. The vegans were mentioned earlier and the fish tapeworm can be remembered for the final examination!

PA is a disease of later life, most cases arising over the age of sixty years. There is a strong familial tendency. It is due to a failure to secrete gastric intrinsic factor, probably as a result of an autoimmune atrophic gastritis. Evidence for this aetiology comes from the association with other autoimmune diseases and the production of antibodies to both parietal cells and intrinsic factor in serum and gastric juice.

PA has an insidious onset. After total gastrectomy the anaemia develops over a period of three to four years; following partial gastrectomy it may appear after 10 to 15 years due to chronic gastritis developing in the gastric remnant. There is pallor with an icteric tinge. Glossitis occurs and there may be symptoms suggestive of gastric carcinoma—anorexia, nausea, vomiting and weight loss—due to the gastric atrophy alone. Furthermore PA carries with it an increased liability to cancer of the stomach which is reported to occur in 10 per cent of cases. Another sinister complication of PA is the development of peripheral neuropathy and subacute combined degeneration of the spinal cord. Heart failure may also occur. Despite these dramatic and devastating changes, many cases go unrecognized for years before referral to hospital, perhaps with a note to the effect that the 'elderly lady has been gradually failing, she cannot be bothered to do anything for herself, has lost interest in food, she has had difficulty in walking and eventually took to her bed nine months ago etc. etc. . . . I do hope you can help her'. Let it be remembered that when someone is cracking up like this, an early medical vetting is required, to forestall the inevitable irretrievable breakdown.

DIAGNOSIS OF PERNICIOUS ANAEMIA

The diagnosis of pernicious anaemia is based on the finding of a macrocytic anaemia with a raised MCV (110–140 fl or cubic microns, normal range 75–95 fl), a low serum B$_{12}$, usually less than 100 ng/l and a megaloblastic marrow. The ability to absorb B$_{12}$ from the gut, only when given with an oral dose of intrinsic factor, is confirmed by the Dicopac double radioisotope test. A histamine or pentagastrin test for achlorhydria is rarely needed to clinch the diagnosis.

TREATMENT OF PERNICIOUS ANAEMIA

Hydroxocobalamin (Neo-cytamen) is the treatment of choice (cyano-cobalamin is much more rapidly excreted in the urine and is therefore the form of B_{12} used in the Dicopac test), and initially 1,000 micro-grams should be injected intramuscularly on five occasions at two-day intervals to replenish the body stores. Oral or parenteral iron will be required also, if there is evidence of iron deficiency. Even if there is no evidence of iron deficiency at the outset, it may develop later as the marrow rapidly increases the production of red cells. A reticulocyte response should be looked for after the fifth day. Maintenance injections of hydroxocobalamin must be given throughout the patient's life; 1,000 micrograms every two to three months. As with chronic iron deficiency anaemia, blood transfusion is best avoided altogether. Sudden death is liable to occur at the start of treatment in the very severe case. Long-term follow-up by the primary care team is required to ensure adequate treatment.

FOLATE DEFICIENCY

Folic acid deficiency is commonly seen in elderly anaemic patients and there is considerable overlap with the other major haematinic

Table 17.5. Causes of folate deficiency

Inadequate intake
Malabsorption
Gastrectomy
Jejunal resection
Gluten-sensitive enteropathy
Increased utilization
Haemolytic anaemia
Malignant disease
Collagen disease
Infections
Folic acid antagonists
Methotrexate
Anticonvulsants
Trimethoprim

deficiencies (Fe and B_{12}). In contrast to B_{12}, lack of intake of folic acid is an important cause of deficiency. Good sources of folate are green vegetables and liver. Re-utilization of folate is less efficient than for B_{12}. Whenever cell turnover increases (e.g. haemolytic anaemia or leukaemia), so folate requirements increase, up to ten times normal and this increase cannot be met if the dietary intake is inadequate. Folate deficiency (Table 17.5) is yet another example of the central theme of geriatric medicine—multifactorial aetiology. Folate deficiency is particularly common in elderly patients with dementia. In a study of demented patients in the Cambridge geriatric unit, about two thirds of the patients had low serum folate levels but one-half of the other (non-demented) patients also had low levels. Treatment with folic acid and later with vitamin B_{12} made no difference to the mental state. This particular study was carried out to see if B_{12} and folate status were especially relevant to senile dementia. No relevance was demonstrated.

DIAGNOSIS OF FOLATE DEFICIENCY

The haematological changes are indistinguishable from B_{12} deficiency. A low red cell folate is the best measure of folate deficiency and it is an indication of the folate status at the time the red cell was made. The serum folate level is much more labile and reflects folate absorption and utilization in the previous 24 h or so. Folic acid absorption is difficult to assess satisfactorily. Of the tests used the technique using tritium-labelled folic acid is preferred when appropriate radioisotope facilities exist. However, investigation of folate deficiency beyond the estimation of serum and red-cell levels is not undertaken routinely.

TREATMENT OF FOLATE DEFICIENCY

Folic acid tablets 5 mg are given orally twice or thrice daily. One tablet daily is sufficient for maintenance. Parenteral folic acid is rarely needed but is available for subcutaneous, intramuscular or intravenous injection in a dose of 5–15 mg daily.

Before any treatment is begun it is wise to have taken blood from the patient for estimation of the serum levels of B_{12}, folate and iron. When necessary, all three haematinics can be started while waiting for the results. Folic acid without B_{12} must not be started unless the B_{12} status is known because in B_{12} deficiency there is the risk of precipitating subacute combined degeneration of the spinal cord. It is best to avoid combined iron and vitamin tablets and multiple vitamin preparations until the nature of the haematological disorder is clear.

When to use folic acid requires more thought than the use of any other haematinic. The following have been suggested as appropriate indications:

1 Low red cell folate.
2 Megaloblastic anaemia with normal B_{12} status.

3 Epileptics on anticonvulsants.
4 Malabsorption states.

Marrow failure

Aplastic or hypoplastic anaemia is rather a rare disorder which can be seen at any age. The marrow is unable to keep up with the demands made upon it so that even though it might look active one or more of the cellular elements of the blood falls progressively. It is not an 'all or none' phenomenon as was once thought; the haemoglobin level may stabilize at around 8–10 g/dl without there being any apparent cause and despite all types of therapy. This relatively mild type of hypoplasia is fairly common in the elderly patient with underlying disease. Thrombo-cytopenia, agranulocytosis, pure red-cell aplasia or pancytopenia may be the predominant presentation in marrow failure. The lack of platelets and white cells, pose the major threat to the patient, because of the risk of bleeding and infection.

In at least half the cases, there is no identifiable cause and in the others, although one or more possible causes are evident, it might well be impossible to prove that the association is causal rather than casual. Innumerable drugs and chemicals have been implicated and most geriatric patients will have had one or more of these noxious substances. Of course some drugs regularly produce marrow depression; e.g. cytotoxic drugs. Other drugs are unpredictable in this respect; e.g. chloramphenicol, sulphonamides (antibacterial more than antidiabetic), phenylbutazone, anticonvulsants, penicillin and phenothiazines. Marrow replacement may occur in diseases such as myelofibrosis, myelo-matosis, leukaemia and secondary carcinoma. Exposure to ionizing radiations, even many years previously, may be relevant. Marrow failure in renal disease, and malignancies not involving the bones, have already been mentioned.

PROGRESS AND TREATMENT

Most of the older patients with marrow failure run a chronic course, with symptoms and signs of increasing anaemia, and sooner or later thrombocytopenic purpura and infection. Any possible causal agent must be removed and no further drugs of any kind given unless strongly indicated. The standard haematinics are always justified after blood has been taken for the proper investigation of iron, B_{12} and folate status —because deficiency of one or more of them is so common. Prednisone 20–30 mg daily may be given, particularly if haemolysis or other autoimmune processes are suspected. The possible benefits of steroids have to be weighed against their undoubted longterm adverse effects including a further increase in risk of infection. The anabolic steroid oxymethalone (Anapolon), in high dosage (up to 5mg/Kg body weight), may induce a remission in some cases of hypoplastic anaemia. Prostatic carcinoma or hyperplasia and incipient cardiac failure are contraindications because of the androgenic and fluid retention effects. If there is a complete failure to respond after three or four weeks, there is little point in continuing these treatments. However the longer the patient survives the better the prospects of ultimate recovery. Patients presenting with an acute, severe, systemic type of illness usually go quickly downhill and die. In the more chronic cases, repeated blood transfusion may be necessary over a period of months or years to keep the haemoglobin in the 8·5–10 g/dl range. When such a case is admitted to hospital for transfusion she should be accommodated in a well ventilated single room to minimize the risk of infection.

Leukaemia

The leukaemias are characterized by clones of malignant haemopoietic cells. The aetiology is largely unknown but immunosuppression or exposure to ionizing radiations from the natural background, atomic warfare, and medical treatment are implicated in some cases. Phenylbutazone is suggested as an aetiological factor in a number of reports. The overall incidence of leukaemia is fairly low, in the UK only about one tenth of that of carcinoma of the lung, but it is slowly rising. The elderly are affected by all the main types but especially by the more common chronic lymphatic and to a lesser extent acute myeloid leukaemia.

Acute leukaemia

This commonly starts with a period of vague ill health, followed by a rapidly worsening illness with anaemia, enlarged lymph nodes and thrombocytopenic purpura. The liver and spleen may be palpable but are not usually grossly enlarged unless there has been a preceding chronic leukaemia. Examination of the blood reveals a raised, normal or depressed leucocyte count (about a third of patients have WBC less than $10 \times 10^9/l$ (10,000/mm^3) when first seen. The differential count will reveal large numbers of cells of a primitive type—'blast cells'. It may be difficult to decide the particular stem line; viz. lymphoblast, monoblast or myeloblast. The platelet count is usually lowered and often falls below $50 \times 10^9/l$ (50,000/mm^3). This leads to a prolonged bleeding time and poor clot retraction. The marrow should be examined. It will be highly cellular with one primitive type dominating the picture.

Acute leukaemia in the elderly is rapidly fatal, irrespective of treatment. Ninety per cent die within four weeks of the diagnosis being made. A wide variety of chemotherapeutic agents is used but no details will be given here.

Chronic myeloid leukaemia (CML)

CML affects middle-aged to elderly people and presents with weakness refractory anaemia, haemorrhage, infection and modestly enlarged lymph nodes. The spleen may attain great size and cause discomfort by dragging on its pedicle or on account of infarction and perisplenitis. There may be leukaemic deposits in the skin, viscera, brain and bone.

The blood shows a very high leucocyte count 100 $\times$ 10^9/l or even more especially segmented neutrophils. The marrow is infiltrated with these cells.

The mean survival time from diagnosis is about two years in older patients. Busulphan (Myleran) is used in a dose of 2–6 mg daily to depress the leucocyte count. When near normal levels are reached, the dose is reduced to the minimum maintenance level to keep the count from rising. An acute myeloblastic transformation is a common terminal event. Infections are less of a problem than with chronic lymphatic leukaemia.

Chronic lymphatic leukaemia (CLL)

This type is seen almost exclusively in late middle and old age. The onset is very insidious and indeed many cases are picked up on routine haematology in the course of some other illness. The patient suffers weakness, repeated infections, enlarged lymph nodes and perhaps serous effusions. Symptomatic zoster may be the presenting feature.

The haemoglobin is often normal, when the diagnosis is first made, but later a normochromic anaemia develops. The WBC is raised to 50–100 $\times$ 10^9/l (50–100,000/mm^3). It can be normal and is less than 10 $\times$ 10^9/l in 10 per cent of cases. Over 90 per cent of the leucocytes are lymphocytes. The marrow examination will reveal a preponderance of lymphoid cells but it is not essential for making the diagnosis. Some of the patients with a low WBC count will have a partial picture of CLL due to underlying lymphosarcoma. All gradations exist in the lymphoproliferative spectrum CLL—lymphosarcoma. Other patients with low counts simply have a 'latent' or 'benign' CLL which requires no treatment.

Hypogammaglobulinaemia frequently occurs and so intercurrent infections are particularly common. There may also be a variable but usually mild degree of autoimmune haemolytic anaemia and thrombocytopenia may also occur.

CLL is the most benign of the leukaemias, and patients may be followed over many years without specific treatment eventually to die of some totally unrelated disease. Alternatively death may result from leukaemic infiltration (as in lymphosarcoma), intercurrent infection, thrombocytopenic purpura or a haemolytic crisis. Only if the disease is progressive is drug treatment required. Chlorambucil (Leukeran) 2 mg and 5 mg tablets in a dose of 0·2 mg per kg per day is given to suppress the white count and when this comes under control the dose is reduced to a minimum maintenance level. If this fails, cyclophosphamide (Endoxana) 10 mg and 50 mg tablets in a dose of 2–5 mg per kg per day initially is used in like manner. If autoimmune phenomena are a problem (e.g. haemolysis or thrombocytopenia) prednisone 10–15 mg thrice daily is used in an attempt to suppress them. Intercurrent infections are treated by appropriate antibiotics.

Polycythaemia vera

This rather rare disease occurs in late middle age and over half the cases will be age 60 years or more at the outset. There is overactivity and extension of the haemopoietic tissues of the bone marrow with an outpouring of red cells, white cells and platelets into the circulation. Occasionally there is progress to chronic myeloid leukaemia or to myelofibrosis. A markedly raised blood viscosity is the nub of the problem clinically. Hypertension often develops and there is vascular disease with liability to thrombosis (e.g. stroke or myocardial infarct) or haemorrhage especially from the gastrointestinal or renal tracts. A florid cyanosed facies is characteristic and the spleen is usually enlarged and palpable.

Specialist investigation and treatment is necessary for these patients to give a good life expectancy. The haemoglobin is in the range 16–20 g/dl and further examination of the blood reveals marked elevation of cell counts as well as the haematocrit and blood viscosity. The total red cell mass is increased. Treatment is by repeated venesection (to give temporary respite) followed by IV radioactive phosphorus or chemotherapy using busulphan (Myleran) as in CML.

Other causes of raised haemoglobin

Relative erythrocytosis is due to haemoconcentration, and secondary erythrocytosis is a physiological response to chronic anoxaemia or high levels of erythropoietin. The treatment is that of the underlying disorder.

Multiple myeloma

Abnormal proteins (paraproteins) can be found at any age but especially in the elderly. These paraproteins are formed by the plasma cells. They occur in a variety of diseases but pre-eminently in multiple myeloma or myelomatosis. For detailed information about para-proteinaemia the reader is referred to the standard textbooks on haematology.

Myelomatosis is a malignant disease of plasma cell precursors usually associated with paraproteinaemia. It is more common than CLL and like that disease affects mainly the elderly. The maximum incidence is in the seventh and eighth decades. As with so many diseases it may be picked up by finding a very high ESR or rouleaux formation on routine haematological screening of a patient complaining of vague ill health. Alternatively it may present with skeletal pain due to widespread osteolytic lesions. Pathological fractures may be found affecting ribs, femora and vertebrae. The latter may give rise to paraplegia. Mental disturbance, nausea and vomiting may be secondary to the hyper-calcaemia which occurs in advanced cases with extensive skeletal destruction. Peripheral neuropathy affects some patients.

The haemoglobin level is normal in about one third of cases, when the diagnosis is first made, but later anaemia develops. This is usually normochromic and normocytic. Plasma cells are rarely present in the blood film except as a terminal event. The ESR is usually (but not invariably) markedly raised due to changes in the serum proteins. Levels over 100 mm/h are common but occasionally the elevation is quite modest. Proteinuria is common and in about 50 per cent of cases it will be of the Bence-Jones type. B-J protein is virtually, but not absolutely, specific for myeloma. The total serum protein level may be very high (8–10 g/dl) and usually it is the beta or gamma globulin which is present in excess. Paraprotein if present is often only 2 g/dl or less. IgG and IgA being the most common. A sternal marrow smear will confirm the diagnosis by showing a great excess of plasma cells.

Often the clinical diagnosis is not straightforward. The patient may present with a severe chest or urinary infection or with heart or renal failure. Increasing uraemia indicates a grave prognosis. The renal insufficiency is due to deposition of protein in the tubules, but is often made worse by the presence of anaemia, hypercalcaemia, plasma cell infiltration and amyloidosis. The heart is also affected by amyloid deposition. Osteolytic lesions have to be distinguished from metastases, secondary to cancer especially of the lung and breast. Skeletal pain, high ESR and anaemia may also be features of rheumatoid disease (which may be complicated by amyloidosis). Diffuse myelomatosis, solitary myeloma and extramedullary plasmacytoma are uncommon variants.

The life expectancy at the time of diagnosis, is on average, less than a year but if the diagnosis is made on the basis of paraproteinaemia in the premyelomatous phase, the life expectation can be very much longer. Amyloidosis is reported in about a quarter of cases and involvement of blood vessels, heart and kidneys commonly occurs. Pyelonephritis is often present. Death may be due to chronic renal failure. At post-mortem many viscera will be found to be infiltrated with plasma cells.

Specific treatment is often unrewarding and special attention must be given to the relief of symptoms. Relief of pain is especially important and the reader is referred to Chapter 20 for details of medical treatment in terminal illness. Deep X-ray therapy may give relief to bone pain and pathological fractures usually heal normally. Mental confusion, nausea and vomiting may resolve when the hypercalcaemia is treated by means of prednisone 15 mg thrice daily, together with rehydration. Blood transfusion is used if the anaemia becomes severe and infection is treated with an appropriate antibiotic. Melphalan (Alkeran) 2 mg and 5 mg tablets is the drug usually used to damp down the plasmacytosis, but it is contraindicated in the presence of amyloidosis and renal failure. It is given in a dose of 5 mg daily, initially for two or three weeks, and the effects on the WBC and the platelet count are then assessed. Thereafter a maintenance dose is given, on the basis of the response, and it is usually around 2 mg daily. Clinical improvement with respect to pain, a trend towards normal in the serum protein electrophoretic pattern and an improvement in the X-ray appearances often occurs. Prednisone may enhance the response to melphalan as well as controlling the hypercalcaemia. It also has a beneficial effect on the patient's sense of well being.

Cancer in the aged

One of the major factors determining the incidence of cancer is age. Thus, for the average young male medical student reading this text, the probability of developing malignant disease within the next five years is less than 1 in 700 but for the average male aged 65 years the probability is increased fifty-fold to 1 in 14. Various theories have been put forward to explain the general increase in the incidence of cancer with age.

1 Carcinogenesis may be stimulated by changes in hormonal control consequent upon ageing.

2 Immunological surveillance mechanisms may fail with ageing. In younger people abnormal clones of cells are more readily destroyed.

3 The longer life allows a longer exposure to environmental factors likely to produce malignant change. Thus the elderly may have experienced a much longer and bigger total exposure to carcinogens; e.g. cigarette smoke, affecting the bronchial mucosa or actinic light affecting the skin.

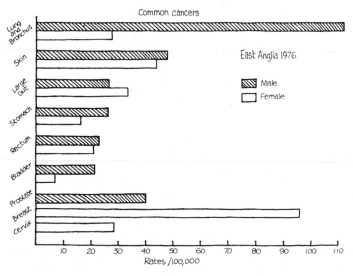

Fig. 17.2

As will be seen from Fig. 17.2, cancer of the lung and bronchus tops the list of common cancers in East Anglia as in the UK as a whole. It shows a marked predilection for the male, and the male incidence is still rising, but the incidence in the female has more than doubled over the past fifteen years. These trends are general for carcinoma of the bronchus in the UK. In both men and women the age of peak incidence has steadily increased over the past 25 years. This increasing incidence persists, until around the age of seventy-five for men and then declines sharply (Fig. 17.3). This sharp deline in incidence, after age seventy-five, is not seen with all epithelial cancers (e.g. stomach). Thus, the epidemiology of lung cancer suggests that, a cohort of persons especially liable to the disease is moving through the population. The most probable environmental factor responsible is thought to be cigarette smoking. Bladder cancer also has its main incidence in the elderly and this has more than doubled in the male over the past fifteen years. There have been smaller increases in the female, *pari passu* with the changing epidemiology of cancer of lung and bronchus.

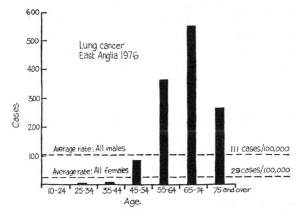

Fig. 17.3

Almost all malignant disease is more common in the older patient, apart from a few malignancies such as Hodgkin's disease and acute leukaemia. Even these can occur in old age. Polycythaemia is also seen in the elderly but less often than in middle age. Myelofibrosis is a rather rare disease, seen almost exclusively in the elderly. Cancer of the lip and tongue are not common and affect mainly the elderly. Their frequency is diminishing. Carcinoma of the stomach is also on the wane, but is still quite common. It also affects predominantly the elderly. Prostatic cancer is almost exclusively a disease of the elderly (Fig. 17.4).

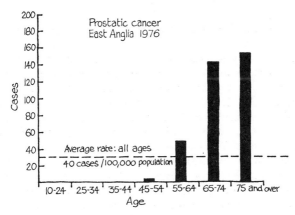

Fig. 17.4

Cancer of the lung, skin, gut, breast and prostate account for the great
majority of all malignant disease in geriatric patients.

Cancer in old age is much more common in men than in women,
largely due to the high incidence of cancer of the lung, skin, stomach,
bladder and prostate. In middle age the incidence in the two sexes is
reversed, because of the high rates affecting the female breast and
reproductive organs. The peak incidence of carcinoma of the breast
has moved from around age 50 to around age 60 during the past 20
years. Deaths due to this disease rise steadily with age (Fig. 17.5).

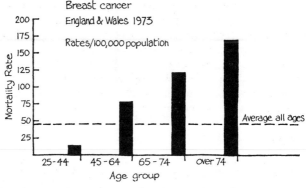

Fig. 17.5

Clinical significance

Because of the very high incidence of so many different forms of cancer
in old age, the geriatrician must regard malignant disease as an ever-
present possibility. The clinical relevance of the cancer may vary
enormously. It may be lethal and is the second commonest cause of
death after cerebro-vascular disease. On the other hand the malignancy
may simply pose a potential threat to the patient. Thus the common
basal cell carcinoma in its earlier stages will cause no systemic upset,
may not be noticed by the patient and responds well to radiotherapy.
Many internal cancers also constitute little threat to the patient's well
being, some other pathology (stroke, ischaemic heart disease) posing
the major problem. With each type of cancer (lung, breast, stomach, or
prostate) there exists a very wide range of biological potential. Some are
highly invasive and have already metastasized when first suspected. At
the other extreme are cancers of similar histological type which are
relatively benign. In hospital cases coming to autopsy it has been found
that many malignancies in the elderly (over 50 per cent) have not been
recognized clinically. In many cases the undiscovered cancer explains
much of the ante-mortem illness. Often, however, it is clear that the

cancer is just an incidental finding unrelated to the terminal illness and death. These incidental cancers are seen in about one-third of all old people at autopsy. The likely sites in order of frequency are prostate, kidney and colon. In about 10 per cent of elderly cancer patients multiple primary growths occur.

Cancer registration figures must give a gross underestimate of the true incidence of malignant disease in the elderly when one realizes that only the minority of the elderly dying in hospital and an infinitesimal proportion of those dying at home come to autopsy.

The presence of cancer in an old person is easily missed clinically, because the symptoms and signs are so vague and occur in a patient suffering from a plethora of pathology. The old (and possibly already chronically ill and disabled) person is just not doing so well, and her relatives note simply the increasing ill health and failure to thrive. In this situation a careful search for signs of the more likely malignancies is indicated, viz. lung, breast, gastrointestinal tract, prostate, uterus and bladder. However the patient with other serious disease may die before the cancer plays havoc with the body's economy.

Presentation

As with so much in geriatric medicine, the doctor needs 'a good nose' or a high index of suspicion to make a proper analysis of the case. Multiple pathology must be regarded as the norm if the cancer is to be diagnosed because some alternative explanation for the presenting symptoms and signs so often exists. For example anorexia, nausea and vomiting are commonly due to drug treatment and so the gastric cancer is missed. Gastrointestinal blood loss is commonly due to hiatus hernia and diverticular disease and so the carcinoma of colon is missed. Rectal bleeding is assumed to be due to the (obvious) haemorrhoids and so the rectal cancer is missed. Anaemia without bleeding may also occur due to multiple factors including haemolysis, impaired iron metabolism, depressed haemopoiesis and occasionally marrow infiltrations as described earlier in this chapter.

When the presentation is completely nondescript and the patient is observed to be 'falling apart at the seams' the general decline may be attributed naively to senility. Psychiatric presentations occur; e.g. mental depression, toxic confusional state or dementia as a 'metabolic' complication or because of cerebral metastases. Other non-metastatic neurological presentations also occur as described in Chapter 13.

Investigations

Despite the evident difficulties, a careful clinical examination supplemented by a few simple special examinations will often reveal the diagnosis. The rectal examination must not be omitted. In the male the prostate, and in both sexes the rectum, are fairly common sites of malignancy. Fifty per cent of colorectal cancers are within reach of the examiner's finger and about 75 per cent within range of the sigmoido-scope. Haematology and plain X-ray of chest, abdomen and bone may be required. Prostatic secondaries show a predilection for the lumbar spine and pelvis.

How much further to proceed with special investigation is often a matter for debate. The doctor must steer a middle course between missing a readily treatable cancer (e.g. operable colonic growth) and pushing ahead with attempts to clinch a diagnosis when no likely benefit will accrue; e.g. of bronchial neoplasm by bronchoscopic biopsy when surgical resection is clearly impracticable. Obviously each case must be decided on consideration of all the circumstances. Never-theless in general it is preferable to have a full diagnosis in each case as an aid to overall management including prognosis, type of drug treat-ment, advice to patient and relatives. The prognosis in each case is a complex function of many variables of which the stage at presentation is dominant. The interaction between tumour and patient is an in-calculable factor and in some cancers (e.g. breast and prostate) no one therapeutic regime is clearly 'superior' to the others. Thus a search for distant as well as local spread is an essential prerequisite to the decision to treat the primary growth. Nowadays, bone and organ scanning for metastases are, for the patient, relatively simple and dignified, proce-dures which give valuable information to help make a prognosis and on which to plan treatment. However in some cases a complete diagnosis may be obtainable only at a cost (in human as well as monetary terms) which makes its pursuit unreasonable.

Having made a tentative or definite diagnosis of cancer, the next problem is to decide whether or not to treat, and whether treatment should aim at cure or palliation. In an elderly patient with a reasonable life expectancy and a readily curable lesion the decision is easy; for example a well woman in her sixties or seventies with a basal cell carcinoma of the face will be urged to have radiotherapy—a treatment which is both effective and easily tolerated. On the other hand an elderly patient with diminished cardiorespiratory reserve and carcinoma of the bronchus cannot be offered effective treatment for the cancer. Unless the patient is very fit a lobectomy carries a high mortality. The patient who survives may be left a respiratory cripple and the possibility of cure is remote. Palliative radiotherapy might be valuable to deal with painful secondary deposits in bone or superior vena cava obstruction due to encroachement on the great vessels. The adverse effects of radiotherapy can be mitigated by the use of small-field, split-dose techniques incorporating rest periods as part of the treatment plan.

A sound, balanced decision needs to be taken on the basis of as much fact and expert opinion as is readily available to ensure that treatment is given only with the genuine hope and intention of helping the patient. In general cytotoxic chemotherapy is ill tolerated by the elderly and immunosuppression occurs all too readily. Too often complex, expensive treatments which are tiresome for the patient are given merely to satisfy the urge of doctors, nurses and relatives that 'something must be done'. Doing nothing in a technical sense might well be far and away the most appropriate treatment.

CHAPTER 18 · SKIN, TEETH, AND
SPECIAL SENSES

'In the days of my youth' Father William replied
'I remembered that youth could not last;
I thought of the future, whatever I did,
That I never might grieve for the past.'

ROBERT SOUTHEY 1774–1843

As the title of this chapter suggests, it consists of those items of geriatric interest which do not fit neatly under any system. Nevertheless, there can be no doubt about their importance or frequency.

The hands

The main function of this section is to call for caution in the interpretation of signs which are usually of sinister importance in younger patients. In the elderly, the same changes are sometimes completely innocent, and occur in the absence of disease.

Wasting of the small muscles

This is a common finding in many geriatric patients in whom it may be of no clinical significance. The actual cause is not definitely known, but changes in the cervical spine are sometimes thought to be responsible.

Liver palms

A peripheral ring of erythema around the palmar surface of the hand is frequently described as a liver palm. However, in old age, this finding is common but rarely associated with liver disease. In some cases, it will be found in connection with rheumatoid arthritis. In other patients it seems to be of no diagnostic relevance.

Clubbing

If bilateral, this sign has the same value in old as in young patients.

However, in stroke victims clubbing may be found only on the hemiplegic side, and is of no clinical importance.

Senile purpura

This condition is described in the section on skin changes. It is of no diagnostic value, but does seem more common in frail, ill elderly subjects, and also in those with exaggerated thinness of the skin on the dorsum of the hand.

Ulnar deviation

Laxity of the metacarpophalangeal joints can result in this deformity without evidence of rheumatoid arthritis. This can be particularly misleading when associated with small muscle wasting and the joints appear enlarged by contrast.

Dull, brittle nails

These are common in old age and not necessarily indicative of iron deficiency.

Finger varicosities

Dilated veins occur on the palmar aspects of the fingers (but not on the tips or pulps) in over half of geriatric patients. There is no apparent connection with venous abnormalities elsewhere in the body.

The feet

Mention will only be made of the importance of examination of the toe-nails, and the need to search for callosities, onycogryphosis and pedal deformities. Such topics may seem trivial, but they can play an important role in preventing mobility in the elderly. The pain from these lesions can be severe and disabling and expert chiropody should be sought without delay.

The mouth

The fact that just over half of geriatric patients have not seen a dentist for 10 or more years demonstrates the extent to which the mouth and its contents are neglected. When complaints are made about this area, they are usually of a sore tongue, sore mouth, sore lips or difficulties with dentures. The absence of pain in the presence of gross caries is quite remarkable.

Glossitis

Tongue changes are common amongst geriatric patients, and affect about one-third. A sore red tongue may be due to vitamin B_{12} or folate deficiency and should alert the observer to the possibility. Severe atrophic glossitis may, however, be due to iron deficiency. A benign chronic migrating superficial glossitis (geographical tongue) is also common in old age.

Sore buccal mucosa

Lesions to be searched for in this condition are the white areas of Candida infection. The bullous eruptions of pemphigus and pemphigoid may start in the mouth and areas of lichen planus may become ulcerated. Also the elderly are not immune to the common complaint of aphthous ulceration.

Angular stomatitis

This occurs at the rate of about 10 per cent in geriatric patients, but does not have the close association with iron and vitamin deficiency found in younger subjects. In the elderly, it is more likely to be due to leakage of saliva from the corner of the mouth. This may be secondary to lax musculature or poorly fitting dentures. The saliva alone may cause local maceration, but in addition, the presence of Candida can worsen the situation. Both water repellant ointments and anti-fungal preparations may therefore be needed for treatment.

Dentures

As up to 95 per cent of geriatric patients are edentulous, it is more appropriate to talk about dentures than teeth. When original teeth are present they are usually in poor condition with equally unhealthy gums.

Surveys have reported one third to two thirds of patients as being dissatisfied with their dentures. The commonest complaints are of looseness or soreness. Poor fitting usually results from atrophy of the supporting tissues, and soreness is most usually due to Candida, plus minor trauma. Although allergic reactions are often blamed, proof is rarely found.

Twelve per cent of patients supplied with dentures never wear them, so great care is needed in patient selection before time and money is expended on their new fitting. It should always be ensured that it is the patient and not her relations or attendants who is requesting the new teeth.

Hair

With increasing age hairs become greyer, thinner in diameter and fewer in number. Scalp hair loss is much more obvious in men, but some is lost from both the temporal and vertical areas in women. An increase in facial hair will affect almost half the women in the population after the age of 60 years. Body hair, like scalp hair, diminishes with age. It disappears in the reverse order to its aquisition—trunk, pubic and finally axillary, although the loss is rarely complete.

Skin

The visible age-changes in skin are familiar to all observers. The wrinkling, thinning, increased fragility and transparency are secondary to changes in the dermis, the epidermis hardly changing even in old age. Not only is the dermis thinner but it contains less water and the elasticity of the collagen is reduced.

In addition to these normal changes pathological skin conditions are very common in geriatric patients (over 90 per cent). In Caucasians in sunny climates there is an increasing incidence of rodent ulcer and epithelioma with age, but this is due to the rising total duration of exposure to sunlight. As skin diseases rarely kill, it will be realized that all of those acquired during a long life may persist into old age. Here, attempts will only be made to give some details of those skin conditions which tend to be restricted to the elderly or are particularly troublesome in this age group.

Benign lesions

Seborrhoeic warts become increasingly common on ageing. They appear as brownish papules up to 1 cm in diameter on the head and trunk. Frequency, darkness and size all tend to increase in old age and the presence of a malignancy elsewhere may accelerate such changes.

Senile seborrhoeic adenoma are firm yellowish nodules, sometimes with a central depression, commonly found on the forehead or cheeks of old people.

Malignant lesions

Basal cell carcinomas are the most frequent form of skin malignancy. The initial lesion is nodular but the central area becomes ulcerated as it enlarges—thus developing into the familiar rodent ulcer. The commonest sites are on the face—especially the cheeks. Although distant spread is very rare treatment is required because of the invasive nature of the lesions. When small they can be dealt with by simple curettage and cautery but larger ulcers need excision or radiotherapy.

Malignant melanoma can sometimes be mimicked by rapidly enlarging deeply pigmented seborrhoeic warts. However, whenever the more serious diagnosis is a possibility the only course is to biopsy and treat extensively only when there is no histological doubt.

Pemphigus and pemphigoid

The main feature in both these conditions is the presence of a bullous eruption. They differ, however, in the site of origin of the blisters.

In pemphigus, the lesions start as splits in the epidermis. The blisters, therefore, tend to be thin walled and fragile. The crusts resulting from burst lesions may sometimes be more evident than actual blisters. Although the initial lesions may be localized, for example, in the mouth, generalized spread will occur. Apparently normal skin between bullae may also be lost when subjected to minimal friction. Due to the considerable fluid loss from the lesions and the high risk of secondary infection, death will result if treatment is not given promptly. The use of corticosteroids has fortunately transformed the prognosis of the condition. In slowly progressing forms, it is sufficient to apply steroid topically. In the more virulent varieties, large doses of oral steroids will be required and even then, some patients will still be lost.

Pemphigoid is more closely restricted to the elderly than pemphigus, 80 per cent of patients being over 60 years of age. The lesions are deeper, arising from below the epidermis. The blisters are less fragile and subsequently more abundant in their undamaged state. Although less frequently fatal, treatment with steroids is still required, and as with pemphigus, a life-long maintenance dose is likely to be needed to prevent recurrence.

Senile purpura

This consists of haemorrhagic areas, sometimes several centimetres in diameter, which are located on the forearms or the back of the hands. Since purpuric lesions by definition are not more than 5 mm across, the term senile purpura is a misnomer. It is a very common and benign condition which steadily increases with age. It is thought to be due to a reduction in supporting tissues, secondary to age changes in collagen. Many geriatric patients are grateful when reassured of the lack of significance of the lesions.

When true purpura occurs in the elderly, it is more likely to be due to thrombocytopenia than a capillary defect. Examination of the peripheral blood film, bone marrow or drug chart will usually reveal the cause. Malignancy or iatrogenic causes are most common.

Scurvy is a rare cause of purpura, but when it occurs, it is usually in an elderly person, especially a widower living alone. The lesions are perifollicular and sometimes associated with curled body hairs. More extensive haemorrhagic lesions known as sheet haemorrhages may also be seen especially on the legs.

Pruritus

Generalized itching can present as a frequent and difficult problem in old age. When no rash is visible apart from the results of constant scratching, an internal disease must be sought. Hepatic disorders will need to be considered, and it should be remembered that itching may precede jaundice. Pruritus may be the first clue to the presence of uraemia or malignant disease. Disorders of the haemopoietic system such as anaemia, polycythaemia and lymphomata can all be associated with itching. Dirt, scabies and other infestations are unfortunately common-place in some sections of the elderly population. Fungal infections are also an important irritation.

Excessive dryness of the skin in old age is by far the commonest cause of itching. The dryness is initially due to the reduced sebaceous activity which occurs with ageing. Further aggravation may be provided by excessive washing especially if detergents or other potent cleansing agents are used. The skin will become not only dry, but criss-crossed by fine reddened fissures which may lead to scaling. Conservation of the natural oils and supplementation where necessary, with oily creams containing lanolin or similar substances should combat the process.

Herpes zoster

See Chapter 13.

Intertrigo

Intertrigo is a form of seborrhoeic eczema—usually found in skin folds. The obese are especially vulnerable, and sore, red, moist, smelly areas

are common under large pendulous breasts, in groins and in transverse
abdominal folds. It is said that fat ladies with myxoedema are immune
from intertrigo.

Cleanliness is the first essential of prevention and treatment. It is
important that the areas are thoroughly dried after washing—a hair drier
can be very useful. Secondary infection is common, especially with
monilia, and nystatin will be required locally. If the macerated areas
show evidence of bacterial infection then neomycin or fucidic acid
may be applied. Steroid creams are best avoided but in severe cases they
may be used in a short course, in low concentration.

Leg ulcers

Most leg ulcers are due to impaired venous drainage, which may itself
be secondary to several factors. Varicose veins, which affect one fifth of
our adult population play an important role. Immobility, usually due to
osteoarthritis, and especially when associated with obesity, also aggre-
vates the stasis. On account of these factors, the ulcer once established
may fail to heal. Furthermore there may be a variable degree of arterial
insufficiency.

The region usually affected is just around and above the medial
malleolus. The first change is the development of an area of varicose
eczema, the skin later becoming congested, swollen, cyanotic and
pigmented with a weeping, scaly or sticky surface. Once the skin's surface
has been broken, the resulting ulcer may become extremely extensive
and even completely encircle the ankle. Chronic infection and crusting
will usually be present, and be a further hindrance to healing. When
arterial insufficiency is the most important aetiological factor, the
ulcers are more frequently situated on the anterior-lateral aspect of
the ankle and lower part of the shin.

The suggested methods of treatment for these leg ulcers are legion, a
state of affairs which can usually be taken to indicate the poor success
rate. However, the basic requirements to enable ulcers to heal are
simple—abolish local tissue swelling and eliminate infection from the
ulcer base. If tissue swelling is due to generalized fluid retention,
diuretics will be helpful; if due to relative immobility, firm bandaging
after positional drainage will be more appropriate. Infection should be
eliminated by local antiseptics and Eusol remains far and away the
favourite. Antibiotics should not be used, either locally or systemically,
unless there is evidence of cellulitis spreading beyond the ulcer crater.
In such circumstances the second route of administration is preferable.
Other local applications are also best avoided as local allergic reactions
may result. Once clear of infection and free of debris, the ulcer base
should be kept healthy by protecting it with sterile, moist, non-adherent

dressings such as tulle gras. The ulcer should be disturbed as infrequently as possible, for, just as a plant will not grow if persistently dug up for signs of progress, an ulcer will not heal if its peace is repeatedly interrupted. Steroids are not indicated unless there is a generalized arteritis as a contributing factor—a rare occurrence. Even minor degrees of anaemia should be corrected in an attempt to achieve healing, and vitamin C supplements should be given if there is any suspicion of dietary insufficiency. Plastic surgery may sometimes be of value.

In spite of much devoted work by the community nursing service and ulcer clinics, many fat old ladies persistently retain their leg ulcers. Their lesions act as a life-line, providing some contact with their community, forming a topic of conversation and ensuring continued attention and care.

Pressure sores

See Chapter 9.

Eyes

Just under 70,000 people over the age of 65 years are registered in the UK as blind, but many more with equally severe eye problems are not included.

The aim of this section is not to give a comprehensive list of ophthalmic conditions, but to provide information about common eye problems seen in geriatric practice. The natural history and description of diabetic and hypertensive retinopathy are omitted as they are well described in standard texts. The other common difficulty not considered here is the problem of refraction but elderly people should be freely referred for sight testing.

Common changes in old age

Presbyopia is difficulty in focusing on near objects, as in reading. It affects all people to varying degrees as they age, and is due to loss of elasticity of the lens capsule. Increased rigidity of the iris is thought to be responsible for the small pupil so often found in the elderly. Dilatation of these pupils is sometimes dangerous, as they can be associated with a shallow anterior chamber. The small pupil is one of the reasons why the elderly have difficulty in seeing in poor light.

Disorders of the eye-lids are also common in old age. In entropion, the lower lid becomes turned inwards, so that the lashes irritate the cornea and conjunctiva. If the lid becomes folded outwards this is known as ectropion, and control of tear drainage becomes impaired. Both conditions can be corrected by simple operations which can be carried out under local anaesthesia.

The painful eye

CLOSED ANGLE GLAUCOMA

When glaucoma is due to sudden closure of the angle of the anterior chamber of the eye, the block in drainage leads to severe pain. The pain may be sufficiently bad to precipitate prostration and vomiting. In about half the cases, however, there are earlier attacks of less severe and transient pain which are usually associated with blurring of vision, and also a halo effect around images.

The affected eye feels tense, the pupil is irregularly dilated and fixed to light, the cornea congested and the conjunctiva reddened.

Once the diagnosis has been made, expert ophthalmological management is required. Emergency treatment consists of eserine or pilocarpine drops to constrict the pupil, and potent analgesics.

OPHTHALMIC HERPES

When the ophthalmic division of the fifth cranial nerve is the site of herpetic infection, the eye may be endangered. The presence of the characteristic rash makes the diagnosis easy. For treatment see Chapter 13.

Slow loss of vision

OPEN ANGLE GLAUCOMA

In this condition the pressure within the eye rises gradually, and without an obvious reason. Initially the diagnosis can only be made by the detection of raised intra-ocular pressure, and for this reason, measurements should always be made with a tonometer when the visual acuity of the elderly is tested. Later a white-cupped optic disc will be seen on ophthalmoscopy but by this time a scotoma will have started to develop. Only when it reaches a large size and starts to encroach on central vision will the patient become aware of her failing sight.

In the early stages, progression may be prevented by the use of pilocarpine drops; if not, a drainage operation will be required. In all cases, management should be in the hands of an ophthalmologist.

CATARACTS

Lens opacities occur in two separate varieties, peripheral and central. The peripheral type consists of 'spikes' of opaque lens radiating from the edge to the centre, and interference with vision does not occur until a late stage. However, patients with the central type become aware of visual impairment much sooner.

Cataract extraction is a simple operation but is only necessary when the lesions are restricting the patient's life. The operation should, however, only be carried out in those patients mentally able to cope with the inevitable psychic and physical trauma. The patient also needs to be informed of the inadequacies of the lenses she will require, to correct her aphakic state. Her field of vision will be restricted and peripheral images will be distorted.

MACULAR DEGENERATION

This condition is almost restricted to old age, apart from some rare familial forms. The changes seen at the macula on ophthalmoscopy may seem slight, but the effect on vision will be disastrous. Accumulations of pigment and exudates are most common, but cysts and haemorrhages may also be seen. Recent work has revealed that these changes are secondary to neovascularisation in splits between the membrane layers of the retina. The value of this knowledge is that photocoagulation might be capable of preventing progression of early lesions. Also, involvement of the other eye occurs in 12 per cent so that close follow up of patients with unilateral macular degeneration may mean that total loss of vision can be prevented. These techniques are at present in their very early stages, but do at last offer the possibility of treatment in a previously irremediable condition.

Sudden loss of vision

Apart from retinal detachment the causes of sudden visual loss are vascular. Such causes become increasingly common with ageing.

ARTERIAL OCCLUSION

Whether the loss of vision in the affected eye is partial or complete, will depend on the site of blockage. Central retinal artery occlusion will cause complete loss, but if only a branch is obstructed the visual loss will be less. The arterial lumen may lose its patency due either to thrombosis or embolism. The ischaemic area of retina will appear grey, and the site of the block, if in a branch, may also be visible. Treatment needs to be rapid and expert as after four hours, the retinal changes are usually irreversible. If an embolus is responsible for the occlusion, it may arise from the carotid artery or heart. It may consist of fibrin, cholesterol, platelets or an infected clot, efforts must be made to avoid a repeat episode.

GIANT CELL ARTERITIS

This is the underlying cause for central retinal artery thrombosis in some cases. Evidence of this possible aetiology must always be sought as prompt treatment with large doses of steroids (Prednisone 20 mgs three times daily) may prevent further episodes. It is of course even better to start treatment before the onset of visual loss. Details of the generalized symptoms and signs of giant cell arteritis are given in Chapter 9.

VENOUS OCCLUSION

Hypertensive and arteriosclerotic patients are at risk not only from retinal artery thrombosis, but also from venous occlusion. Other high-risk groups are those with increased blood viscosity, for example, patients with polycythaemia or macroglobulinaemia, and also patients with neoplastic disease. In venous occlusion the visual loss is not always sudden, but may take several days, and it is usually not complete.

When the central vein is blocked, the optic disc becomes swollen, red and congested. The veins are distended, the arteries are seen to be buried in the swelling and flame-shaped haemorrhages radiate from the disc. Occlusions of branch veins usually occur at arterio-venous crossings.

Once occlusion has happened, treatment seems ineffective, but any precipitating factors should be corrected, if possible, in order to protect the other eye.

IATROGENIC EYE DISEASE

Many drugs used in the treatment of chronic diseases have potential serious effects on the eyes. The phenothiazines have been reported as causing corneal and lens opacities, and in some cases, retinopathy. Antimalarials used in the treatment of rheumatoid arthritis, are also known to cause severe retinopathy. Long-term steroid treatment has caused cataracts in some patients, and their use will sometimes produce a rise in intra-ocular pressure. More recently the β blocker, practalol, has caused considerable concern, because of the complications of dry eye and corneal damage and is no longer used for long-term treatment.

Ears
Hearing

Just over one-eighth of a million people in this country over the age of 65 years are registered deaf or hard of hearing. Probably ten times as many have difficulty with their hearing, but have not bothered to register either through ignorance or indifference to their symptoms. The important causes of deafness in old age will be discussed in order, according to their frequency. Impaired hearing is a significant disability, not only for the obvious social disadvantages, but also because of its association with mental disorders. The elderly deaf are those most likely to suffer from paranoid psychosis.

PRESBYCUSIS

Hearing naturally becomes impaired with ageing, and this process is known as presbycusis. It starts at the age of about 30 years, but only becomes noticeable after 30 to 40 years of gradual deterioration. High frequency sounds become increasingly difficult to hear, and in normal speech, this especially affects the consonants s, f, and z. It also makes it more difficult to listen to female voices, as compared with those of men. Recruitment also occurs, which means that noisy surroundings are less well tolerated and make concentrated listening more difficult. Recruitment can therefore be a severe handicap in noisy out-patient departments or in the X-ray examination room. The hearing impairment is generally greater in men than women and this might be a reflection of their greater exposure to noise damage during their working life.

Both ears are normally equally affected, and air conduction is most impaired so that it comes closer to bone conduction. When sufficiently severe to cause inconvenience a hearing aid can be used to compensate for the changes of presbycusis.

WAX

It is very important to remember wax as a cause of deafness. Frequently it is responsible for impaired hearing in old age, where its combination with presbycusis can result in considerable deafness. Wax tends to become harder in the elderly, and its natural and spontaneous elimination from the external meatus is less efficient.

Detection of this cause for deafness is simple and treatment easy. After a 3- to 4-day period of softening with olive oil drops, the wax can usually be syringed away without difficulty.

MIDDLE-EAR CATARRH

This is usually the cause when someone complains of a worsening of her usual deafness after an upper respiratory tract infection. Fortunately, spontaneous resolution is the common outcome, but if this does not occur, expert drainage by myringotomy will be needed to allow the trapped fluid to escape.

OTOSCLEROSIS

This should be suspected in the 'young old' with a degree of deafness too severe to be accounted for by presbycusis; the deafness will be bilateral, and bone conduction will be more effective than air conduction. Expert confirmation of the diagnosis will be required, and also consideration of stapedectomy.

PAGET'S DISEASE

A full description of this condition is given in Chapter 9. It needs, however, to be mentioned here as deafness is often a feature of Paget's disease, due to bony compression of the auditory nerve. Improvement in hearing following treatment with calcitonin has been reported in some cases.

IATROGENIC DEAFNESS

Antibiotics of the aminoglycoside group are well known for causing permanent damage to the eighth cranial nerve. Those most likely to cause deafness are neomycin and kanomycin. High doses of the potent diuretic ethacrynic acid have also resulted in hearing impairment. Any toxic drug is most likely to cause damage in patients with reduced renal function, and many elderly patients are therefore at extra risk.

'Dizziness'

'Dizziness' is certainly a very frequent complaint in geriatric medicine, but one which unfortunately often eludes accurate diagnosis. In many cases, the cause is out with the vestibular mechanism. Such examples are postural hypotension, cardiac irregularities and anaemia where dizziness is not associated with vertigo. Vertigo, an abnormal sensation of rotation, occurs as part of 'dizziness' when the fault lies in the inner ear or its connecting pathways. The cause, however, may still be distant, for example, cervical spondylosis causing vertebrobasilar ischaemia on neck movement. The latter and other conditions are discussed in Chapter 10 which is concerned with instability.

'MÉNIÈRE'S SYNDROME'

If a history is obtained of severe episodic vertigo and tinnitus and progressive deafness, starting in middle age, then the diagnosis of Ménière's disease can fairly confidently be made. In these patients, the cause is increased fluid pressure in the vestibular apparatus.

More commonly, these symptoms arise for the first time in old age, with any of the three being the most troublesome. The mechanism is thought to be vascular in origin, and many will, in addition have hypertension, diabetes or evidence of widespread atherosclerosis. Treatment is usually unhelpful, and the sedatives and tranquillizers used in many cases are sometimes responsible for increasing the patient's unsteadiness.

IATROGENIC VESTIBULAR DAMAGE

Streptomycin and gentamycin are the preparations most likely to lead to persistent dizziness. The risks are greatest when there is renal impairment as in so many geriatric patients.

Communicating with the deaf

Patients who have become deaf in their old age will not have developed the skills of sign language or expert lip reading. Nevertheless, gestures can still be used as a supplement to speech and the position of the interviewer should be such that the patient has a good view of his lips. A quiet room without auditory or visual distractions is a definite advantage and sessions of questioning should be kept as short as possible.

A clear, slow voice should be used, and the patient asked if she can hear, and the voice should then be adjusted if necessary. Shouting is rarely helpful.

If the patient has a hearing aid, make sure that it is used. Check that the ear-piece is in place, that the amplifier is switched on and tuned properly. It is sometimes best to speak directly into the microphone, but again important not to shout.

When the patient does not have an aid of her own, but seems to need one, a temporary apparatus can be used. The simplest is a flexible ear trumpet, which may be successful if the hearing defect is not severe. This instrument, however, often causes embarrassment to both the patient and interviewer. Battery-operated microphone and ear-piece sets are available and are simple to use. The ear-piece may either be held in place, or be incorporated into a head-phone set. If all else fails, there is no alternative to the tedious and laborious process of writing down each question. In all situations, considerable patience and sympathy are required if the desired information is to be obtained from any deaf patient.

CHAPTER 19 · TREATMENT:
MEDICAL AND SURGICAL

I do not wish two diseases. One nature made and one
man made.

NAPOLEON I, 1769–1821

Medical treatment of the aged patient

Until comparatively recently the medical attitude to diseases in the
aged was one of ataraxy and neglect. Nowadays, the introduction of
new and potent pharmaceutical remedies and the burgeoning of the high
technological approach to common medical problems have produced a
danger that neglect of the elderly might give way to overzealous
investigation and frenetic efforts at treatment. These are the extremes
of a wide range of attitudes to geriatrics. The authors believe that the
middle way will prove to be the path to therapeutic success in the
majority of cases. It is of paramount importance to realize that although
there is no medical treatment which will combat senescence *per se*,
very many diseases in the elderly do respond satisfactorily to appropriate
treatment. Details of these treatments are given throughout the book.
This chapter simply aims to give some additional guidelines to medical
and surgical treatment.

Table 19.1. Principles of drug
treatment

Accurate diagnosis
Improve quality of life
Minimum drug schedules

The keystone of medical treatment is accurate diagnosis. Repeatedly
the reader's attention has been drawn to the difficulties in making an
accurate diagnosis. These include an inadequate history, the presence
of multiple pathology (and in consequence polypharmacy) and the
altered reaction to disease, so often observed in the elderly. A lack of
appreciation or a stoical indifference to pain, the weak response of the
body to infection and the striking interplay of psychosocial factors are
all worth bearing in mind. Also the elicitation and interpretation of

physical signs is difficult and time-consuming. These difficulties not-withstanding, much of the problem is the doctor—his attitudes, knowledge and skills. Universal application of good geriatric practice would produce an immense improvement in the care of the elderly. That is why this book came to be written.

Sensible prescribing

Having made the diagnosis the doctor should aim to improve the quality of the patient's life using the minimum number of drugs in the simplest possible way. Not all medical problems are amenable to drug treatment. If in doubt, no drug is usually better than just any drug selected by inspired guesswork. A placebo (e.g. vitamin C tablets) might suffice if the doctor feels that the urge to prescribe is irresistible. In many

Table 19.2. Limitations of drug treatment

Loss of organ reserve
Lack of patient compliance
Adverse side effects
Drug interaction
Senescence

patients with anxiety, mild to moderate depression and restricted mobility, social and physical rehabilitation may be more appropriate than medicines. If drugs are used, it is important that they should be taken by the patient, precisely as prescribed by the doctor. Patient compliance in this respect, is notoriously poor and it gets worse as the frequency of doses and the multiplicity of drugs increase. To help obviate some of the difficulties, many geriatric units now make an attempt to familiarize the patient with taking her own drugs prior to discharge. Obviously, the utmost simplicity of prescribing is required, and supervision of the drugs by a sensible, concerned relative or friend or the community nurse, may be essential, if adequate home treatment is to be provided.

Adverse drug reactions

Adverse drug reactions (ADR's) are much more of a problem in the elderly than in the young, the incidence in the eighth decade being some seven times that in the third. The elderly tend to be exposed to bigger total drug burdens and are less tolerant of them than the young. This latter phenomenon appears to be due in part to generally higher blood levels of the drugs and in part to impaired homeostasis so that even the milder ADR is less well tolerated. For example a tendency to hypotension, increased body sway or cerebral impairment might all be tolerable in a young person yet be disabling to an old lady. There is little evidence of enhanced tissue sensitivity in the elderly although this probably exists with respect to nitrazepan and warfarin. However it has to be admitted that a great deal of the pharmacology of the aged remains to be worked out.

The generally high blood levels of drugs in the elderly relate to reductions of body weight, lean body mass, metabolic activity and renal function. Additionally more free drug is available in the blood if the plasma binding sites are reduced in number as happens in hypoalbuminaemia commonly seen in ill old people. Absorption of drugs from the gut is usually by passive transfer and therefore not commonly impaired.

The kidney is the major route of drug excretion and renal function falls progressively with age even in the absence of overt disease. Thus it can be assumed that, with drugs dependent upon this route of excretion and possessing a low therapeutic ratio (i.e. ratio of toxic to therapeutic blood levels) toxic effects are likely unless an appropriate reduction in dosage is made. Indeed drugs in this category are best avoided altogether—e.g. the aminoglycosides, digoxin, nitrofurantoin, chlorpropamide and the biguanides. Luckily the indications for them in geriatrics are few and shrinking year by year.

The adverse effects of drugs may be more burdensome to the patient than the original disease. They are so numerous that whole books have been written about them. Some are mentioned in a little detail in this section to press home the point that the prescriber must retain a highly critical approach to his activities. Ideally he should know (not just hope) that the drug he prescribes will do good and that the likely adverse effects will not be worse than the disease to be treated. In the patient with multiple pathology, the urge to treat each and every 'treatable' complaint must be firmly resisted. There must be cogent reasons for every single drug used. The liability of the elderly to mental confusion, giddy spells, falls, postural hypotension and incontinence has been mentioned repeatedly in different chapters. These upsets are often due to drug treatment. Common offenders are the psychosedatives, anti-Parkinson drugs, antidepressants and diuretics. These matters are dealt with in the appropriate chapters.

FLUID AND ELECTROLYTE BALANCE

Fluid and electrolyte balance may be upset with deleterious effects on the patient. The classic example of hypokalaemia, due to diuretic therapy, causing digitalis toxicity must always be kept in mind when using these drugs. A less dramatic adverse effect of hypokalaemia is lassitude and muscle weakness. Many elderly patients have a low body potassium even before medical treatment begins; the lack being due to reduced intake or excess loss on account of gastrointestinal or renal disease. The plasma concentration of potassium, represents only about 2 per cent of the total body potassium, and accurate assessment of total body potassium is available only in a few specialist centres using a whole body counter. Therefore for clinical purposes, the context of the complaints coupled with a low-serum potassium level must suffice in the recognition of the deficit. The use of diuretics is detailed in Chapter 14 but let it be said here that the dose and type of preparation should be tailored to the patient's needs. Massive diuresis is usually not required and might precipitate acute retention of urine or acute hypotension and circulatory collapse.

Sodium and fluid retention also results from a number of other drugs. For example the adrenal corticosteroids especially cortisone and fludrocortisone—the latter being used to treat postural hypotension associated with hypovolaemia. Prednisone and prednisolone have less effect on salt and water metabolism. The sex hormones used especially in the treatment of breast and prostatic cancer are particularly liable to cause oedema, cardiac failure and hypertension. Similar effects may be seen with phenylbutazone and oxyphenbutazone. The sex hormones have another calamitous adverse effect in the increased incidence of thromboembolism which accompanies their use even in small doses.

PHOTOXICITY

The prevailing passion for sunbathing is shared by some elderly patients, and so it must be remembered that many of the commonly used drugs can make the skin abnormally sensitive to sunlight. This may occur in a matter of hours or days after first taking the drug. The resultant phototoxicity allows bright sunlight to provoke a severe sunburn on the exposed skin. The damage is usually superficial and resolves when the causative agents are withdrawn. Less often photo-allergy occurs; this takes two to three weeks to develop or comes on after repeated courses of the drug. It lasts for months or years and the whole thickness of the skin is affected. Itching and eczematous changes are common. Drugs likely to cause solar sensitivity include tetra-cyclines, phenothiazines, antihistamines, nalidixic acid, the thiazide diuretics, sulphonamides (antibacterial and antidiabetic) oestrogens and barbiturates.

Drug interactions

Drug interaction may occur when two or more drugs are given con-currently. The pharmacological effects of the drugs may be enhanced or diminished by the interaction. For example, trimethoprim and sulphamethoxazole exhibit synergism, making the combined preparation a more valuable antibiotic than the simple sum of its two parts. On the other hand aluminium hydroxide binds with oral tetracycline to form an inabsorbable complex and so deprives the patient of the antibiotic. Drugs may interact at the receptor sites in the tissues; barbiturates and antihistamines appear to potentiate the effect of alcohol in this way. This can be dangerous. The CNS depressant effects of alcohol plus antihistamine are very much greater than a simple summation of their separate effects would suggest. The monoamine oxidase inhibitors (MAOIs) when used concurrently with an adrenergic agonist can cause catastrophic hypertension and several deaths have been reported. The long list of drugs and foodstuffs contraindicated in the presence of MAOIs make these preparations so hazardous that they should not be used in geriatrics.

Many drugs circulate firmly bound to the plasma proteins especially the albumin but only the free drug is pharmacologically active. Many naturally occurring substances are also bound in this way (Table 19.3). These two groups of agents vary in their binding potential and may thus displace one another. For example phenylbutazone will displace sulphas (antidiabetic as well as antibacterial) and the coumarin anti-coagulants and so enhance their pharmacological activity. The dangers of overdose (with hypoglycaemia or bleeding in these two examples)

Table 19.3. Substances bound to plasma proteins

Physiological	Pharmacological
bilirubin	penicillins
bile acids	tetracyclines
porphyrins	barbiturates
fatty acids	sulpha drugs
uric acid	phenylbutazone
vitamin C	warfarin

will be apparent. This is especially so with long-acting drugs like warfarin and chlorpropamide. Hypoglycaemia is life threatening, and in the case of chlorpropamide potentiated by phenylbutazone, even if it is corrected by glucose, it may recur hours later despite stopping all drug treatment.

DRUG METABOLISM

The majority of drugs undergo some metabolic change in the liver prior
to excretion by the kidney. Therefore hepatic metabolism governs to
some (variable) extent both renal excretion and the plasma half-life
(T/2). Phase I hepatic reactions, include oxidation, reduction and
hydrolysis and phase II reactions include conversion to sulphates,
glucuronides and mercapturates. If the enzyme systems in the liver are
depressed by treatment or disease, the effects of certain drugs will be
enhanced; e.g. alcohol, pethidine and barbiturates. The monoamine
oxidase inhibitors have this depressant effect on the microsomal enzymes in the liver in addition to widespread suppression of the monoamine
oxidases. This depressant effect persists for weeks after the MAOI has
been stopped. Some drugs stimulate the liver enzymes (a process known
as induction) and thus accelerate drug metabolism and thereby diminish
the pharmacological effects of the inducing drug and of other drugs given
concurrently. The best-known example is the barbiturates which induce
the microsomal enzymes to cause an accelerated biotransformation of
warfarin, phenytoin, phenylbutazone and the barbiturates themselves.
Because of the diminished pharmacological activity of the more rapidly
destroyed drug, the dose must be increased to provide an adequate
therapeutic response, but with the danger of overdose when the inducer
is stopped. For example, the danger of bleeding when a patient stabilized
on warfarin and also taking barbiturate is persuaded to stop the latter.
Many other drugs activate the microsomal enzymes in this way,
including glutethimide (Doriden), meprobamate (Miltown) and chloral
hydrate. The enzyme induction is non-specific and it increases the
metabolism of bilirubin also. This fact has been used therapeutically in
unconjugated hyperbilirubinaemia, to reduce the icterus.

NEED FOR PRUDENT PRESCRIBING

From what has been said it will be realized that drug treatment
intended to be beneficial can be very hazardous. Elderly patients are
more than usually prone to adverse drug reactions because of their
generally more extensive previous drug exposure and their bigger
schedule of current drugs on account of multiple pathology. Additionally
they often have some degree of renal failure and a rather small lean
body maas. Erosion of cerebral reserve compounds the difficulties and
the patient may get into a frightful muddle with her numerous tablets.
Furthermore, if she takes the tablets, they may very likely make her
more mentally confused!! To use a transatlantic expression the patient
has been put into a 'no win situation'. Clinical pharmacology is a
complicated business and polypharmacy produces mind-stretching

pharmacokinetic possibilities. The physician needs to have a good working knowledge of the pharmacology of a few drugs best suited to his practice. He should use them sparingly, discreetly and with consummate skill.

Surgical treatment in old age

In surgery as in medicine, the crux of the matter is diagnosis, followed by prudent treatment. As always, there may be problems of multiple pathology and additionally there is the problem of reduced tolerance to shock. The concomitant medical disorders may to a variable degree make surgery difficult, increase the likelihood of post-operative complications and even preclude operation. Especial attention must be given to the recognition of these incidental medical problems, viz.: intellectual failure, ischaemic heart disease, cerebrovascular disease, diabetes mellitus, renal failure, skin infections (especially intertrigo), chronic bronchitis and emphysema. Anaemia and dehydration related to the surgical disease are commonly present in patients requiring urgent operation. Furthermore surgical emergencies (at all ages) do less well than elective cases, the mortality increasing four-or five-fold. A mortality rate of 30 per cent might be expected in emergency abdominal surgery with peritonitis. With the patient in very poor shape pre-operatively the likelihood of death will be very much higher.

Assessment for operation

An assessment of the patient's attitude to the proposed procedure is of cardinal importance. Is the patient keen or at least willing to have the operation? The elderly patient should practically never be pushed into surgery and certainly there must be no brow-beating. A simple explanation of the clinical problems, an outline of the courses open and an indication of the likely prognosis with and without operation is all that is required. However, if the patient is too ill to decide, then the doctor (preferably after consultation with the relatives) must decide. The prognosis without operation must be most carefully considered, to see if it is really so much worse a prospect than the prognosis after successful surgery. Additional factors to be considered are the manifest risks of the operation and its likely complications.

A particularly careful history and physical examination is required. Some simple psychometric tests must always be used (see Chapter 8). Failure to do this will allow the patient with considerable dementia to go for operation unrecognized. This can have disastrous results partly because of the increased mental disturbance post-operatively and partly because the degree of dementia may be sufficient to negate the value of surgery. A great deal of upset is caused, but to little avail; the patient and her relatives being completely dissatisfied with the whole affair.

Table 19.4. Assessment for surgery

Mental and physical state
Prognosis without operation
Patient's attitude to surgery
Hazards of surgery
Prognosis if operation successful

The chest X-ray and ECG will be part of the routine work-up. Unsuspected neoplasm, tuberculosis, cardiac enlargement or hiatus hernia may be spotted on the former. The electrocardiogram may show evidence of gross and previously unsuspected myocardial damage. Lack of mobility leaves the cardiovascular system undertaxed and so the ischaemic heart disease is silent. Whether normal or abnormal the ECG is most useful for comparison with later records should there be a post-operative collapse. Myocardial infarction following operation can be a most difficult diagnostic problem and the doctor needs all the help he can get. Evidence of recent myocardial infarction and the presence of congestive failure would favour deferment of the operation for at least six months. Even after a good recovery these cases represent substandard risks.

The patient's drug history needs to be known. Previous sensitivities must be recorded and a note made of the current drug schedule to help the anaesthetist with his choice of anaesthetic and pre- and post-operative medication. To avoid the risks of interaction the minimum number of drugs should be used. Pre-operative sedation of the type used in younger patients may cause restlessness and mental disorientation. A test dose a day or two before operation might be helpful to see how the patient reacts. In any event the actual doses should be kept down to the minimum.

Priorities for surgery

Cases considered for surgery fall into three broad categories with regard to priority:
1 Urgent
2 Imminent
3 Elective

In the urgent category are those surgical emergencies which brook no delay. They require speedy pre-operative assessment and preparation and operation within hours. Perforated peptic ulcer, strangulated hernia, acute appendicitis, popliteal embolus and fractured femur (usually) come into this category.

In the imminent category are those patients who will soon require surgery but a period of observation and medical treatment over days rather than hours would be reasonable. Subdural haematoma or gangrene of the foot would fall into this category.

In the elective category come the majority of ailments potentially treatable by operation. The need for surgery is not urgent in terms of hours, days or even weeks and indeed the need for surgery may be debatable. In these cases much depends on a comparison of the life expectancy and burden of disability with and without surgery. In this context it is as well to remember that a man aged sixty years and in average health can expect to live for a further fifteen years and a well women of the same age can expect to reach eighty years. Even the seventy-year-olds can expect to live ten and twelve years respectively. Thus in a well person, a surgical condition which may give rise to trouble at a later date should be dealt with, while the going is good, because the results of emergency surgery when the crisis comes, will be very much worse than with the elective procedure. Two common examples are the hernia which causes discomfort and may strangulate and the gall-bladder with stones which has already produced one or two attacks of acute cholecystitis. Uterine prolapse, rectal prolapse, haemorrhoids and troublesome varicose veins might also be dealt with in the fit old person. The aim of surgery being to add life to years—just the same as in medicine.

The possibilities for surgery range from the highly desirable to the totally unreasonable. The range is wide and which case falls where in the spectrum is often debatable. Surgery of election should normally be attempted for resectable cancer of the colon and upper rectum when continuity of the gut can be made good. But if the growth is such that a permanent colostomy is required that is quite a different matter. It takes a year or more for a willing and fully competent person to adjust to the colostomy life. This may well prove beyond the capacity of the aged person. A permanent colostomy is certainly not worth contemplating as a palliative measure and may indeed be questionable as part of a curative procedure in many patients. Similar arguments apply to operations on the upper gut. A gastrectomy which is curative (e.g. for persistent or recurrent bleeding from a peptic ulcer or an apparently operable cancer) is advisable. A gastrostomy for cancer of the oesophagus is not advised. Palliative resection of the cancer is a practical procedure in the fitter patients. The aim being to restore normal swallowing until death. However, the operative mortality is about 20 per cent and in many cases the patient will not be fit for the operation. In this situation the lumen can be maintained by the insertion of a Celestin tube through the narrowed gullet using an oesophagoscope and with a small incision in the stomach to pull through the pilot bougie. For the least fit patients, the Soutar's tube is still used but it provides a smaller lumen than the Celestin technique. In the elderly patient with bronchial carcinoma, lobectomy is an operation which usually falls into the unreasonable category. Nevertheless even in the seventy-year-olds, if the general health and lung function are good, lobectomy is a practical proposition. Only the squamous-celled growths are submitted to surgery. The oat-celled variety does badly whatever treatment is given.

Preparation for operation

As already mentioned mental and physical fitness is often defective in some respect and any pre-operative decrement in health worsens the post-operative prognosis. In the non-urgent case there is ample time in which to improve physical fitness by the correction of anaemia, control of diabetes and treatment of infection. The undernourished patient will benefit by improved nutrition and the obese by weight reduction. A course of graded physical exercise, including breathing exercises, will help further to improve physical fitness. In the emergency case, swift pre-operative resuscitation is required to give the surgeon a reasonable chance of success. The usual blood tests are performed—haemoglobin, PCV, urea and electrolytes, blood-grouping and cross-matching. Once the blood has gone to the laboratory an attempt must be made to correct the dehydration, hypovolaemia and anaemia according to the needs of the case. Intravenous fluids will be required. The type of fluid given intravenously will depend on the type of fluid loss viz.:

Acute blood loss—replace with whole blood.
Chronic blood loss—give packed cells.
Diarrhoea and vomiting—give sodium chloride solution (150 mmol/l) and potassium supplement.

Acidosis will require correction with sodium lactate or sodium bicarbonate solution (each 167 mmol/l).

If the dehydration is at all severe, several litres of fluid (2 litres of sodium chloride to 1 litre of sodium lactate) should be run in during the first few hours. The central venous pressure (CVP) should be monitored using a simple manometric device and the pressure kept below 10 cm. A check on the patient's urinary output is required together with the usual observation of pulse, respiratory rate, blood pressure and auscultation of the lung bases. If fluid overload occurs the infusion must be stopped and a potent loop diuretic administered intravenously. Bacteraemic shock will fail to respond to this type of resuscitation. Large doses of hydrocortisone intravenously (100 mg 4 hourly) as well as antibiotics should be given.

Post-operative management

Restlessness and mental confusion are common and invite the prescription of psychosedative drugs which may make matters worse. A remediable cause may be found; e.g. dehydration and electrolyte imbalance, distended bowel from flatus or faeces, pain from the operation wound or pressure sores and drugs. Acute toxic psychosis may follow the use of anticholinergic drugs (e.g., atropine and propantheline). The dehydration and electrolyte imbalance require correction.

Table 19.5. Post-operative restlessness and confusion

Dehydration and electrolyte imbalance
Drugs
Pain
Distension of bowel or bladder
Underlying dementia
Infection or infarction

Sufficient fluid must be given to ensure a urinary output of one litre every 24 hours. Parenteral fluids one litre every 8 hours with monitoring of CVP will be required if the patient is unable to drink adequately. Morphine and barbiturates can be lethal in aged post-operative patients and are best avoided altogether. Both make the patient much less co-operative. Morphine depresses respiration and the cough reflex and frequently makes the patient vomit. If morphine is used the dose should be as small as possible (5–10 mg subcutaneously). Diamorphine (heroin) in similar doses causes less sedation and much less nausea but the risk of respiratory depression is as great. The main effects of morphine last up to six hours after subcutaneous injection. Heroin has a shorter action. Both drugs are potentiated by the phenothiazines. If respiratory depression occurs, nalorphine 5–10 mg or levallorphan 0·2–2 mg should be given intravenously to counteract the opiate. Chlorpromazine 25–50 mg twice or thrice daily will help to quell nausea and vomiting if the patient is unable to swallow.

In the early hours after the operation (and indeed during the operation) the patient will be at risk of developing pressure sores. These must be prevented if at all possible by frequent turning (see Chapter 9). A pressure sore will add greatly to the patient's distress and to her length of stay in hospital. Deep breathing, coughing and movement are all to be encouraged as soon as possible. Even after major abdominal surgery it should be the aim to have the patient standing up by the side of her bed (well supported) and sitting out in a chair within 24 hours. Thereafter she is encouraged into increasing physical activity. This is so important that the ward sister and the ward doctor should personally supervise it.

Chest and heart complications commonly follow operation in the elderly, no doubt due to the fairly high incidence of pre-existing chest and heart disease. The reported incidence varies from 10 to 50 per cent according to the selection of cases and the thoroughness of pre-operative assessment. Flare-up of chronic bronchitis, bronchopneumonia, segmental or lobar collapse, pulmonary infarction and pleurisy all commonly occur; also myocardial infarction, cardiac dysrhythmias and heart failure. Wound sepsis and dehiscence is more common in older patients. Perhaps the most common serious post-operative complication is deep-vein thrombosis and the commonest cause of post-operative death is pulmonary embolism.

DEEP-VEIN THROMBOSIS

Early ambulation and the prevention or early correction of dehydration do much to reduce the incidence of deep-vein thrombosis (DVT). The thrombosis begins in the venous plexus of the calf and may be impossible to detect clinically. Later the thrombus spreads to the popliteal and femoral veins causing increased risk of pulmonary embolism. In the minority of cases there is some ankle oedema with pain and tenderness in the calf. Special techniques are available to detect and localize the thrombus but they are not in general use; e.g. the intravenous injection of radio-iodine labelled fibrinogen which becomes incorporated into the thrombus and can be located by a portable monitor; also the use of ultrasound (Sonicaid) to detect reduced flow in the vessels. The introduction of these tests has underlined the magnitude of the problem of post-operative DVT; this complication being detectable by these techniques in one-quarter to one-half of major abdominal surgical cases.

DVT commonly results in pulmonary embolism and it may permanently obstruct the venous drainage from the limb. Pulmonary emboli may be small and recurrent and produce a clinical picture suggestive of bronchopneumonia. Attacks of pleurisy and haemoptysis, or intractable heart failure with hypotension may develop. A large embolus is usually rapidly fatal.

Treatment of DVT requires immediate anticoagulants. Heparin is given intravenously 10,000 units every six hours and warfarin 20–25 mg as a loading dose is given orally. The dose of the latter is varied in response to the results of the Thrombotest. When the patient is stabilized on the warfarin the heparin is stopped. (Some authorities prefer the extended use of heparin monitored by control of whole blood-clotting times as opposed to the early switch to warfarin.) The warfarin is given once daily and maintenance doses will be advised by the laboratory. Adjustment of the dose must be made carefully because it is a long-acting drug and therefore has a cumulative action.

So dangerous and so common is DVT post-operatively that new ways of dealing with the problem are always under consideration. A case has been made for low-dose prophylactic heparin given sub-cutaneously. Excellent results have been achieved with treatment started two hours before operation and continued for seven days or until the patient is fully mobilized. The dose used is 5,000 units every six hours. There is less DVT and embolism and no increase in haemorrhage. Another prophylactic treatment still under trial is the use of drugs (e.g. aspirin and dipyridamole (Persantin)) to reduce platelet adhesiveness. The treatment is started the day prior to the operation in an attempt to prevent the formation of platelet—thrombin complexes which adhere to the venous endothelium and initiate the thrombotic process. With dipyridamole and aspirin taken together a reduction greater than 50 per cent has been found in the incidence of DVT following general surgery. Additional prophylactic measures are correction of hypovolaemia, minimum sedation and early physical activity.

HAZARDS OF WARFARIN THERAPY

The heparin–warfarin treatment described is standard practice in the UK and, together with general prophylactic measures, is the best we can do to reduce the risk of pulmonary embolus in cases of deep-vein thrombosis. These drug treatments are not without considerable risk especially in geriatric practice. Difficulties in control correlate with increasing age and debility, liver disease, renal failure and changing concomitant drug treatment. Interference with normal drug metabolism may take place at various points along the pharmaco-kinetic pathway (Fig. 19.1). Many drugs interact with warfarin; phenylbutazone, salicylates and broad spectrum antibiotics enhance the anticoagulant effect by displacement from plasma albumin. Pheno-barbitone and some other sedatives depress it due to enzyme-induction (already described under drug interaction). Distalgesic (dextro-propoxyphene and paracetamol) is also reported to enhance the hypo-prothrombinaemic effect of warfarin. Apparently it does not displace the warfarin from the plasma binding sites but may compete with it for metabolism by the liver microsomal enzymes that hydroxylate the warfarin. Certainly dextropropoxyphene causes plasma warfarin levels to rise. Paracetamol alone appears to be innocuous in this context and so it is the analgesic of choice in this situation.

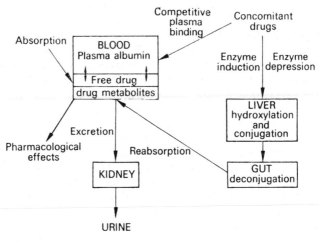

Fig. 19.1. Warfarin pharmacokinetic pathways

Patients on anticoagulants are at risk from spontaneous bleeding, e.g. into the skin, muscles, renal tract and gut. Spontaneous intramural haematoma affecting the gut particularly the jejunum, may occur. Also the mesentery may fill with blood and there may be haemorrhagic serous effusions. The symptoms relating to the gut consist of abdominal discomfort or intestinal colic, intestinal obstruction and bloody diarrhoea. Usually a long single segment of gut is involved but the haematomata can be multiple. They usually subside after stopping the anticoagulant and any potentiating drug (e.g. aspirin, tetracycline or phenylbutazone). General supportive measures will be required including nasogastric tube, parenteral fluids and possibly transfusion of fresh blood. Surgical intervention will usually not be required. Intramural bleeding must be

Table 19.6. Warfarin control difficult in the presence of

Renal failure	Dextropropoxyphene
Liver disease	Antibiotics
Phenylbutazone	Phenobarbitone
Indomethacin	Salicylates

differentiated from segmental mesenteric vascular occlusion because of the therapeutic implications. In the former there is usually other evidence of bleeding and the Thrombotest result is low. In the latter the reverse obtains.

Some common surgical conditions

It is beyond the scope of this book to go into details of the innumerable surgical conditions which afflict the elderly. What follows is a simple review of some of the very common problems to give the student an insight into the opportunities provided by the surgical approach.

Gallstones

Gallstones occur in epidemic proportions in the UK. The incidence increases steadily with age so that about one quarter of the over seventies have them. Mostly the stones are silent for very long periods of time but if the patient lives long enough there is an even chance of developing symptoms and these are likely to be more serious in the elderly. Attacks of biliary colic, cholecystitis or obstructive jaundice may necessitate operation. With elective surgery in a well person the risks are low—below 1 per cent in expert hands. In emergency surgery the risks are greater. Thus there is good reason to advise elective cholecystectomy whenever gallstones are discovered and especially if one or more acute attacks have been experienced, unless the general condition of the patient contraindicates surgery. The younger the patient the more valid the argument.

Prostatic hyperplasia

About one-fifth of surgical emergencies in patients over the age of seventy years are due to acute retention of urine. Prostatic hyperplasia is the commonest cause, but some cases will be due to other causes (see Chapter 11). In the male with a previous history of prostatism and a palpably enlarged prostate the diagnosis is certain, but the precipitating factor may have been enforced recumbency, on account of some other illness, or the use of anticholinergic drugs. It is urgent to relieve the distended bladder, and this may occur if pain can be relieved and the patient sat in a warm bath. Failing this a narrow gauge catheter should be passed using closed drainage into a plastic bag. It is important to maintain sterility because this reduces post-operative morbidity.

Early surgical consultation is indicated and age is no barrier to operation—even the ninety-year-old can come through satisfactorily.

The peak age incidence for prostatectomy is in the seventh decade. Transurethral resection (TUR) is used increasingly. Over 75 per cent of prostatectomies in Cambridge are of this type and the post-operative mortality is around 3 per cent. Urine flow is much improved by surgery —this being the main purpose of the exercise. Frequency of micturition is usually not improved and the patient must be warned of this to spare unnecessary disappointment. Some cases fail to recover continence. This is especially so in those with dementia. These cases are best managed by permanent catheterization.

CARCINOMA OF THE PROSTATE

This relatively common cancer is essentially a disease of old age as was illustrated in Chapter 17. The incidence and mortality increase rapidly after middle age. Over 75 per cent of cases present with retention of urine or urinary infection, 15 per cent present with symptoms due to metastases, particularly bone pain, but in some of these cases also obstruction is present. Others are picked up when investigating general debility or some similar nondescript complaint. The prostate may be generally enlarged or nodular. Approximately 50 per cent of all hard nodules of the prostate are carcinomatous. The growth may spread locally outside the prostate to the seminal vesicles, to block off a ureteric orifice or produce a more extensive local spread—the 'frozen pelvis'. Histological diagnosis can be obtained by needle biopsy. This is a quick, cheap and relatively painless procedure. Haematuria occurs if the bladder is inadvertently entered. The aggressiveness of the cancer (as with most cancers) varies a lot from case to case but in general terms 85 per cent of untreated and 60 per cent of treated cases will be dead in three years. Overall less than 15 per cent survive five years and the treated cases do just a little better. The older patients appear to suffer from a generally less aggressive illness so that often some other disease causes death.

Secondary deposits occur in lymph nodes, lungs, liver, adrenals and bones. Prostatic carcinoma shows a marked predilection for the lumbar vertebrae, pelvis and femur but any bone can be involved and the full extent may only be revealed by bone scan. Spread via the vertebral plexus of veins is said to account for this particular distribution. The skeletal metastases are osteoblastic and produce dense sclerosis readily recognizable on X-ray and also elevation of the serum alkaline phosphatase (normally below 100 IU/l). The prostatic epithelium also secretes acid phosphatase and this property may be maintained by the tumour to produce an elevation of the serum acid phosphatase (normally below 6 IU/l). However not all prostatic cancers produce elevation of acid and alkaline phosphatases and not all elevations of these enzymes are due to prostatic cancer. In the past physicians have attached too much significance to the acid phosphatase level in making the diagnosis. High levels due to other causes (e.g. rectal examination and benign prostatic adenoma) can be misleading.

TREATMENT OF PROSTATIC CANCER

It is impossible to be dogmatic about the management of this common but capricious cancer. It exhibits an amazing range of aggression in different patients. The main lines of treatment available are TUR, oestrogens, castration, radiotherapy and radical or total prostatectomy. Combined procedures may be employed. The exhibition of oestrogens, often in very high doses, enjoyed great popularity until it was discovered that the hazards of treatment were greater than those of the disease; namely thromboembolic disease and fluid retention sufficient to tip the elderly patient into congestive cardiac failure. Furthermore there is no good evidence that large doses of stilboestrol are any more valuable than small doses in the control of the cancer. Painful gynaecomastia is an irritation to the patient and adds to his burden.

Table 19.7. Treatment of
cancer of the prostate

Masterly inactivity
Transurethral resection
Hormones
Castration
Radiotherapy
Radical prostatectomy

The use of oestrogens in every patient with carcinoma of the prostate is unnecessary and potentially harmful. Many patients require no treatment of any sort when first seen. Oestrogens are indicated when there is advanced local disease or distant metastases. Stilboestrol 1 mg thrice daily will achieve suppression of plasma testosterone to 'female' levels; i.e. a pharmacological castration. Even with these small doses fluid retention may occur and a diuretic will be required. If the stilbo-estrol is ill tolerated or ineffective, alternative preparations are available to suppress testosterone secretion; e.g. fosfestrol (Honvan) 100 mg thrice daily or ethinyloestradiol 50 μg twice daily. Chlorotrianisene (Tace) is a synthetic pro-oestrogen given in a dose of 24 mg (one tablet) daily. It is said to be beneficial in prostatic cancer but it does not depress plasma testosterone levels. If drug therapy fails orchidectomy might be justified. Adrenalectomy, hypophysectomy and cytotoxic drugs have all been tried and found wanting.

If obstruction to urine flow persists despite hormone therapy then a transurethral resection must be considered. The alternative would be permanent catheter drainage. Radiotherapy is reserved for extensive local growth or painful bony metastases not responding to oestrogens. Radical resection of the whole prostate for a malignant nodule with no evidence of metastases has its advocates—but not in Cambridge. Impotence and incontinence are common and unacceptable complications of this operation for a lesion which in these selected cases probably has a relatively benign prognosis.

Gastrointestinal cancer

As was seen in Chapter 17 there are some common cancers of the gastrointestinal tract affecting the elderly. They are all regarded as surgical diseases. Cancer of the large gut including rectum is the second commonest cause of death from malignant disease in the UK. Cancer of the stomach ranks third. Cancer of the stomach is a gloomy business in most cases, less than 5 per cent (all ages) remaining alive five years after diagnosis. Colon and rectum have overall five-year survivals of just over 20 per cent of all cases. Treated cases of large bowel cancer do rather better overall than do the untreated cases with average five-year survivals of about 30 per cent. This could in large part be due to selection for surgery of the earlier cancers in the fitter patients. Information such as this leads one to believe that in most cases these patients have disseminated disease before resection of the primary growth. Matters of diagnosis and medical treatment are dealt with in Chapter 15. About a third of patients with cancer of the stomach who come to surgery will have an apparently operable growth. When gastrectomy is performed as a 'curative' procedure the five-year mortality is still around 75 per cent. Furthermore the patient needs to be pretty fit to withstand this sort of operation which might involve total gastrectomy and splenectomy. Clearly only the minority of elderly patients should be submitted to this sort of ordeal when the likely gain is so small. Radiotherapy and cytotoxic drugs offer nothing better.

Cancer of the large bowel much more often comes to surgery with an operable lesion. In other words these cancers present earlier in terms of recognizable local and distant spread. Thus the prognosis is better overall than for the stomach. Surgical resection with the restitution of continuity of the gut is usually recommended. As already explained colostomy must be avoided in the older patient and should never be used as a palliative measure. It presents an insufferable burden to the old person. With advanced rectal growths fulguration may offer worthwhile palliation. Cytotoxic drugs and radiotherapy are of little avail in these cases.

INTESTINAL OBSTRUCTION

Many of these obstructions are of a simple mechanical nature so that early diagnosis and treatment really does effect a cure. On suspicion of the diagnosis immediate surgical consultation is required. Mortality rates are acceptably low for the otherwise fit elderly person presenting to the surgeon with early uncomplicated intestinal obstruction. With delay (often in the hands of the physician who tends to prevaricate and over-investigate) complications develop and the mortality rises steeply.

Acute obstruction of the small gut is usually due to a femoral or inguinal hernia. A thorough examination of the groins and abdominal wall is required. The scar of a previous abdominal operation, may be the clue to the diagnosis in those cases which are due to adhesions or visceral hernia.

Carcinoma of the left side of the colon is one of the commonest causes of obstruction of the large gut. Volvulus especially of the sigmoid but also of the caecum is also seen. The site of the obstruction can usually be determined by examination of plain X-ray films of the abdomen taken with the patient upright and supine. Rapid pre-operative resuscitation is required to correct fluid and electrolyte loss while the stomach is kept empty by suction and concomitant medical conditions are treated at the same time. However, time is of the essence because delay increases the risk. For example the overall mortality from strangulated hernia is low but rises steeply if gangrenous bowel has to be resected. Large bowel obstructions usually allow more time for preparation but here again delay can spell disaster. The twisted bowel may become gangrenous, peritonitis follows and the outcome very often is death.

Fractures

The incidence of fracture increases with age, due to a decrease in the mechanical strength of the bone, and the greatly enhanced liability to fall. Fractures of hip, wrist, and vertebral body are most common but any bone may be involved. Treatment is designed to relieve pain, secure adequate reduction and fixation and to restore normal function. The patient with fracture presents as a surgical emergency and so commonly is in an unsatisfactory state for surgery. Full pre-operative assessment and preparation as described earlier will be required for all the major cases.

The common fracture at the wrist due to a fall onto the outstretched hand may require reduction under a general anaesthetic and a period of immobilization in a plaster-of-Paris cast. The fingers must be left free and the hand used by the patient right from the start. When there is little displacement of the distal fragments a simple cock-up splint is all that is required.

FRACTURED FEMUR

Fractures of the upper end of the femur present a formidable problem. These are mostly fractures requiring major surgery and are, as it were, self-selected unfit patients. These patients suffer from all the ills that the elderly are heir to. There are three main types of upper femoral fracture:

    1 undisplaced subcapital.
    2 displaced subcapital.
    3 trochanteric.

In Cambridge the undisplaced subcapital fracture is usually fixed using Moore's pins. It is the least common of the three types, suffers much less surgical trauma and carries a much better prognosis for survival than the others. The displaced subcapital fracture is the most common type and was called the 'unsolved fracture' because of the high failure rate with internal fixation. There is much debate regarding the most appropriate treatment. The Cambridge orthopaedic surgeons currently use a Thompson type of hip replacement for all of these cases. The operative mortality is of the order of 12 per cent which compares very favourably with other hospitals offering a district general service. The trochanteric fracture can be readily fixed with a nail and plate combination (locally a sliding device is used) which relieves pain and allows early mobilization.

The overall mortality for fractured neck of the femur remains high despite phenomenal advances in anaesthetic and surgical technique. The innumerable hazards of emergency major surgery in a (usually) unfit old person pose insuperable problems. Nevertheless there is always room for improvement and new approaches are constantly under trial. The mortality in the better units is well below the national average. Early operation is best if the medical conditions allow. Hence the aphorism—'never let the sun set twice before operation on a fractured femur!' Another maxim is 'never allow stasis in the calf muscles'. The natural calf muscle pump must be kept at work and even during the operation an assistant will flex and dorsiflex the patient's feet every five minutes to keep the blood flowing. The affected limb should be kept elevated to improve venous return. In the ward the foot of the bed is raised for the same reason. Various mechanical devices are available to give intermittent calf pressure and stimulate calf blood flow. Anticoagulants and antiplatelet drugs have been used but without such clear advantages as in general surgery. In dealing with a fracture of a major bone haemostasis cannot be achieved as in general surgery.

Anticoagulants introduce the risk of bigger blood loss from the raw bone ends; they are not used routinely in the Cambridge orthopaedic department.

Having regard to the manifold difficulties involved in these cases the results are surprisingly good and inestimably better than those provided by the old 'rest-in-bed' and 'wait-and-see' line of management. Truly, orthopaedic surgery is in the van of the battle to salvage these severely disabled elderly people.

Hip replacement surgery

Another big contribution of orthopaedic surgery is in elective surgery for osteoarthritis of the hip. The older operations of osteotomy, arthroplasty and arthrodesis are giving way to total hip replacement. This newer operation gives relief from pain and stiffness with preservation or even increase in mobility. There are many special types available but the important central feature is the high density plastic cup to replace the acetabulum and a strong biologically inert metal head and neck. The combination gives minimal wear and hence very long life to the prosthesis unlike the all-metal types. In Cambridge the Charnley (especially) or a variety of the McKee prosthesis is used.

A controversy rages around the use of cement (made from a plastic material) to help fix the prosthesis in position. Its use appears to be associated with increased mortality in the older patients but whether this is due to a sensitivity reaction to the cement or to enhanced risk of fat embolism is a matter for debate.

A less dramatic but none-the-less important contribution of orthopaedics to geriatrics is the use of surgery to help the patient with end-stage arthritis or severe flexion contractures from whatever cause. Patients who cannot sit or lie down in comfort may have their appalling disabilities diminished. In these cases, appropriate surgery brings benefit not just to the patient, but also to those who care for her. Appropriate surgery ranges from manipulation of a joint under a general anaesthetic, through tendon lengthening (or simply severing) operations to total hip replacement. Even if the patient will never walk again the total hip replacement operation can in selected cases make a world of difference to her comfort and ease of nursing.

Anaesthesia in old age

The risks of anaesthesia (as with surgery) rise with age and emergency surgery carries the highest risk of all. Nevertheless, in an individual case, if it is deemed appropriate to operate the anaesthetist will never reject the case on grounds of age alone. The timing of the operation will be decided jointly by the surgeon and the anaesthetist. The combined effects of adequate preoperative preparation and control during the anaesthetic can achieve wonders for the poor risk case, viz. the benefits which accrue from a careful review of drug treatment, correction of anaemia, dehydration and electrolyte imbalance, tracheal and bronchial toilet and oxygen therapy. ADR can be a problem during anaesthesia and the anaesthetist must be given full information concerning the patient's current and previous drug treatments especially with respect to steroids, anticoagulants, antihypertensives, betadrenergic blockers, antidepressants including MAOIs and antidiabetics.

General anaesthesia is mostly used for major surgery in UK although in some countries spinal and epidural techniques are widely employed. For all types of technique generally lower doses of anaesthetic agent are required e.g. for an epidural block the initial dose would be about half that for a younger patient. The maintenance of adequate blood pressure is absolutely vital because of the need to maintain adequate cerebral perfusion (see also Chapter 12). Frugal pre and post operative sedation and analgesia is required to maintain a course between uncontrolled anxiety and pain on the one hand and disastrous hypotension and respiratory depression on the other. A single thoughtless prescription of an over large dose of post operative sedation can annul much of the painstaking good work of both anaesthetist and surgeon. Small doses of analgesic (e.g. pethidine 10–15 mg) given early and repeated at short intervals are better than too much, too late. The patient must never be left unattended until she is fully able to protect her own airway. Even though she has apparently recovered consciousness, she may be unable vigorously to cough and reject secretions or vomit from larynx and respiratory tract.

Space does not allow an adequate chronicle of the contribution of medical and surgical treatments to the care of old people. Even so it is hoped that from this restricted and somewhat arbitrary selection the reader will have gained some insight into the highs and lows of therapeutic endeavour. The range of possibilities is vast, stretching from the simple replacement of a missing haematinic or hormone to the employment of very sophisticated radiotherapeutic, chemotherapeutic or surgical techniques. The doctor needs to know what is available and (more important still) how to select the treatment which will serve his patient best.

CHAPTER 20 · CARE OF THE DYING

Men fear death, as children fear to go in the dark; and as that natural fear in children is increased with tales, so is the other.

SIR FRANCIS BACON

Medical attitudes to death

Death is an essential ingredient of life. It affects everyone eventually and except in sudden death the doctor is almost always involved. The doctor, therefore, must be well prepared if he is to cope adequately. Good medical care for the dying is just as important as good medical care for any other suffering person. Yet often the medical management is patently inadequate and the dying patient, her relatives and attendants all suffer more than necessary. Possibly the doctor's own fear of death is the barrier to good care for the dying—this fear preventing him from grappling with the patient's problems in the same logical and practical way that he routinely employs in the management of non-fatal illness. Maybe he sees death as some kind of medical failure and is embarrassed by it, preferring not to talk about it. With patients, their relatives and even with other members of the professional team he may play charades and avoid the central issue. Little wonder that the medical management of death can leave the patient acutely anxious, frustrated, resentful and suffering intolerable physical distress.

Positive approach to the dying

A positive approach is important once it is realized that the end is in sight. The dramatis personae have clearly defined roles. The patient has the dual role of continuing to live while manifestly dying. She needs to keep up her interest in family, friends and surroundings while actually taking leave of life. The relatives and friends have a parallel dual role of continuing to live their own lives while supporting the patient and allowing her to withdraw from them. The care practitioners —doctors, nurses and social workers—have to use their own resources of understanding, knowledge, tact and techniques to help the patient and her relatives act out their separate roles. This enabling function of care is the key to successful medical management.

Death the prerogative of the elderly

Death can occur at any age but increasingly it is the prerogative of the elderly. In Cambridgeshire 76 per cent of all deaths in 1977 occurred at the age of 65 or over. The main causes of death are heart disease, malignant disease and cerebrovascular disease (Table 20.1).

Table 20.1. Deaths in Cambridgeshire 1977

Total deaths 5,403	Males 2,726
	Females 2,677
Main causes of death	Ischaemic heart disease 26%
	Malignant disease 22%
	Cerebrovascular disease 13%
Deaths age 65 years and over 76%	

At all ages up to 74 the male death rates are higher but inevitably thereafter there is an excess of female over male deaths (Fig. 20.1). The majority of elderly persons dying in hospital do so on the general medical wards. Nevertheless the active geriatric department carries a proportionately heavier burden of death (Table 20.2) but despite this manages to be a relatively cheerful place in which to work, live and die!

Table 20.2. Chesterton Hospital, Cambridge 1978

Geriatric beds—117			
Admissions 1,082	Source of cases — Emergency	504
Discharges 822	Elective (WL)	360
Deaths 266	Relatives respite	78
	Transfer	130

Unrelieved distress

Observations in general hospitals have shown that the dying suffer from much more unrelieved distress than do other patients with serious but non-fatal illness. Similar observations in geriatric wards have shown that some 20 per cent of dying patients suffer unrelieved distress but this tends to be less severe in the older patients. As might be expected, mental distress at the prospect of dying is much less acute in the elderly. Depression is more common than anxiety in both young and old and both these symptoms are more common and severe against the background of prolonged and intense physical suffering. Anxiety is particularly associated with breathlessness. If there is no physical discomfort the older patient usually has no mental distress. Clearly the onus on the doctor and nurse is to relieve the physical discomfort of the dying. Secondary benefits may well be relief from mental distress in both patient and her relatives and a big boost to the morale of both parties. As death approaches in elderly patients, mental confusion becomes increasingly common and loss of consciousness ensues for a variable period (measured in hours or days) in about 50 per cent of cases.

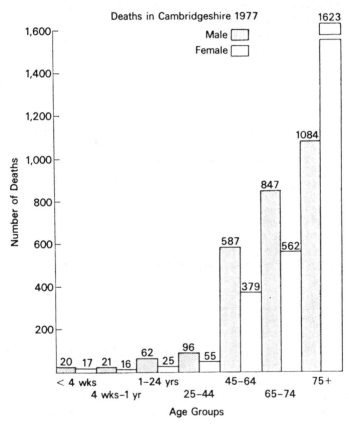

Fig. 20.1

Domiciliary care

It is commonly said that it is best for the patient to die in her own bed at home with her family and friends. Many elderly patients plead—'Don't send me into hospital to die, doctor' and relatives state categorically—'we wouldn't dream of allowing mother to be put away to die'. Yet the facts speak otherwise and show that there is an inexorable trend towards death in hospital, nursing home and residential care home, with only about one-third of deaths occurring at home. There is a similar trend towards birth being a wholly hospital activity. 'What next?' you might ask when turning over in the mind a quotation from T. S. Eliot—'Birth, copulation, death—there's nothing else when you get to brass facts.' All ready made munitions for those who battle against the 'over-medicalization' of our lives.

A study by Isaacs of all deaths at age 65 and over in Glasgow in 1968 showed that only 35 per cent occurred at home and 55 per cent were in hospital. Another study in Wales showed only 24 per cent of deaths at home. The average age at death was 72 years. Despite the high utilization of the hospital a third of the patients suffered incomplete relief from distress and many were never free from distress. Experiences such as these suggest the requirement for better medical management of the dying. Failure to provide this will increase the demand for 'mercy killing'; an idea abhorrent to most doctors.

Plans for home care

Home care for the elderly person who is dying is often possible, and indeed preferable to hospital care, if a well-thought-out plan of action is conducted by the primary care team under the leadership of a suitably skilled and motivated person (general practitioner, health visitor or social worker) (Table 20.3). The plan must have in it mechanisms for

Table 20.3. Plans for home care

Mobilize help	Relatives and friends
	Clergy
	Voluntary agencies (Age Concern, Fish Scheme, Youth Action)
	Financial—Local offices of Social Security and Social Services
Deploy domiciliary support services	Community nurse
	Home help
	Good neighbour
	Incontinent laundry service
Clarify medical needs	Diagnosis
	Drug treatments
	Special procedures (e.g. insertion of plastic tube in carcinoma of oesophagus)

dealing with the medical aspects (especially relief from physical and mental distress) and also mechanisms for mobilizing support for the patient through her relatives, friends, the clergy and the innumerable voluntary and statutory agencies. This is a statement of the obvious, yet all previous studies in the UK of the care of the elderly at home spell out the gross underutilization of existing resources in terms of financial help, special equipment and the deployment of personnel. It is all too often a case of too little, too late and with a total lack of a logical plan.

Prolonged pre-death dependence

Terminal care for the elderly can be a very protracted affair with a period of pre-death dependence lasting for months or years. The length of this dependence rises as a function of age and is usually characterized by decreased mobility, mental disturbance and persistent incontinence. To permit home care, special attention must be given to alleviate these symptoms especially the associated sleep disturbance and to make some social life possible for the supporting family. Careful attention to these details may make the difference between success and failure. Too ready acceptance of the supporting relative's claim that she will manage somehow without outside assistance, might pave the way to disaster. An eye must be kept on the situation by the family doctor to ensure that help is given before the burden becomes too great to support.

On the other hand too ready acquiescence in arrangements for long-term hospital care also must be avoided, if the hospitals are to be allowed to offer a full range of services, and if the emotional needs of patients and relatives are to be satisfied. This is not to say that help should not be sought from the geriatric department; quite the contrary. An early referral for medical assessment, as an out-patient or by the consultant meeting the family doctor (and often the practice nurse) in a domiciliary consultation, can prove invaluable in helping to formulate a suitable care pattern. A short spell of in-patient care may be indicated initially for full clinical assessment and later intermittent admission offered to give essential relief to relatives. The hospital should provide longer-term care only when the needs of the patient are clearly beyond the resources of the primary care team. In essence, the pattern for terminal care should allow all parties (carers and cared for) to get the help and support they require with due regard to their emotional as well as their physical needs.

ALLEVIATION FACTORS

A check list of important factors which must be alleviated to permit home care is given in Table 20.4. These factors or problems do not necessarily have to be cured or wholly resolved but they must be considered and some practical help given. Sleep disturbance which is very common and faecal incontinence which is much less common are both particularly ill-tolerated by the relatives. Urinary incontinence is also very common but generally is comparatively well-tolerated. Practical advice is given on these and related matters in the appropriate sections of this book.

Table 20.4. Factors to be alleviated to allow home care (after Sanford)

Sleep disturbance	Ill tolerated
Urinary incontinence	Better tolerated
Restriction of social life	Need planned breaks
Immobility	Need special aids
Faecal incontinence	Ill tolerated

These factors are listed in order of frequency.

SOCIAL NEEDS OF RELATIVES

Restriction of social life is also extremely well-tolerated by relatives but lack of early complaints about this must not lull the doctor into the belief that no problem exists. The stress is there and if not relieved the supporting relatives will crack and demand hospital admission. They may never be persuaded to accept a similar burden of care ever again. Thus they will resist the patient's return home when their consciences would tell them otherwise. This disastrous degree of overload must be avoided whenever possible by a nicely balanced use of resources. Well-planned holiday relief, weekends off, days off, nights off etc. will allow relatives to give maximum support to the dying old person while continuing to live and develop their own lives. Lack of sensitivity to the needs of the relatives may secure short-term home care at the expense of a very long terminal phase in hospital together with great emotional distress to patient and relatives alike. Most old people readily agree to a sojourn in the local geriatric department, to allow their relatives a holiday, especially when they see that this will allow them to achieve their wish to live out their lives, and ultimately to die, at home.

RELIEF OF ANXIETY IN THE RELATIVES

The importance of simple help cannot be overemphasized. Just having someone there, not necessarily all the time but on an informal 'pop-in' basis can transform the situation for a sick old person at home. Obviously as the needs increase more help will be required, but in the earlier stages, and on occasion right up to the time of death, it is not so much what is happening that is insupportable, but the prospect of what might happen. 'What happens if she gets an attack of pain or vomiting while I'm out shopping or collecting the children or when I am at work?' asks the daughter. Unrelieved anxiety of this nature may well erode the supporting relative's ability to cope and the sick person's wish to remain at home. Simple visiting, and the provision of an alarm system of some sort, might be all that is required in the earlier stages of terminal care. But unless there is a workable practical approach to the problem—('what happens if . . . ?') the resultant anxiety will precipitate premature hospital care.

Anxiety in the relatives may be due to feelings of inadequacy, including possibly the feeling that the dying person would get more and better attention in hospital. In many cases the reverse would be true because the main need is for love and a sympathetic understanding attendant to be available, to help with simple household tasks and with personal care—bathing, feeding and toilet. In these matters understanding relatives and friends may be able to do much more for the patient than would be possible in hospital. Even a well-staffed hospital ward cannot provide on duty a nurse–patient ratio of $1:1$. Yet at home the attendant–patient ratio may be better than $1:1$ for much of the 24 hours. Furthermore intimate knowledge of the patient's likes and dislikes is more likely to be possessed by those who know her well. For intermittent and not too frequent specialist nursing tasks (e.g. an enema change of catheter) help on a modest scale can be provided through the district nursing service.

PEACE AT THE LAST

Anxiety is also a problem to the patient facing death and to her relatives in other ways. The older patient worries more about her symptoms and what will happen to her possessions and pets than she does about the imminence of death. Many of the aged actually regard the coming of death with tranquillity. As William Hunter the surgeon put it 'If I had strength enough to hold a pen, I would write how easy and pleasant a thing it is to die.' This sense of peace at the last should be readily achievable, certainly for the period immediately before death, in cases where death is regarded as inevitable and imminent. Less readily achievable but well worth attempting is comfort and succour to patients, relatives and carers for the long period of pre-death dependence so commonly suffered by the elderly.

Anxiety may be due to pain—especially the pain of pressure sores, flexion contractures, arthritis, neuralgia and less often malignant disease. Relief of the pain relieves the anxiety. Drug treatment may suffice or recourse may be had to the more esoteric techniques of an anaesthetist, radiotherapist or surgeon specializing in pain control.

Ambivalent attitudes

Relatives are often ambivalent in their feelings and attitudes, worrying because the patient manifestly is getting more ill yet dreading the prospect of her recovery and the need for her to die all over again. They may resent meddlesome interference by doctor and nurse, demanding a withdrawal of 'all those tubes and things' yet allege neglect and callous indifference to the death of a loved one. They may urge the doctor to do something to 'get it all over'. These reactions are all perfectly normal and understandable. The patient's professional attendants must not take offence—yet, hand on heart, how many of us as doctors and nurses can honestly say that we never do! We should simply discuss with the relatives what is happening and why. Anxiety, hostility and resentment must be met with empathy, tact and humanity to achieve good standards of medical care.

Telling the patient

'Am I going to die, doctor?' This is a question which is often on the patient's mind in the weeks or months before death. Yet usually it is not put into words, and if it is verbalized, most often the person to be asked is not the doctor at all but a relative, a friend, the ward maid or the nurse. Maybe the doctor is too remote, too hurried in his visit or possibly the patient feels the doctor would be embarrassed by the question so intent is he and his colleagues on cure or (more usually) salvage activities of some sort. Certainly many doctors are embarrassed and brush the question aside with a gentle rebuke and a facile reassurance based on a totally unrealistic appreciation of the patient's predicament.

To the question 'Am I going to die, doctor?' there can be no pat answer but the doctor must not attempt to stifle the patient's curiosity. To keep the dialogue under way he might answer 'Well yes, of course, you will die eventually, we are all going to die—there can be no exceptions! However, you are not just dying at the moment. What in particular are you worried about?' This will give the patient the chance to unburden and to set her thoughts in order. Rarely is it a matter of the doctor telling the patient anything. Mostly it is a question of allowing the patient to tell the doctor of her anxieties and other problems. The doctor should let the old person decide the pace at which the relevant information is to be shared. When the direct question comes he must answer clearly and with compassion—giving sufficient information to satisfy the patient but still leaving room for hope. He should avoid telling lies. Deception is very difficult to maintain and once discovered destroys trust more effectively than anything else. When death is imminent the patient is usually unaware or so overwhelmed by some symptom in urgent need of relief (e.g. breathlessness) that the question is not put. Even when death is not imminent, anxiety about symptoms or less often about the mode of dying are of greater moment to the patient than the contemplation of death itself.

Drug treatment for the dying

The aim is to secure relief from distress while allowing the patient to remain mentally alert and in maximum control of herself at least until death is very near as measured in hours or days. The doctor should employ the minimum drug schedule necessary to achieve the aim. As death approaches the patient's future telescopes into a very short space of time and the intermediate short-term gain from treatment becomes paramount while the question of the long-term hazards of the drugs used is irrelevant.

Tackle physical problems first

In the medical approach to the patient's problems it is usually better to attempt relief from physical distress first and to tackle the problems of mental and emotional distress later. The mental and physical symptoms are, of course, inextricably interlinked, but in practice drug treatment of the physical symptoms, coupled with good overall management, often produces in the patient and her relatives a striking relief from emotional turmoil. Relief from pain, breathlessness, abdominal distension or cough can allay anxiety, restlessness and insomnia. Yet the use of hypnotics or tranquillizers might make matters worse if the underlying physical symptoms go on unabated.

The dying dement

In dementing elderly patients mental confusion, inane repetitive shouting, banging on furniture and nocturnal restlessness are frequently precipitated or exacerbated by physical discomfort. An overloaded rectum or a distended bladder are commonly responsible. These and other physical discomforts must be looked for and relieved, exemplifying, once more, the need to tackle the physical aspects of the patient's distress before the mental. Thus, this principle holds good, even in the presence of established mental illness in old people. Nowhere is it more important than in the care of the dying demented old person yet it is just in this context that it is all too easy to ignore completely the patient's physical distress.

Pain control

Pain is not just a physical phenomenon; there is always an emotional component. The person's tolerance of pain varies with her outlook, morale and level of anxiety. The general measures already mentioned will raise the threshold for pain. The doctor needs to be familiar with a number of pain-relieving drugs and some are now mentioned in order of ascending potency. 'Don't use a sledge-hammer to crack a nut' is a traditional maxim but remember also that for the dying patient the doctor must be able to ensure consistent relief from pain. The next dose of the pain-reliever is to be given before the analgesic effects of the first dose have worn off.

MILD PAIN

Soluble aspirin 300–900 mg thrice daily after food. Dextropropoxyphene 32·5 mg and paracetamol 325 mg (Distalgesic) 2 tablets thrice daily or every four hours. Also available as a soluble preparation. Benorylate (Benoral) an ester of aspirin and paracetamol is useful because it needs to be given only twice in the day. Each 10 ml contains 2·2 g aspirin and 1·8 g paracetamol.

MODERATE PAIN

Dipipanone 10 mg and cyclizine 30 mg (Diconal) 1–2 tablets every four hours.

SEVERE PAIN

Diamorphine and cocaine elixir BPC.
    The diamorphine and cocaine are present at a dose of 5 mg of each in 5 ml of the standard preparation but the prescriber can alter the doses up or down as required. The medical use of diamorphine is illegal in some countries because of its addictive properties. In terminal care it is an excellent drug. Morphine can be substituted in identical doses. Indeed, diamorphine in solution hydrolyses spontaneously to morphine over the course of a few days. The cocaine is intended as a euphoriant but it may cause restlessness and hallucinations. In most cases the diamorphine with a phenothiazine is sufficient.
    The dose of the elixir containing 2·5–30 mg diamorphine (heroin) and 5–10 mg cocaine must be given regularly to secure total control of pain. This usually means every four hours if the pain is severe. A phenothiazine syrup e.g. prochlorperazine (Stemetil) 5 mg in 5 ml or if extra sedation is required, chlorpromazine (Largactil) 25 mg in 5 ml

can be given along with the diamorphine and cocaine elixir. The phenothiazines potentiate the analgesic effects of the heroin and damp down anxiety, nausea and vomiting.

In cases of intractable vomiting, intestinal obstruction or when, for any reason, the patient is unable to swallow, injections of morphine subcutaneously or intramuscularly every four hours should be substituted for the elixir. Starting with half the previous oral dose of heroin the dose is gradually increased until control of pain is secured. Diamorphine injection BP is available in vials of 5, 10 and 30 mg to be made up with water for injection immediately prior to use. Morphine suppositories are available (strengths: 10–60 mg) and may be used as an alternative to injections. Elderly patients seem not to need very big doses but for each patient the actual dose must be found by titration against the patient's pain. A start should be made with a low dose but increasing it fairly quickly until total relief from pain is achieved. Once a pain-free state is achieved it is sometimes possible to reduce the heroin content of the elixir or the parenteral dose of morphia while maintaining the four hourly frequency of administration. Despite the undoubted addictive properties of diamorphine this proves not to be a problem in terminal care measured over weeks and even months.

NAUSEA AND VOMITING

The phenothiazines are most useful and generally adequate for the control of nausea and vomiting. If they prove inadequate, cyclizine tablets BP (Valoid) 50 mg or metoclopramide tablets 10 mg (Maxolon) orally twice or thrice daily given half to one hour before food should be tried. Cyclizine 50 mg in 1 ml water for injection can be given thrice daily by intramuscular injection if the oral route proves to be impracticable.

With malignant large bowel obstruction, stool softeners are useful until the obstruction is complete, e.g. dioctyl sodium sulphosuccinate (Dioctyl-Medo) as tablets or syrup given in a dose of 100–200 mg thrice daily with plentiful fluid.

COUGH

Codeine linctus BPC with 15 mg codeine phosphate in 5 ml is the most generally useful preparation; 5–10 ml is given as a dose especially at night or alternatively, methadone linctus 5–10 ml. The diamorphine and cocaine elixir is, of course, an effective cough suppressant.

CONSTIPATION

This is a common problem with elderly patients and often made much worse by the use of the drugs described for the relief of other symptoms, e.g. dextropropoxyphene, codeine, diamorphine. An adequate oral fluid intake, stool softeners (*v. supra*) and a stimulant of peristalsis are all required. For the latter we use Senokot as tablets, granules or syrup, starting with a low dose and gradually increasing it to produce satisfactory bowel motility.

Problems of drug treatment for anxiety, insomnia and mental depression are dealt with elsewhere.

Euthanasia

Although suicide has been legal in the UK since 1961, accessaries to the deed are criminal. Many people would like some modification of the law, to allow those who wished to have their lives terminated, to secure the necessary medical help (lethal injection or whatever). The Voluntary Euthanasia Society exists to promote this concept and to have the necessary legal machinery created. The whole notion of euthanasia (in the sense of being medically assisted suicide) bristles with ethical, legal, social and moral problems and the authors would not wish to act in the role of executioners.

On the other hand the literal concept of euthanasia as a gentle and easy death (as opposed to proleptic mercy killing) is at the heart of good medical practice. It is the doctor's vocation to cure sometimes, relieve often, and comfort always, even in death.

Some legal implications of incapacity

The Court of Protection

In the United Kingdom the Court of Protection is concerned with the protection of the property of all persons who are mentally incapable of managing their own affairs. The Court exists to protect the property (including all moneys) of patients but not to exert control over the patients themselves although, of course, in practice financial control inevitably results in some degree of control of personal freedom. It is a question of intent. Many elderly patients at home and in hospital, have intellectual failure of such a degree that they are quite unable to manage their own affairs and they get themselves into a tremendous muddle over simple financial tasks. Bills are paid three times over or not at all! Relatives or well-meaning friends can squander or misappropriate funds through incompetence, deceit or wrongful use of a Power of Attorney.

The Court normally appoints a Receiver, who may be a relative or a friend, a solicitor or some other suitable person to act as the patient's statutory agent. In certain small cases the matter is more simply dealt with by an order authorizing the application of the patient's property for her benefit. Whichever course is adopted it is a relief to all concerned to know that the property is being protected. The powers of the Receiver are strictly controlled and he must work within the guidelines set by the Court. For example he may not (on his own initiative) make loans or gifts, dispose of property or interfere with the patient's investments, but he should see to it that the patient is provided with those little extras that often add so much flavour to life, e.g. special foods, or drinks, books, flowers, toilet articles and clothing. In other words, almost anything within the patient's means, that will add to her quality of life.

The Master of the Court cannot appoint a Receiver until appropriate medical evidence is furnished in the form of a Medical Certificate on the appropriate form to state that the patient is incapable, by reason of mental disorder, of managing and administering her property and affairs. The Chief Clerk, The Court of Protection, Store Street, London WC1E 7BP will give full details to anyone who needs them.

POWERS OF ATTORNEY

A person of normal testamentary capacity may if she wishes appoint some other person to act for her. This legal right to act for another is readily achievable if the principal (the patient) is in a fit state of mind to appoint an agent. This is all quickly arranged through a local solicitor and for a patient incapacitated by physical illness it is the obvious solution to the practical difficulties of managing her own affairs. However, it is an arrangement fraught with danger in the case of frail elderly persons with insidious intellectual failure and bouts of mental confusion which so often accompany physical illness.

Thus the Power of Attorney may be valid when it is given but months or years later when it is no longer valid it is still being acted upon. This happens time and time again with elderly patients. This results in the agent acting illegally since he no longer has the valid consent of the patient. In this way relatives and others may relieve the elderly patient of her fortune when (if the facts were known) the Power of Attorney would be revoked. There is a clear duty on the part of the doctor to protect his patient. He can do this by agreeing to his patient signing a Power of Attorney instrument only if there is no doubt about her testamentary capacity and by maintaining vigilance to ensure that the instrument is revoked when her intellect fails. If the relatives or solicitor fail to make application to the Court of Protection when the time is ripe then the doctor should write to the Chief Clerk (*v. supra*) giving the necessary general particulars for the Court to act. The law on the matter is quite clear—'Where such a change occurs to the principal (patient) that he can no longer act for himself, the agent whom he has appointed can no longer act for him' (Lord Justice Brett, 1879).

CHAPTER 21 · THE AGEING PROCESS

> And namely whan a man is old and hore,
> Than is a wif the fruit of his tresore;
> Than should he take a yong wif and a faire
> On which he might engendren him an heire

From 'The Marchante's Tale' by GEOFFREY CHAUCER

Reference has been made, throughout the preceding pages, to many of the structural and functional changes associated with ageing. The fundamental nature of the ageing process itself has, until recently, been shrouded in mystery. Current gerontological research is achieving considerable advances, which will provide the geriatric medicine of the future with a sound theoretical foundation. Numerous theories of ageing have been propounded, and the following selection represents some of the most promising lines of thought. Explanations of the process can be attempted at different levels, so these hypotheses are not mutually exclusive, but may indeed all contain elements of the truth. Ageing may even be of multifactorial causation.

Ageing—the mathematical model

Gompertz regarded ageing as an increase in the probability of death, the probability approximately doubling every eight years after the age of thirty. This diminishing resistance to death is a simple and incontrovertible mathematical expression of the ageing process.

Ageing as an evolutionary adaptation

The cycle of ageing, death and rebirth permits the gradual remodelling of the species as a process of evolutionary adaptation. Furthermore, death is a social necessity, for without it, the world's population crisis would by now have assumed even more alarming proportions. As we can no longer rely upon the benevolent intervention of the plague bacillus to solve the crisis for us, there has to be an inbuilt or 'programmed' mechanism to ensure mortality. The ageing process provides this mechanism. Birth is the new investment which enables the species to adapt and remain viable: but the mortgage is heavy, for ageing is the interest, and death the capital repayment. To parody the ancient adage, 'While there's death, there's hope'.

This necessity of ageing and death for progress can also be seen at tissue level, and those who postulate a 'biological clock' can point to the tail and gills of the tadpole, whose death is necessary for the development of the frog.

Loss of irreplaceable cells

Most of the cells of the animal body continue to be replaced throughout life. Other cells—notably neuronal cells—are incapable of division, so that once they are destroyed, they cannot be replaced. Heart muscle cells also have to last a lifetime. It is possible that senescence is due to a gradual, random fall-out of these cells due to a variety of micro-environmental insults. Theories dependent on random cell death are known as 'stochastic' theories to distinguish them from theories based upon intrinsic programming. A number of possible types of insult can be postulated, and inadequate supplies of nutrients caused by arterial disease are among the likeliest.

The production of unsound cells in later life

According to the 'error catastrophe' theory associated with the name of Orgel, cellular ageing occurs through the accumulation of errors in the proteins and enzymes synthesized by the cell. These defects are self-reproducing, so there is eventually an exponential rise in their production. Sooner or later, damage occurs to the genes and chromosomes. The errors can occur through template failure due to abnormalities of DNA or RNA, compared by Comfort to the scratched photographic negative which will always produce faulty prints. The alternative mechanism is transcription failure, in which the negative is perfect but the wrong chemicals are used and the print is blurred.

It is probable that the original errors arise through mutations, induced, perhaps, by mutagenic stimuli. These stimuli may be chemical (e.g. drugs) or physical (e.g. radiation), so that this explanation also has a stochastic basis. Among the mutagens which can affect DNA are the free radicals such as the superoxide and hydroxy-radicals, and antioxidants have been shown to extend the life span of rodents. Implicit in error accumulation is not only error production but also defective functioning of the normal mechanisms for error removal.

Limited capacity for division

Until a few years ago, it was thought that healthy tissues were potentially immortal. Hayflick has studied the ageing of fibroblasts in tissue culture. He concludes that normal human and animal cells have a finite capacity for division *in vivo* and *in vitro*, and that this capacity is inversely related to the age of the donor. In those cases where the cultures acquired apparent immortality, he found that they had also acquired many of the attributes of malignant cells—notably aneuploidy (varying chromosome numbers).

Auto-immunity

The incidence of auto-immune disease rises in old age, and Burnet has speculated that auto-immunity is the basis of ageing itself. Two processes might contribute to this mechanism, of which the first is impaired immune surveillance due to a decline in the population of thymus-mediated (T) lymphocytic cells which normally mop up abnormal and neoplastic cells. It is certainly true that in the aged, a diminution in the function of the immune system is accompanied by an increase in the incidence of malignant disease as well as infection. The other contributory factor would be the presence of new antigens arising from the mutation of somatic cells.

Colloid ageing

Attention has hitherto been focused on the cells, but it is possible that senescence is caused by changes in the intercellular matrix of the connective tissues. These changes involve the collagen and elastin fibres, and comprise chemical cross-linkages between adjacent parts of macro-molecules, together with altered physical properties. Comfort points out that it is these physical properties which mainly enable us to distinguish between veal and beef, and that we are familiar with similar changes in perished rubber and old glue and plastic. It is of interest that penicillamine has been shown to reduce the formation of these cross-linkages.

Accumulation of waste products

Lipofuscin granules are bodies of intracellular pigment with character-istic staining properties. They are to be seen in many tissues (nervous tissue, muscle, liver, kidney), especially in the elderly. The exact derivation of this material is uncertain, but is possibly from intracellular membranes attacked by free chemical radicals. According to the 'clinker' hypothesis of ageing, the function of the cell deteriorates as inert debris accumulates within it. Extracellular debris such as amyloid also accumulates over the years and may interfere with organ function.

The rate of ageing

It is a commonplace observation that the rate of ageing appears to vary widely, both between one individual and another, and in the same individual, from one time to another. In this context, the rate of ageing is a rather loose descriptive term which encompasses the various mental and physical attributes which the observer imagines to correlate with chronological age. Among the elderly, in particular, this variation is very striking, and over the age of 75 the apparent 'biological age' correlates very poorly with chronological age.

At one end of the scale, the attainment of 113 years seems to be the world's record for longevity. There are abundant claims well in excess of this, but none sufficiently well documented to stand up to careful scrutiny.

At the other end of the scale is a group of rare and bizarre conditions known as the premature ageing syndromes.

Premature ageing syndromes

The outstanding feature of these conditions is the appearance of premature ageing. The archetype of these syndromes is **progeria**, the first to be described (in 1904). Failure to thrive can usually be observed within the first year of life, the characteristic appearance develops within the second year, growth decelerates severely towards the end of the first decade, and survival beyond the sixteenth birthday is exceptional. The features of precocious ageing include the shedding of scalp and body hair, generalized loss of subcutaneous fat, and a dry, atrophic, wrinkled skin. The nose is beaked, the frontal tuberosities prominent, and the chin recessed. The joints are stiff and prominent due to peri-articular fibrosis. Mental development is normal, but puberty is delayed, usually indefinitely. There is severe generalized atherosclerosis including the coronary and cerebral vessels, and myocardial fibrosis is also usual.

In **acrogeria,** the changes are more pronounced in the skin of the hands and feet than elsewhere, and the cardiovascular system is spared. In **pangeria** (Werner's syndrome) there is greying of the hair in child-hood, juvenile cataracts, osteoporosis, atherosclerosis, and a high incidence of malignancy: hypogonadism is typical. Patients with **metageria** are tall and thin and live rather longer despite early athero-sclerosis. The other related disease is **total lipodystrophy,** in which the lack of subcutaneous fat gives an aged and wizened appearance, and there is usually hyperlipidaemia.

Do these diseases represent an acceleration of the ageing process, or merely a cruel parody of it? Despite their rarity, progeria and Werner's syndrome are important models, because there is growing evidence linking them with some of the theories discussed. In particular, cultured fibroblasts from these patients only undergo from two to ten doublings instead of the normal twenty to forty—the 'Hayflick limit' is reduced. They have abnormal collagen, probably with extensive cross-linkages: and finally, the tissues show abundant and widespread lipofuscin deposition. These observations suggest that the diseases *are* premature varieties of ageing, and that further advances in our knowledge of the ageing process can be anticipated.

APPENDIX
'FAILURE TO THRIVE' OR
'GOING-OFF SYNDROME'

Hours/Days

Abdominal crisis
Atrial fibrillation – and other
   dysrhythmia
Cardiac failure
Dehydration
Hypotension
Hypothermia
Myocardial infarction
Pneumonia
Pulmonary thromboembolism
Respiratory failure
Septicaemia
Subdural haematoma
Urinary tract infection
Virus infections

Weeks/Months

Addison's disease
Anaemia
Constipation
Dementia
Depression
Diabetes
Dilutional hyponatraemia
Drugs – including alcohol
Gastric ulcer
Hypokalaemia
Hypothyroidism
Malabsorption
Malignancy, lymphoproliferative
   disorders, myeloma etc.
Myopathy – all causes
Parkinson's disease
Polycythaemia
Polymyalgia rheumatica
Pyelonephritis
Subacute bacterial endocarditis
Subdural haematoma
Thyrotoxicosis
Tuberculosis
Uraemia
Vitamin deficiency – including
   osteomalacia

INDEX

Doxycycline   235, 270
Drop attacks   147
Dropped beats   223
Drugs, adverse reactions to   316–319
  and confusion   105, 111–12
  anticoagulant   327
  anticonvulsant   190–1
  antileukaemic   290, 291
  antiplatelet   180, 327
  butyrophenones   203
  causing extrapyramidal disorders   203
  causing postural hypotension   208
  diamorphine and cocaine elixir   343
  folic acid   287
  fluid and electrolyte disturbance from   317
  fludrocortisone   208
  high blood levels in the elderly   317
  idoxuridine in herpes zoster   210
  in cerebrovascular disease   190
  in epilepsy   190–1
  in parkinsonism   197–201
  post herpetic neuralgia   210
  in terminal care   346–8
  interactions   319
  iron preparations   282–3
  limitations of   316
  metabolism of   320
  morphine, postoperative   325
  phenothiazines, cause of extrapyramidal disorders   203
  postoperative   325
  phototoxicity, due to   318
  plasma binding of   319
  renal excretion of   317
  tetrabenazine in hemiballismus   202
  thiopropazate in hemiballismus   202
  toxic effects on marrow   228
Duodenal ulcer   243
Dying patient, care of   337–50

drug treatment for   345–8
  needs of relatives   342–3
  pain control   346
  (see also Death)
Dyskinesia, tardive   203
Dysphagia   241
  due to cerebrovascular disease   189

Ectopic beats   222, 223
Ectropion   308
Elderly, definition   9
  not a homogeneous group   10
  in institutions   22, 51–9
Elderly mentally infirm (EMI)   55, 118
Elderly severely mentally infirm (ESMI)   55
Electroconvulsion therapy (ECT)   122
Electrolyte imbalance   140
Emboli, pulmonary postoperative   326
Embolism, arterial   230
  pulmonary   233–4
Emphysema   236
Enabling approach   2
Endocarditis, bacterial or infective   229
  non-bacterial thrombotic   229
Endogenous depression   120
Engagement, social   5
Entropion   307
Epilepsy   190–1
Erythrocytosis   292
Erythrocyte sedimentation rate (ESR)   280
Ethambutol   237–8
Euthanasia   348
Examination of aged patient   99
  neurological   192
Exercise, and atheroma   217
Expectation of elderly   19
  of life   13
Extrapyramidal disorders   193–204
  drug-induced   203
  rigidity   152

Mesenteric vessels, disease 219
Metabolism, drug 320
Metastases, cerebral 206
Metformin 259
Metoclopramide 248
Mexiletine 223
Microemboli, cerebral 177
Micrographia, in Parkinson's disease 195
Middle ear catarrh 312
Miliary tuberculosis, cryptic 237
Mithramycin 131
Mitral valve disease 227, 228
Mobile day units 48
Mobile units for foot care 48
Moditen 117
Monoamine oxidase inhibitors (MAOIs) 121, 319
Morphine, postoperative use 325
Motivation 88, 108
Motor neurone disease 211–12
Mucoid degeneration of mitral valve 228
Multifocal atrial rhythm 223
  tachycardia 223
Multi-infarct dementia 114
Multiple myeloma 292–3
Muscle fasciculation in motor neurone disease 211
  rigidity in parkinsonism 195
  wasting small hand muscles 192
Myelofibrosis 288, 291
Myelomatosis 292–3
Myocardial infarction 148, 218, 220
Myopathy 137
  of malignancy 206
  thyrotoxic 261
Myxoedema 137, 151, 229, 262–4
  madness 111

Nalidixic acid 270
National Assistance Act 119
Nephropathy, analgesic 271
  obstructive 270
Neuralgia, post-herpetic 210
  trigeminal 213

Neurofibrillary tangles 113
Neurofibromatosis, acoustic neuroma in 206
Neurogenic bladder 164
  claudication 231
Neurological norms in the elderly 192
Neuroma, acoustic 206
Neuronal fallout 113
Neuropathy, diabetic 212
  entrapment 214
  of malignancy 206
  peripheral 212
Neurosis 123
  anxiety 123
  institutional 123
Neurotic pseudodementia 109
Neurotransmitters 114
Nifedipine 221
Night sitting 50
Nitrofurantoin 270
Noradrenalin 120
Normal pressure hydrocephalus 112
Nuclear medicine 70
Nurse, community 48

Occupational therapist 84–7
  domiciliary 49
Occupational therapy in parkinsonism 199
Oedema 225
  pulmonary 226
Oesophageal stenosis 242
Oesophagitis 242
'Old old', the 14
Old peoples' homes 52
Oliguria, differential diagnosis 269
'On-off' or 'Yo-yo' effects in parkinsonism 199
Operation, surgical, assessment for 321
Ophthalmic herpes 210, 308
Osmoreceptor function 268
Osteoarthritis 132
Osteoid 129
Osteomalacia 31, 128, 151, 247
  incidence 32, 129

368 INDEX

INDEX 369

Valve disease 226–7, 228
Varicella virus in herpes zoster 209
Varicose ulcers 306
Vasodilators, cerebral 115
Vasopressin, in dementia 116
Vegans 276
Venous thrombosis 141, 326
 in fractured femur 334
 in hemiplegia 186
Venous ulcers 306
Ventricular tachycardia 223
Venturimask 235, 237
Verapamil 221, 222
Vertigo 146, 152, 312
Vibration sense 101
Visiting Schemes 43
Visual field defects 145
Vitamin B12, daily requirement 276
 deficiency of 249, 285
 treatment 286
Vitamin C deficiency 31
Vitamin D, deficiency 31, 129
 sources 31
 treatment 130

Vitiligo 263
Voluntary services 50
Volunteers 43

War pensions 33
Wards, geriatric 65–7
Warden controlled flatlets 51
Wardens, flying 50
 street 50
Warfarin therapy 327–9
Wasting, of small muscles of hand 192
Wax in ears 311
Weakness 136
Welldorm 117
Wheezing, differential diagnosis 234–6
Women, elderly, preponderance of 15

Xylose test 254

Youth Action 17
'Yo-yo' or 'on-off' effects in Parkinson's disease 199